# Immunology of Endocrine Diseases

# IMMUNOLOGY AND MEDICINE SERIES

## IMMUNOLOGY
· SERIES · SERIES · SERIES · SERIES **AND** SERIES · SERIES · SERIES · SERIES ·
## MEDICINE

# Immunology of Endocrine Diseases

**Edited by**
## Alan M. McGregor
Senior Lecturer and Honorary Consultant Physician,
Department of Medicine, University of Wales College of Medicine,
Heath Park, Cardiff

**Series Editor: Professor W. G. Reeves**

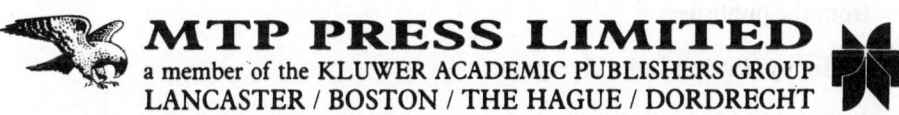

## MTP PRESS LIMITED
a member of the KLUWER ACADEMIC PUBLISHERS GROUP
LANCASTER / BOSTON / THE HAGUE / DORDRECHT

Published in UK and Europe by
MTP Press Limited
Falcon House
Lancaster, England

**British Library Cataloguing in Publication Data**

Immunology of endocrine diseases. —
   (Immunology and medicine series)
   1. Endocrine glands — Diseases —
   Immunological aspects
   I. McGregor, A. M.     II. Series
   616.4′079         RC649

   ISBN-13: 978-94-010-8352-2     e-ISBN-13: 978-94-009-4171-7
   DOI: 10.1007/978-94-009-4171-7

Published in the USA by
MTP Press
A division of Kluwer Academic Publishers
101 Philip Drive
Norwell, MA 02061, USA

**Library of Congress Cataloging-in-Publication Data**

Immunology of endocrine diseases.

   (Immunology and medicine series)
   Includes bibliographies and index.
   1. Endocrine glands — Diseases — Immunological
aspects. I. McGregor, A. M. (Alan M.), 1948—
II. Series. [DNLM: 1. Autoimmune Diseases.
2. Endocrine Diseases — Immunology.   WK 100 I33]
RC649.I46   1986       616.4′079       86–14381

ISBN-13: 978-94-010-8352-2

Typset by Witwell Ltd., Liverpool.

# Contents

This book is dedicated to:

Duncan D. Adams
Deborah Doniach
Ivan M. Roitt
Noel R. Rose

whose publications 30 years ago in 1956,
and contributions since have shaped our
understanding of the organ-specific,
autoimmune endocrine diseases.

# Preface

Nineteen eighty-six is a most appropriate year in which to be writing about developments in the organ-specific, autoimmune endocrine diseases. It celebrates the publication 30 years ago in 1956 of the classic papers of Roitt and Doniach and their co-workers[1], and of Rose and Witebsky[2] and Adams and Purves[3].

These three sets of fundamental observations provided the initial building blocks upon which much of what has been established in the field in the last 30 years was built.

No publication of this nature on endocrine autoimmune disease can cover every aspect of the subject. I have chosen to highlight the organs (thyroid and pancreeas) which have attracted the most attention, and the areas of work within these fields within which most research effort is currently focused. There are still some gaps; the insulin and TSH receptors are not considered, nor in any detail are the role of cytotoxic mechanisms in mediating gland destruction. Molecular biology will undoubtedly in the next few years clarify once and for all the controversy that surrounds the structure of the TSH receptor and T cell cloning, the role of cell-mediated cytotoxicity. The pathogenetic mechanisms underlying autoimmunity are increasingly well understood and the search for the aetiology has begun. In this context, the role of the immune system itself (and abnormalities within it) in the development of autoimmunity is still unresolved; is their an organ-specific suppressor T cell defect?[4], what of epithelial cell HLA-DR expression?[5], what of the anti-idiotypic antibody?[6]. The role too of the environment in the development of autoimmune disease likewise remains uncertain. Can iodine be implicated in the development of thyroid disease?[7] and what of infectious agents causing disease in genetically-predisposed individuals?[8]. All these are questions for the future.

In this monograph, I have chosen to highlight areas which have been associated with important developments or are areas of considerable current interest. The authors selected are currently working in these areas and their contributions enhance our understanding of their field of expertise.

*Alan M. McGregor*
*Cardiff, May 1986*

## References

1.   Roitt, I. M., Doniach, D., Campbell, P. M. and Hudson, R. V. (1956). Autoantibodies in Hashimoto's disease (lymphadenoid goitre). *Lancet*, **2**, 820–1

2.  Rose, N. R. and Witebsky, E. (1956). Changes in the thyroid glands of rabbits following active immunisation with rabbit thyroid extracts. *J. Immunol.* **76**, 417–27
3.  Adams, D. D. and Purves, H. D. (1956). Abnormal response in the assay for thyrotrophin. *Proc. Univ. Otago Med. Sch.*, **34**, 11–12
4.  Volpé, R. (1981). Autoimmunity in the endocrine system. *Monographs in Endocrinology*, **20**, 1–187
5.  Bottazzo, G. F., Pujol-Borrell, R., Hanafusa, T. and Feldman, M. (1983). Role of aberrant HLA-DR expression and antigen presentation in the induction of endocrine autoimmunity. *Lancet*, **2**, 1115–18
6.  Cooke, A., Lydyard, P. M. and Roitt, I. M. (1983). Mechanisms of autoimmunity: a role for cross-reactive idiotypes. *Immunology Today*, **4**, 170–5
7.  Hall, R. and Köbberling, J. (1985). Thyroid disorders associated with iodine deficiency and excess. *Serono Symposia Publication Volume 22*. (New York: Raven Press)
8.  Onodera, T., Tonionlo, A., Ray, U. R., Jenson, A. B., Knazek, R. A. and Notkins, A. L. (1981). Virus-induced diabetes mellitus *XX*. Polyendocrinopathy and autoimmunity. *J. Exp. Med.*, **153**, 1457–73

# Series Editor's Note

The modern clinician is expected to be the fount of all wisdom concerning conventional diagnosis and management relevant to his sphere of practice. In addition, he or she has the daunting task of comprehending and keeping pace with advances in basic science relevant to the pathogenesis of disease and ways in which these processes can be regulated or prevented. Immunology has grown from the era of anti-toxins and serum sickness to a state where the study of many diverse cells and molecules has become integrated into a coherent scientific discipline with major implications for many common and crippling diseases prevalent throughout the world.

Many of today's practitioners received little or no specific training in immunology and what was taught is very likely to have been overtaken by subsequent developments. This series of titles on IMMUNOLOGY AND MEDICINE is designed to rectify this deficiency in the form of distilled packages of information which the busy clinician, pathologist or other health care professional will be able to open and enjoy.

*Professor W. G. Reeves, FRCP, FRCPath*
*Department of Immunology*
*University Hospital, Queen's Medical Centre*
*Nottingham*

# List of Contributors

**S. BAEKKESKOV**
Hagedorn Research Laboratory
Niels Steensensvej 6
DK 2820 Gentofte
DENMARK


**A. H. BARNETT**
Department of Medicine
University of Birmingham and
  East Birmingham Hospital
C/O East Birmingham Hospital
Bordesley Green East
Birmingham B9 5ST
UK


**M. CHRISTIE**
Hagedorn Research Laboratory
Niels Steensensvej 6
DK 2820 Gentofte
DENMARK


**H. A. DREXHAGE**
Laboratory for Clinical Immunology
Department of Pathology
Free University Hospital
De Boelelaan 1117
1081 HV Amsterdam
THE NETHERLANDS


**P. A. EALEY**
Department of Chemical Pathology
University College Hospital
Gower Street
London WC1E 6AU
UK

**R. D. VAN DER GAAG**
Laboratory for Clinical Immunology
Department of Pathology
Free University Hospital
De Boelelaan 1117
1081 HV Amsterdam
THE NETHERLANDS


**R. JANSSON**
Department of Internal Medicine
University Hospital
University of Uppsala
S-751 85 Uppsala
SWEDEN


**A. KARLSSON**
Department of Internal Medicine
University Hospital
S-751 85 Uppsala
SWEDEN


**Y. M. KONG**
Department of Immunology and
  Microbiology
Wayne State University
  School of Medicine
540 East Canfield Avenue
Detroit
MI 48201
USA


**L. F. KUMAGAI**
Department of Internal Medicine
Division of Endocrinology
University of California
Davis
4301 X Street
Building Folb II-C
Sacramanto, CA 95817, USA

IMMUNOLOGY OF ENDOCRINE DISEASES

**A. B. KURTZ**
The Middlesex Hospital
Mortimer Street
London W1N 8AA
UK

**Å. LERNMARK**
Hagedorn Research Laboratory
Niels Steensensvej 6
DK 2820 Gentofte
DENMARK

**M. E. LUDGATE**
Department of Medicine
University of Wales College
  of Medicine
Heath Park
Cardiff CF4 4XN
Wales
UK

**N. J. MARSHALL**
Department of Chemical Pathology
University College Hospital
Gower Street
London WC1E 6AU
UK

**A. M. McGREGOR**
Department of Medicine
University of Wales College
  of Medicine
Heath Park
Cardiff CF4 4XN
Wales
UK

**S. NAGATAKI**
The First Department of
  Internal Medicine
Nagasaki University School
  of Medicine
7-1 Sakamoto-machi
Nagasaki 852
JAPAN

**R. M. POPE**
Department of Medicine
University of Wales College
  of Medicine
Heath Park
Cardiff CF4 4XN
Wales
UK

**H. TAMAI**
Department of Psychosomatic
  Medicine
Faculty of Medicine
Kyushu University
3-1-1 Maidashi
Higashi-ku
Fukuoka 812
JAPAN

**A. P. WEETMAN**
Department of Medicine
Royal Postgraduate Medical School
Hammersmith Hospital
Du Cane Road
London W12 0HS
UK

# 1
# The Mouse Model of Autoimmune Thyroid Disease

Y. M. KONG

## INTRODUCTION

The autoimmune nature of human thyroid disease was described nearly three decades ago[1a,b] and, several years later, such immunological manifestations were observed in familial clusters[2]. However, only in the past 10 years has our understanding of the autoimmune mechanisms taken a big leap forward. The gain in new insight is a logical consequence of two parallel developments, the rapid advances in our knowledge of the immune network and the use of animal models which simulate various components of the multi-faceted autoimmune thyroid disease. The closest human counterpart that these models represent is Hashimoto's thyroiditis. Recently, two major reviews have described the various animal models, including the rabbit, guinea pig, rat and mouse, in which autoimmune thyroiditis is inducible, and the Buffalo strain of rat and obese strain of chicken, in which the disease arises spontaneously[3,4]. The comprehensive review by Weetman and McGregor[3] further compares and aligns certain features found in both animal models and clinical disease. The intent of this chapter is therefore not to duplicate existent overviews of findings in various animal models. Rather, it is to illustrate the recent applications of immunological concepts, as they became formulated, to systematic investigations of the regulatory mechanisms of autoimmunity.

The mouse was chosen for these studies because its genetic composition was the best analysed through the development of recombinant strains. Its immune system was also the most easily manipulated due to the early availability of multiple inbred strains and immunological markers identifying lymphocyte surface antigens. More importantly, observations on the immunobiology of the mouse have generally found correlates and provided clues to immune functions in the human. For example, our emerging understanding of the contribution of the human HLA complex to the immune response is based primarily on numerous studies of the immunogenetic and molecular aspects of the mouse H-2 complex. Experimental autoimmune thyroiditis (EAT) in the mouse has certain features reminiscent of Hashimoto's thyroiditis; its induction with mouse thyroglobulin (MTg) is genetically based and it exhibits characteristic autoantibody production to MTg and mononuclear cells in the thyroid infiltrate.

By incorporating knowledge gained over the past 10 years on immunoregulation in the mouse, we have designed experimental approaches to: (1) analyse the genetic basis for the recogitory and controlling parameters in EAT by using recombinant strains; (2) demonstrate the importance of T-cells autoreactive to thyroglobulin (Tg) and their responses to activation *in vitro*; (3) examine the pathogenic mechanisms mediated by T-cells; and (4) explore the suppressor mechanisms which maintain self-tolerance or unresponsiveness to self-antigens. These approaches will be discussed in turn below. The use of an induced rather than spontaneous model of EAT has provided the opportunity to dissect the normal regulatory events which interfere with the triggering of autoimmune responses of autoreactive T-cells in genetically susceptible individuals to the ever-present autoantigens.

## GENETIC ANALYSIS OF SUSCEPTIBILITY TO EXPERIMENTAL AUTOIMMUNE THYROIDITIS

### Mapping the immune response gene for thyroglobulin (Ir-Tg) to the I-A subregion

In 1971, Rose and co-workers[5,6] firmly established that EAT in the mouse can be induced with homologous Tg incorporated in complete Freund's adjuvant (CFA) and that the extent of thyroid damage is linked to the H-2 major histocompatibility complex (MHC). For example, immunized inbred strains of the k or s haplotype develop both MTg antibodies and thyroiditis, whereas those of the b or d haplotype produce autoantibodies with little or no thyroid infiltration. This MHC-based susceptibility to EAT has served as a prototype for linkage studies in the human as well as in other models of organ-specific autoimmune diseases. As the HLA complex became better defined, many autoimmune diseases, including Hashimoto's thyroiditis, have found association with the DR region[7]. Using recombinant strains within the MHC, available in the early 1970s, the Ir-Tg gene encoding susceptibility to EAT was placed at the K end of the H-2 complex, which included both the K region (class I genes) and I-A subregion (class II genes)[8].

In carrying out genetic mapping of the Ir-Tg gene, three considerations were deemed important. One, congenic mice differing only in the MHC must be tested at some point to verify MHC linkage without the influence of background genes. Two, since CFA contains *Mycobacterium tuberculosis* (usually the more virulent human strain of H37Ra is used with autoantigens), it is necessary to ascertain that the MHC linkage is not related to possible immune response genes to mycobacterial antigens. Three, emulsification of an autoantigen in CFA could cause denaturation, and any inadvertent immune responses to denatured MTg epitopes must be minimized or differentiated. Our subsequent finding that lipopolysaccharide (LPS), endotoxin from Gram-negative bacteria, can serve as an adjuvant for MTg without altering the MHC association found with CFA[9] demonstrates that the MHC linkage is indeed to Ir-Tg, removing the second concern[10]. That both MTg and LPS can be given in the aqueous form, 3 hours apart, rules out denaturation due to CFA as a major problem in interpretation. Employing LPS as the adjuvant, we have recently tested congenic mice with the same B10 background genes but different in the MHC[11]. The first concern of possible background genes influencing MHC linkage of the Ir-Tg gene is greatly reduced; the k and s haplotypes, for example, are still susceptible to EAT, whereas the b and d haplotypes remain resistant. The use of other adjuvants, such as polyadenylic-polyuridylic acid complex[12] and muramyl dipeptide[13], further confirms the location of Ir-Tg within the H-2 complex.

Being a less potent adjuvant than CFA, LPS has served as a finer discriminator of responsiveness to MTg; antibody production to MTg is much lower in resistant than in susceptible strains and thyroid infiltration hardly occurs in resistant mice. Subsequent availability of a new recombinant strain, B10.MBR, between the K region and I-A subregion permitted the pinpointing of the Ir-Tg gene[14]. As shown in Table 1.1, although B10.MBR carries the resistant b allele at the K region, it retains the capacity of the prototype, B10.BR, to develop thyroiditis. Comparisons with the other recombinant strains including B10.A(4R) map the Ir-Tg gene to the I-A$^k$ subregion. These observations are supported by in vitro studies showing that sensitization of mouse lymphocytes with thyroid monolayers is under I-A subregion control[15]. The I-A subregion encodes Ia (DR-like) molecules which are responsible for antigen presentation to T-cells bearing the appropriate receptors. The recent demonstration of DR antigens on human thyroid cells[16] has therefore generated immense interest. More than likely, the mouse Ir-Tg gene is involved in the initial recognitory events associated with activation of inducer T-cells ($T_1$). It has been shown that EAT induction requires the presence of T-cells from susceptible, but not resistant, strains[17].

**Table 1.1** Genetic mapping of autoimmune response gene to mouse thyroglobulin (MTg) in H-2 recombinant strains

| Strain | H-2 haplotype | K | A | (J) | E | S | D | TL | MTg antibody titre† (Mean log$_2$ ± SE) | Thyroiditis† Positive/total (%) |
|---|---|---|---|---|---|---|---|---|---|---|
| B10 | b | b | b | b | b | b | b | b | 1.6 ± 0.3 | 4 |
| B10.BR | k | k | k | k | k | k | k | a | 9.5 ± 0.4 | 72 |
| B10.A | a | k | k | k | k | d | d | a | 8.5 ± 0.3 | 52 |
| B10.AKM | m | k | k | k | k | k | q | a | 7.5 ± 0.7 | 52 |
| B10.MBR | bql | b | k | k | k | k | q | a | 7.0 ± 0.4 | 72 |
| B10.A(4R) | h4 | k | k | b | b | b | b | b | 9.3 ± 0.4 | 53 |
| B10.A(5R) | i5 | b | b | k | k | d | d | a | 4.7 ± 0.4 | 20 |

Modified from Beisel et al.[14].

*Within the H-2 complex: K, D and TL regions encode class I antigens; I region encodes class II (Ia) antigens and is subdivided into I-A, (I-J) (its location being re-examined) and I-E subregions; S region encodes class III antigens.

†Data from day 28.

## Influence of D-end and K-end genes

In the early studies on MHC association with EAT[6,8], the a haplotype was found to be intermediate in susceptibility to EAT with reduced thyroid infiltration. Since the a haplotype is a recombinant of k and d haplotypes with the d allele at the D end, class I genes at the K and/or D region may affect EAT susceptibility. To test this hypothesis, we immunized recombinant strains, similar at the I region but different at the D region, with MTg and LPS, and compared their autoantibody titres and thyroid pathology[18]. Table 1.2 shows that, whereas the MTg antibody titres are little affected, reduced thyroid damage is observed in mice carrying the susceptible k allele at the I-A subregion but the b, d or q allele at the D region. This D-end influence is unrelated to the susceptibility status of the parent; the f haplotype is resistant to EAT induction[19], but the $D^f$ genes have little moderating effect on thyroid inflammation.

The D-end genes can also regulate autoantibody production besides thyroid infiltration. When the I-A subregion of recombinant mice contains the susceptible s allele, both autoantibody titres and thyroiditis are reduced by the presence of the $D^d$ genes[18]. Table 1.2 also rules out the TL region, which is adjacent to the D region, as having a role in EAT susceptibility, a finding later verified with congenic mice differing only at the TL region[11]. The sites of action of D-end genes in EAT remain to be elucidated. As will be described in a later section, one area of involvement may be in the destruction of thyroid epithelial cells by cytotoxic T-cells wherein class I antigen restriction takes part[20]. On the other hand, the D-end genes may also modify antibody production to MTg. D-region control has been implicated in resistance to a number of diseases[18] and more recently in levels of enzymatic activities including neuraminidase[21]. Thus, the D region with its complex gene structure may have multiple sites of action in EAT, resulting in the suppression of antibody production and/or thyroid damage.

The influence of the K-end genes in modifying EAT has been studied by us[14], as well as by Cohen and co-workers[22,23], with certain recombinant and K-region mutant strains. These results have been discussed elsewhere[14,24]. Briefly, we have not noted as much influence of the K end in EAT induction as have others. We have reported some differences in the incidence of thyroiditis when certain K-region alleles are superimposed on mice displaying a D-end effect (Table 1.1, B10.AKM vs. B10.MBR). Our use of a less potent adjuvant (LPS rather than CFA) may in part explain the difference in results. That the K end does play a role in effector function[23] is evidenced by the K (class I) antigen restriction in thyroid target destruction by cytotoxic T-cells[20] (see later).

## Influence of non-MHC genes and sex hormones

The contribution of genes outside of the MHC to the overall autoimmune response to MTg was determined by using LPS as adjuvant to examine six H-2 haplotypes originating from four different backgrounds[11]. Whereas the major role played by the MHC is affirmed, the background genes can influence EAT. For example, regardless of the H-2 haplotype, mice of C3H

**Table 1.2** Influence of D-end genes on autoimmune response to mouse thyroglobulin (MTg) in H-2 recombinant strains

| Strain | H-2 haplotype | H-2 complex* | | | | | | | MTg antibody titre† (Mean log$_2$ ± SE) | Thyroiditis† (Mean index ± SE) |
|---|---|---|---|---|---|---|---|---|---|---|
| | | K | A | (J) | E | S | D | TL | | |
| B10.BR | k | k | k | k | k | k | k | a | 11.2 ± 1.0 | 2.2 ± 0.2 |
| B10.AKM | m | k | k | k | k | k⏐ | q | a | 9.8 ± 0.4 | 1.3 ± 0.3 |
| B10.AM | h3 | k | k | k | k | k⏐ | b | b | 9.0 ± 0.3 | 1.1 ± 0.2 |
| B10.A | a | k | k | k | k⏐ | d | d | a | 9.1 ± 0.4 | 0.6 ± 0.2 |
| B10.M (17R) | aql | k | k | k | k⏐ | d | f | a | 10.8 ± 0.5 | 2.2 ± 0.2 |

Modified from Kong et al.[18].
*See Table 1.1 for description.
†Data from day 28; thyroid pathology graded on an index scale from 0 to 4.

background show higher MTg antibody levels and more thyroid involvement than those of B10 background. Other background genes may influence antibody titres only. Given the interplay of class I and class II genes described above, it is clear that selective usage of mouse strains on different backgrounds can reflect multiple genetic influences and expressions of autoimmune thyroid disease. Such multiple controls more than likely exist in polygenic humans.

The preponderance of women, compared to men, afflicted with auto-immune diseases has led to investigations on the role of sex hormones in autoimmunity. In NZB/W F₁ mice, a model for systemic lupus erythematosis, early orchiectomy and oestrogen administration of males increase the severity of disease, whereas ovariectomy and testosterone reduce its severity in females[25]. Castration of thymectomized and irradiated male rats results in the increase in both autoantibody levels and incidence of spontaneous autoimmune thyroiditis, approaching those seen in uncastrated females[26]. The increases are reversible with testosterone. In our study of mice susceptible and resistant to EAT, castration merely increases the autoantibody titres in susceptible males to levels observed in females without affecting the incidence (or severity) of thyroiditis (Table 1.3). This effect is reversed by a testosterone implant[27]. It is possible that sex hormones would exert a more noticeable influence on mouse EAT if recombinant strains showing D-end and/or K-end as well as background effects were used.

**Table 1.3** Autoimmune responses to mouse thyroglobulin (MTg) in sham-operated and castrated susceptible (C3H) and resistant (BALB/c) mice

| Strain | Sex | Operation | MTg antibody titre* (Mean log₂ ± SE) | Thyroiditis* Positive/total (%) |
|--------|-----|-----------|--------------------------------------|--------------------------------|
| C3H | Male | Sham | 10.3 ± 0.9 | 100 |
| | | Castrated | 15.3 ± 0.5† | 100 |
| | Female | Sham | 13.1 ± 0.7 | 100 |
| | | Castrated | 12.5 ± 1.1 | 100 |
| BALB/c | Male | Sham | 5.0 ± 0.7 | 0 |
| | | Castrated | 4.4 ± 0.8 | 14 |
| | Female | Sham | 4.7 ± 0.4 | 0 |
| | | Castrated | 4.5 ± 0.5 | 0 |

Modified from Okayasu et al.[27].
*Data from day 28.
†$p < 0.001$ compared to sham-operated group.

## ROLE OF AUTOREACTIVE T-CELLS AND THEIR ACTIVATION

### Induction of experimental autoimmune thyroiditis with syngeneic thyroglobulin

In the complex environment we live in, the triggering events resulting in auto-reactive T₁ activation and autoimmune sequelae must be quite varied. A model of induced EAT permits the exploration of some of these events. Whereas CFA greatly enhances the immunogenicity of autoantigens, an emulsified autoantigen is far from physiologic. On the other hand, LPS is a product of Gram-negative bacteria and can be derived endogenously or exogenously. It could represent a natural adjuvant providing the necessary signals, similar to factors derived from other infectious agents and polyclonal activators. We have already determined that LPS or CFA injections without MTg into susceptible mice are insufficient to bolster the immunogenicity of endogenous Tg, present in nanogram amounts in the circulation, nor can microgram amounts of MTg given (twice) without adjuvant induce EAT[9].

To examine if adjuvant stimulus is an absolute requirement, microgram amounts of MTg were administered over a period of 4 weeks. As shown in Table 1.4, repeated injections of syngeneic (C3H) thyroid antigens in the absence of adjuvant resulted in low levels of antibody production and 38–57% incidence of thyroiditis in susceptible (C3H) mice. In this and other experiments, 100% of the susceptible mice developed autoantibodies; their levels declined rapidly, soon after the cessation of MTg injections[28]. In the presence of such homoeostatic control, about 50% displayed autoantibodies without thyroid infiltration, as in many humans, whereas the remaining 50% developed prominent thyroid lesions 7–14 days after peak antibody production. In contrast, resistant (BALB/c) mice showed only negligible levels of autoantibodies and no thyroid damage (Table 1.4). Their resistance could be a reflection of strong suppressor mechanisms preventing triggering, or the lack of appropriate Ia molecules or T-cell receptors. These observations provide evidence for the existence of T-cells autoreactive to self-Tg which can be stimulated to override suppressor mechanisms normally present in susceptible mice (see later). An adjuvant in the host appears to reduce the autoantigenic threshold required to trigger Tg-specific T-cells.

**Table 1.4** Induction of autoimmune thyroiditis in susceptible (C3H) mice with syngeneic thyroid antigens in the absence of adjuvant

| Strain | Thyroid extract* (μg) | Thyroglobulin antibody titre (Mean $\log_2$ ± SE) | | | Thyroiditis Positive/total (%) |
| --- | --- | --- | --- | --- | --- |
| | | Day 14 | Day 28 | Day 35 | |
| C3H | 1.6 | <1.0 | 4.0 ± 0.6 | 4.2 ± 1.1 | 38 |
| | 40 | 1.6 ± 0.4 | 5.6 ± 0.2 | 3.7 ± 0.2 | 57 |
| BALB/c | 40 | <1.0 | 1.3 ± 0.5 | 1.0 ± 0.5 | 0 |

Adapted from ElRehewy et al.[28].
*Freshly prepared and injected into syngeneic mice, 16 intravenous doses in 4 successive weeks.

## Differential responses of susceptible and resistant mice to thyroglobulin in vitro

That autoantibodies are produced, after repeated MTg injections, without concomitant thyroid infiltration[28] effectively disqualifies antibodies as sufficient in causing thyroid damage. To initiate pathogenesis, clearly the stimulation of cells besides helper T-cells ($T_H$) that aid only antibody formation is necessary. This additional stimulus is lacking or hindered in EAT-resistant mice which can make MTg antibodies of various immunoglobulin classes indistinguishable from those in susceptible mice[29]. To examine cellular events culminating in thyroiditis, lymph node cells from immunized susceptible and resistant mice were restimulated with MTg *in vitro* and their proliferative responses measured after several days in culture[30,31]. Immune cells from susceptible mice responded to MTg stimulation *in vitro*, whereas those from resistant mice did not, despite the addition of irradiated normal spleen cells to optimize culture conditions and antigen presentation[32]. Moreover, in such MTg-immunized mice, only lymph node cells from susceptible (CBA) mice responded to heterologous human Tg *in vitro* (Table 1.5). When the same strains were immunized with human Tg, both sets of lymphocytes reacted strongly to stimulation with human Tg containing its own specific epitopes, but again only those from susceptible mice proliferated in response to cross-stimulation with mouse Tg.

**Table 1.5** Comparison of T-cell proliferative responses of susceptible (CBA) and resistant (BALB/c) mice to shared epitopes of mouse and human thyroglobulins

| Strain | Immunizing antigen* | [$^3H$] thymidine uptake of lymph node cells (Mean cpm ± SD) | | |
|---|---|---|---|---|
| | | None | MTg 50 μg/ml | HTg 50 μg/ml |
| CBA | MTg | 1420 ± 150 | 11110 ± 320 | 16710 ± 1100 |
| | HTg | 2030 ± 410 | 5490 ± 640 | 45310 ± 2800 |
| BALB/c | MTg | 260 ± 30 | 240 ± 30 | 310 ± 30 |
| | HTg | 180 ± 5 | 280 ± 20 | 35200 ± 6900 |

Adapted from Simon *et al.*[32].
*MTg or HTg, mouse or human thyroglobulin, given in complete Freund's adjuvant.

The above observations demonstrate that cells from EAT-susceptible, but not resistant, mice are activated by shared determinants on mouse and human Tg, as well as by putative MTg-specific epitopes. The proliferating cells are T-lymphocytes bearing the Lyt-1 markers[32], present on $T_I$ (inducer), $T_H$ (helper) as well as $T_A$ (amplifier) and $T_D$ (mediator of delayed hypersensitivity). In this system, blastogenesis is not indicative of the involvement of $T_H$ *per se*, since both immunized susceptible and resistant donors of these lymphocytes are producing autoantibodies. Rather, their response to mouse or human Tg *in vitro* signifies the capacity to develop EAT[31,32]. These T-cells interact with mouse or human Tg presented with Ia molecules[32,33], the presence of monoclonal antibodies to I-A$^k$ (but not to the inappropriate I-A$^d$) abrogates proliferation (Table 1.6). Similar antibodies to DR antigens inhibited the proliferative response of T-lymphocytes from Hashimoto's patients to human Tg[34]. The response to MTg involves recognition by the mouse T-cell receptor; rat monoclonal antibodies to its common region, L3T4, also prevent in vitro proliferation (Table 1.6).

**Table 1.6** Effect of anti-Ia or anti-L3T4 antibody on the proliferative responses to mouse and human thyroglobulins

| Immunizing antigen | In vitro antigen | $[^3H]$ thymidine uptake (Mean cpm ± SD) | | | |
|---|---|---|---|---|---|
| | | None | Anti-I-A$^k$ (10 µg/ml) | Anti-I-A$^d$ (25 µg/ml) | Anti-L3T4 (1:2)† |
| MTg* | None | 1 800 ± 450 | 1 900 ± 50 | 2 700 ± 410 | |
| | MTg | 10 800 ± 3 100 | 1 980 ± 200 | 10 800 ± 5 300 | |
| MTg | None | 4 500 ± 300 | | | 2 200 ± 240 |
| | MTg | 29 600 ± 7 800 | | | 300 ± 60 |
| HTg* | None | 420 + 50 | ND | ND | |
| | HTg | 27 500 ± 3 300 | 1 900 ± 760 | 26 600 ± 5 100 | |

*Modified from Kong et al.[33]; MTg or HTg, mouse or human thyroglobulin, given in complete Freund's adjuvant.
†Culture supernatant of rat monoclonal antibodies to L3T4 (hybridoma GK1.5 of F.Fitch) was added to spleen cells from mice immunized with MTg and lipopolysaccharide.

## Transfer of experimental autoimmune thyroiditis by thyroglobulin-activated T-cells

The possibility of expanding Tg-specific T-cells in vitro will enable the cloning and characterization of these cells. Moreover, the relative contribution of T-cell subsets in pathogenesis can be examined (see later). Several laboratories have determined that the expanded T-cell population can adoptively transfer EAT into normal syngeneic recipient mice[35-39]; one such line has also been used to induce resistance if first irradiated[35]. We are particularly intrigued by the determinants on Tg which can activate these cells to transfer disease, although the chemical structure of Tg has not been delineated. It is not known what epitopes on Tg are autoantigenic for T-cells; three is the estimate for human B-cells of thyroiditis patients[40]. A high percentage of human anti-Tg sera cross-reacts with MTg (unpublished observations). But, it is unknown if any human Tg epitope recognized by human T-cells is shared with MTg, although mouse T-cells do respond to stimulation with human Tg (Table 1.5). Table 1.7 shows that T-cells from MTg-immunized mice can be activated with human Tg, as with MTg, to transfer EAT; characteristics of the thyroid infiltrates are quite similar (Figure 1.1; A, B). From these populations, cytotoxic T-cells are also derived[39] (see later). The least efficient activator for transfer is concanavalin A (Con A), since a higher number of viable cells is required to achieve thyroid infiltration equivalent to that seen with human Tg-activated cells. Although Con A is a strong T-cell mitogen, many of the blast cells evidently are not Tg-specific and do not lodge in the thyroid to initiate damage. We have shown that antigen specificity is required for the adoptive transfer of EAT[39].

**Table 1.7** Transfer of autoimmune thyroiditis with MTg-, HTg- or Con A-activated spleen cells from MTg-immunized mice*

| Exp. no. | In vitro activation | No. cells transferred* | MTg antibody titre† (Mean log$_2$ ± SE) | Thyroiditis† | |
|---|---|---|---|---|---|
| | | | | (Mean index ± SE) | Positive/total (%) |
| 1 | MTg | 10$^7$ | 1.9 ± 0.5 | 1.8 ± 0.1 | 100 |
| | MTg + 1500 R | 10$^7$ | 1.1 ± 0.4 | 0.0 | 0 |
| 2 | MTg | 10$^7$ | 2.8 ± 0.6 | 2.8 ± 0.1 | 100 |
| | HTg | 10$^7$ | 2.3 ± 0.4 | 2.0 ± 0.1 | 100 |
| | Con A | 10$^7$ | 2.6 ± 0.5 | 0.4 ± 0.3 | 40 |
| | Con A | 3 × 10$^7$ | 3.0 ± 0.5 | 1.9 ± 0.1 | 100 |

*Donor mice were immunized with mouse thyroglobulin (MTg) and lipopolysaccharide and their spleen cells were cultured for 3 days: Exp. 1, with MTg and transferred i.v. with or without irradiation into normal recipients; Exp. 2, with MTg, human thyroglobulin (HTg) or concanavalin A (Con A) and then transferred; data adapted from Simon et al.[39].
†Determined 14 days following cell transfer.

Similar to human Tg, bovine or porcine Tg can also activate spleen cells from MTg-immunized mice to transfer EAT (unpublished observations). These findings raise the interesting possibility that conserved regions on Tg may be thyroiditogenic in genetically susceptible mice. However, the heterologous thyroglobulins are not as good as the homologous MTg in inducing EAT by active immunization even with CFA[35,39,41]. Thus, in vivo mechanisms may exist to suppress or lessen the pathogenicity of conserved (shared) epitopes. Apparently, after expansion and differentiation in vitro, this subset of T-cells autoreactive to the conserved regions is no longer susceptible to such suppressor influence. Moreover, lymphocytes from human Tg-immunized mice, activated by either MTg or human Tg (as in Table 1.5), also transfer EAT and develop into cytotoxic T-cells[39] (see later). At present, it is not known if MTg shares the same conserved epitope with all three thyroglobulins.

## PATHOGENIC MECHANISMS MEDIATED BY T-CELLS

### T-cells cytotoxic for thyroid monolayers

Despite the well-known immunological manifestations of autoantibody production and mononuclear infiltration in the target organ of human and animal autoimmune thyroiditis, efforts to understand the pathogenic mechanisms have been hampered by the lack of an appropriate assay for thyroid damage in vitro. Applying recent advances in thyroid culture and monoclonal technology, and taking advantage of our ability to expand the immune T-cell populations with Tg in vitro (see previous section), we have established a cytotoxicity assay for thyroid target destruction[20,33]. Primary thyroid cultures from normal mice were propagated in the presence of

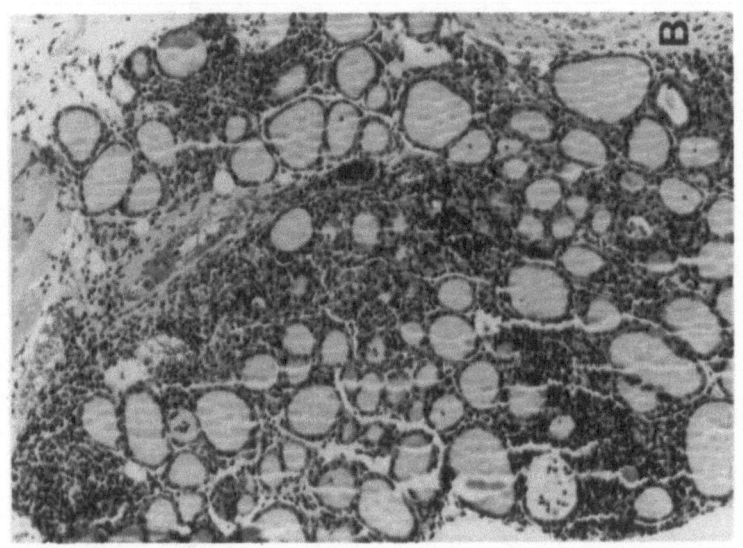

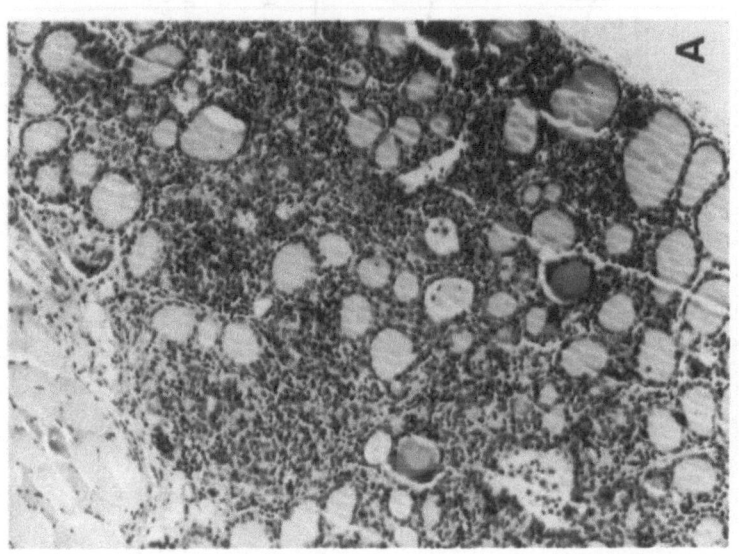

**Figure 1.1** Microscopic sections of the thyroids from recipient mice given *in vitro*-activated spleen cells from donors immunized with mouse thyroglobulin (MTg), showing mononuclear cell infiltrates. Haematoxylin and eosin stain, original magnification × 240. (A) from recipient of MTg-activated spleen cells; (B) from recipient of human thyroglobulin-activated spleen cells

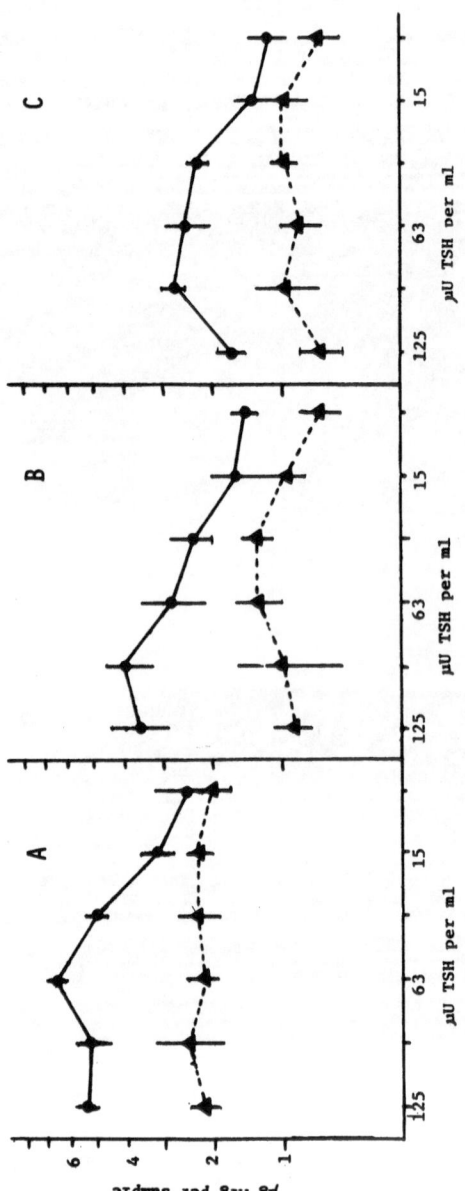

**Figure 1.2** Amounts of mouse thyroglobulin (MTg) in the supernatant of primary thyroid cell cultures at different concentrations of thyroid-stimulating hormone (TSH) with (●) or without (▲) 1 mmol/1 of cAMP. Samples were obtained on day 3 (A), 6 (B), or 9 (C) of culture. Data from Creemers *et al.*[20] p. 563, reproduced by copyright permission of the Rockefeller University Press

thyroid-stimulating hormone (TSH) and dibutyryl adenosine 3′,5′-cyclic monophosphate (cAMP). The *in vitro* synthesis of MTg was assessed to ascertain the functional capability of the thyroid epithelial cells and to optimize cultural conditions. The amounts of MTg in concentrated supernatant samples were determined with enzyme-linked monoclonal antibodies to MTg[42]. Figure 1.2 shows that a combination of TSH and cAMP increased the production of MTg up to 9 days of culture, compared to TSH alone. Such functional thyroid monolayers were labelled with [111]Indium in microculture plates, to which MTg-activated lymphocytes were added after 5-6 days of stimulation[20]. Table 1.8 presents an example of thyrocyte killing measured by the release of [111]Indium. Thyroid cells can also stimulate lymphocytes from MTg-immunized mice to develop cytotoxicity, but are less efficient than added MTg, possibly due to the low amounts of MTg synthesized in culture[33]. Similarly, human Tg generates cytotoxic T-cells ($T_C$) *in vitro* after MTg immunization (Table 1.9). As discussed in the previous section, activation with human Tg also results in the generation of effector cells which transfer EAT[32].

**Table 1.8** Cell-mediated cytotoxicity for thyroid cultures by primed lymphocytes after *in vitro* stimulation with mouse thyroglobulin (MTg) or thyroid cells*

| *In vitro* activation | No. effector cells added | Specific [111]In-release from thyroid target cells (% ± SD) |
|---|---|---|
| MTg, 10 μg/ml | $2 \times 10^5$ | 72 ± 8 |
| MTg, 25 μg/ml | $2 \times 10^5$ | 61 ± 8 |
| Thyroid cells | $2 \times 10^5$ | 20 ± 8 |
| Thyroid cells | $2 \times 10^6$ | 48 ± 9 |
| Thyroid cells | $1 \times 10^7$ | 59 ± 13 |

Modified from Kong *et al.*[33].
*Lymph node cells were collected on day 14 after immunization with MTg in complete Freund's adjuvant and cultured for 5 days prior to cytotoxic assay.

Of further interest is the capacity of human Tg to generate $T_C$ from human Tg-immunized mice (Table 1.9). As mentioned in the previous section, human Tg in adjuvant is less effective than MTg in inducing EAT *in vivo*. However, after *in vitro* expansion of T-cells responding to human Tg, which includes the epitopes shared by MTg, their capacity to cause thyroiditis in recipient mice and kill thyroid targets *in vitro* is greatly enhanced[32]. It appears that priming with human Tg *in vivo* activates $T_I$ and $T_H$ with high levels of antibody production but thyroid damage requires additional T-cell differentiation which is susceptible to suppressor influences. Studies are in progress to determine if such regulation of effector mechanisms is encoded by K- and D-end genes.

Since MTg plus adjuvant induces severe thyroiditis in certain actively immunized strains, it seems capable of providing the additional stimuli to

**Table 1.9** Generation of cytotoxic cells following *in vitro* restimulation with mouse or human thyroglobulin*

| Immunizing antigen | In vitro antigen | No. effector cells | Specific [111]In-release from thyroid target cells (%) |
|---|---|---|---|
| MTg | MTg, 25 µg/ml | $2 \times 10^5$ | 21.0 |
| | | $8 \times 10^5$ | 49.6 |
| | HTg, 50 µg/ml | $2 \times 10^5$ | 15.3 |
| | | $8 \times 10^5$ | 58.6 |
| HTg | MTg, 50 µg/ml | $2 \times 10^5$ | 18.1 |
| | | $8 \times 10^5$ | 51.0 |
| | HTg, 25 µg/ml | $2 \times 10^5$ | 13.9 |
| | | $8 \times 10^5$ | 27.7 |

Modified from Simon *et al.*[32].
*Lymph node cells were collected on day 12 following immunization with either mouse or human thyroglobulin (MTg or HTg) in complete Freund's adjuvant and cultured for 6 days with either MTg or HTg.

overcome regulatory effects. Our *in vitro* studies suggest at least two additional steps in T-cell stimulation and/or differentiation contributing to thyroid damage. The first is the expansion of a Tg-specific, Lyt-1-bearing, T-cell subset demonstrable after immunization. Its proliferative response is blocked by antibodies to L3T4 in the T-cell receptor and is abrogated by prior deletion with Lyt-1 antibodies (see previous section). Within this population are $T_A$, so designated because they amplify and promote the second step in the differentiation of $T_C$ from precursor cells. If the Lyt-1$^+$ $T_A$ are deleted early in culture, insufficient numbers of $T_C$ develop *in vitro* to destroy thyroid monolayers[20], suggesting that $T_A$ provide the lymphokines (e.g. interleukin-2) required for $T_C$ generation.

The characteristics of the cytotoxic response are summarized in Table 1.10 and are the same whether MTg or Con A serves as activator for the primed lymphocytes. Similar to lysis in virally-infected cells by virus-specific $T_C$, Tg-specific $T_C$ exhibit dual recognition of class I antigens and Tg on thyrocytes. Only syngeneic thyrocytes are destroyed and the killing is blocked by prior incubation of target cells with antibodies to K or D antigens. These observations suggest a major role for $T_C$ in pathogenesis; their characteristics have recently been corroborated by others using mouse lymphocytes primed *in vitro* with thyroid cells[43]. However, the relative contribution of $T_C$ *in vivo* and to what extent they initiate thyroid damage remain to be elucidated.

### T-cell subsets in the thyroid infiltrate

In studies on the adoptive transfer of EAT, *in vitro* activation of primed lymphocytes with Tg requires about 3 days[37,39] (see previous section). Although cytotoxicity usually is undetectable at this time, the precursors of $T_C$ are co-transferred and can undergo differentiation in the host. The activated Lyt-1$^+$ T$_A$ may also recruit T$_C$ of host origin to participate in thyroid damage. That the mononuclear cell infiltrate in mice developing EAT contains many macrophages has implicated a role for T$_D$, which produce lymphokine stimulatory for macrophages. The presence of T$_D$ has been described in immunized mice but it does not correlate with lesion development[41]. If the transferred Lyt-1$^+$ subpopulation also contains T$_D$, their actual role in thyroiditis is unknown.

**Table 1.10** Characteristics of cytotoxic response mediated by primed lymphocytes against syngeneic thyroid target cells

| *Immunizing antigen** | *Cell-mediated cytotoxicity* | *In vitro culture with:* | | |
| | | BSA | MTg | Con A |
| --- | --- | --- | --- | --- |
| Saline | Detectable after *in vitro* stimulation | | – | – |
| MTg | Detectable after *in vitro* stimulation | – | + | + |
| | Mediated by Thy-1$^+$ cells | | + | + |
| | Mediated by Lyt-2$^+$ cells | | + | + |
| | Requiring presence of Lyt-1$^+$ cells for differentiation | | + | + |
| | Blocked by treating thyroid targets with antibodies to MTg | | + | + |
| | Blocked by treating thyroid targets with antibodies to class I antigens† | | + | + |

Summarized from Creemers *et al.*[20] and Kong *et al.*[33].
*Mouse thyroglobulin (MTg) or saline given in complete Freund's adjuvant.
†CBA T-cells are cytotoxic for CBA, but not BALB/c, thyroid targets; cytotoxicity is blocked by antibodies to CBA class I (K, D) antigens.

We have begun examining the kinetics of cellular infiltration into the thyroids of mice developing EAT. Suspensions of thyroidal leukocytes and peripheral blood leukocytes (PBL) were compared at varying intervals after immunization with MTg and adjuvant. B (sIg$^+$) cells in both the thyroid and PBL remained constant at <5% and 19–24% respectively[44]. Total T (Thy-1$^+$) cells in PBL fluctuated between 45 and 59%. However, thyroidal T-cells showed a steady decline from 50% to below 30% (day 21). The decline was paralleled by an increase in cells which did not express T or B surface markers, representing primarily macrophages (rather than antibody-producing cells). In the T-cell subpopulations, there was a shift in Lyt-1$^+$: Lyt-2$^+$ ratio from about 7 down to 2 (Table 1.11), as the early predominance of Lyt-1$^+$ subset was followed by the relative increase in Lyt-2$^+$ cells. The T-cell ratios in PBL did not correlate with those observed in the thyroids. Thus, it is essential to examine at intervals infiltrates of the target organ rather than PBL to follow the progression of autoimmune disease. Whether the Lyt-1$^+$ cells contain Tg-specific T$_A$ (and possibly T$_D$) and the Lyt-2$^+$ cells include T$_C$ must await functional analysis, made difficult by the small number of antigen-specific T-cells in mouse thyroids.

**Table 1.11** Distribution of T-lymphocyte subsets in the thyroid infiltrate and peripheral blood of mice developing autoimmune thyroiditis

| Cell source | Day | Leukocytes* (%) | | |
|---|---|---|---|---|
| | | Lyt-1⁺ | Lyt-2⁺ | $\frac{Lyt\text{-}1^+}{Lyt\text{-}2^+}$ |
| Peripheral blood | 13 | 12.3 | <1.0 | 12.3 |
| | 17 | 6.2 | 5.8 | 1.1 |
| Thyroid | 13 | 51.1 | 6.7 | 7.6 |
| | 17 | 29.8 | 12.4 | 2.4 |

Adapted from Creemers *et al.*[44].

*sIg⁺(B) cells: peripheral blood, 19–20% and thyroid infiltrate, 1–2%; positive thyroid pathology, 57–60%.

## SUPPRESSOR MECHANISMS REGULATING AUTOIMMUNE THYROID DISEASE

### Activation of suppressor T-cells by pretreatment with thyroglobulin

The absence of autoimmunity in genetically susceptible individuals cannot be attributed to the absence of circulating Tg or the lack of autoreactive T-cells (see previous section). The use of induced models of rodent EAT has permitted the examination of normal regulation present *prior* to induction. Studies in both the mouse[45] and rat[46] a decade ago demonstrated that autoimmune thyroiditis can arise spontaneously after early thymectomy and irradiation to delete suppressor T-cells ($T_S$). These findings suggest the natural occurrence of $T_S$ which interfere with the trigger of autoimmunity by the ever present autoantigens. Moreover, the very existence of $T_S$ in the adult mouse appears sufficient to safeguard against autoimmune responses, when additional stimuli are introduced in the form of adjuvant; the injection of LPS or CFA without MTg into EAT-susceptible mice does not lead to autoimmune thyroiditis[9]. However, suppressor influences can be overcome in EAT by: (1) the administration of both MTg and certain adjuvants[9,12,13]; (2) repeated injections (16 times) of MTg[28]; and (3) the transfer of *in vitro*-activated effector T-cells[35,37,39].

To determine whether the naturally occurring $T_S$ were antigen-specific and could be stimulated to expand their influence, we applied experiences gained in earlier studies using a foreign antigen in mice. The prior injection of deaggregated bovine γ-globulin activated antigen-specific $T_S$ which suppressed subsequent immunization[47]. Accordingly, EAT-susceptible mice were pretreated with ultracentrifuged MTg 10 and 3 days before immuniz-ation with MTg and CFA[48]. Table 1.12 shows that resistance to EAT induction is reflected in three assays of autoimmunity. Compared to immunized controls, MTg-pretreated mice display no lymphocyte prolifera-tive response to MTg, negligible autoantibody production and mild thyroid inflammation in only 10% of the animals. Lymphocytes from these mice respond to stimulation with Con A and the control antigen, purified protein derivative, present in CFA[48]. The MTg-specific cells are Thy-1$^+$ and suppress the induction of EAT in normal recipients following cell transfer. Thus, prior MTg stimulation strengthens existing tolerance to withstand an immunizing regimen of MTg plus adjuvant. This state of suppression can still be demonstrated after an interval of 73 days (Simon et al., unpublished observations). The existence of both $T_S$ and $T_I$ ($T_H$), which can be selectively activated with a self-antigen, led us to advance the concept of clonal balance to explain the normal maintenance of self-tolerance in genetically susceptible individuals[49].

**Table 1.12** Resistance to induction of autoimmune thyroiditis following pretreatment with mouse thyroglobulin (MTg) as measured by three different assays*

| MTg pretreatment | Lymphocyte proliferative response (Mean cpm ± SE) | MTg antibody titre (Mean log$_2$ ± SE) | Thyroiditis (Mean index ± SE) | Positive/total (%) |
|---|---|---|---|---|
| – | 19 900 ± 200 | 9.8 ± 0.6 | 2.3 ± 0.2 | 100 |
| + | 1 000 ± 60 | <1.0 | 0.0 | 10 |

Modified from Kong et al.[48].
*Susceptible mice were pretreated with 200 μg MTg i.v. 10 and 3 days before challenge with 60 μg MTg in complete Freund's adjuvant; data from day 14.

The activation of $T_S$ by pretreatment with soluble MTg is markedly dose-dependent[48], as further illustrated by recent studies[50]. The extent of suppression begins to increase at about 50 μg (Table 1.13). To determine the fate of intravenously injected MTg (mol. wt. 660 000), the half-lives ($t_{1/2}$) of circulatory MTg were determined by the use of enzyme-linked monoclonal antibodies to MTg[20,42]. An initial rapid clearance rate of $t_{1/2}$ of 3 hours resulted in approximately 1% MTg remaining at 24 hours. However, this was followed by a second (biological) $t_{1/2}$ of about 10 hours. Table 1.13 shows that tolerogenic doses (≥ 100 μg) sustained an MTg level above normal for 2–3 days, whereas subtolerogenic doses (≤ 25 μg) were reduced to baseline levels within 24 hours. The rapid clearance of MTg by the mononuclear phagocytic (reticuloendothelial) system explains the need for the high MTg doses for pretreatment. It is known that at least 2–3 days are required for $T_S$ expansion in vivo. Recently, we have observed that the prior administration of LPS, which interferes with phagocytic uptake 24 hours later, converts a sub-tolerogenic dose of MTg to a tolerogenic dose by extending the initial $t_{1/2}$ to about 5 hours[51]. Possibly, the added time of above-threshold levels of circulating MTg permits more $T_S$ to be stimulated or differentiated.

## Suppressor activation by administration of thyroid-regulating hormones

In the experiments just described, resistance to EAT induction is greatly enhanced by exogenously administered MTg and correlates well with sustained levels of circulatory Tg above baseline for several days. Although the $t_{1/2}$ of this phase is 10 hours, the rapid initial clearance reduces the

**Table 1.13** Effect of pretreatment dose of mouse thyroglobulin (MTg) on circulatory MTg level and enhanced resistance to autoimmune thyroiditis

| MTg dose* | Duration of MTg level | Suppression (%) | |
|---|---|---|---|
| | above normal† | | |
| (μg) | (hours) | MTg antibody‡ | Thyroiditis‡ |
| None | None | 0 | 0 |
| 25 | 15–25 | 40 | 33 |
| 50 | 25–35 | 67 | 67 |
| 100 | 35–40 | 100 | 67 |
| 200 | 45–50 | 100 | 83 |

Adapted from Lewis et al.[50].
*Injected i.v. 10 and 3 days before immunization with MTg and lipopolysaccharide (LPS).
†Circulatory MTg level above upper limit of normal (mean + 2 SD) measured at 2.5, 8 and 24 hours after the first pretreatment dose of MTg.
‡Data from day 28.

sustained Tg level to only 2- to 3-fold above normal limits. We reasoned that this kind of elevation could occur in nature due to fluctuating output of thyroid-regulating hormones, in turn affecting resistance to autoantigenic stimuli. To test the effects of thyroid-stimulating hormone (TSH) and thyrotropin-releasing hormone (TRH), each was injected daily for 14 days into mice and their autoimmune status was determined both before and after EAT induction[48]. As seen in Table 1.14, the injections of TSH or TRH alone did not result in antibody production (preimmunization). Thyroid sampling also showed no infiltration. After immunization, IgG antibodies to MTg were observed in the majority of TSH- or TRH-treated mice, but at levels significantly lower than in immunized controls without hormonal treatment. Furthermore, the incidence of thyroiditis was greatly reduced (0–17% vs. 67%). Interestingly, when LPS was also given in conjunction with TSH and TRH on three occasions, thyroid infiltration was similarly reduced after immunization, and IgG antibodies to MTg were further suppressed to undetectable levels. The data show that hormonal manipulation of endogenous thyroid function can enhance resistance to EAT. The immune response to a control antigen, ovalbumin, was unaffected by hormonal pretreatment, indicating that thyroid stimulation had no effect on the overall immune system[48].

To determine whether resistance could be related to sustained changes in endogenous Tg level, we infused TSH for 7 days with an osmotic pump placed in the peritoneal cavity. Circulatory Tg levels peaked at 2- to 3-fold above baseline within 3 days and then declined. $T_4$ (thyroxine) levels peaked at 24 hours and served to verify the effect of TSH on thyroid function. Ten days after TSH implant, the animals were immunized. Whereas MTg antibody titres were lower than immunized controls in one of two experiments (Table 1.15, Exp. 1), the severity of thyroiditis was significantly reduced by prior TSH infusion. In other experiments, wherein LPS was injected 6 hours after TSH implantation, MTg levels peaked at similar

**Table 1.14** Resistance to induction of autoimmune thyroiditis following pretreatment with daily injections of TSH* or TRH*

| Treatment (dose) TSH or TRH days 0–13 LPS days 1, 8, 15 | MTg antibody titre (Mean log$_2$ ± SE) | | IgG antibody Positive/total (%) | Thyroiditis Positive/total (%) |
|---|---|---|---|---|
| | Preimmunization* | Postimmunization† | | |
| TSH (0.25 U) | <1.0 | 7.7 ± 1.4 | 67 | 0 |
| TSH (0.25 U) + LPS (20 µg) | 1.5‡ ± 0.4 | 5.2‡ ± 0.2 | 0 | 17 |
| TRH (1 µg) | <1.0 | 7.8 ± 0.4 | 83 | 17 |
| TRH (1 µg) + LPS (20 µg) | 1.9‡ ± 0.4 | 5.0‡ ± 0.3 | 0 | 0 |
| None | <1.0 | 13.8 ± 0.4 | 100 | 67 |

Modified from Kong et al.[48].
*Averaged from days 7, 14 and 20 during and after treatment with thyroid-stimulating hormone (TSH) or thyrotropin-releasing hormone (TRH) and lipopolysaccharide (LPS).
†Immunized i.v. with 20 µg each of mouse thyroglobulin (MTg) and LPS on days 21 and 28; data from day 45.
‡Mercaptoethanol-sensitive (IgM).

intervals of 3–4 days but consistently reached higher concentrations of 3- to 5-fold above baseline than in mice given TSH pump alone[51]. After challenge with MTg and adjuvant, both antibody titres and thyroid infiltration were greatly reduced. As discussed previously, LPS could be affecting clearance of MTg, resulting in higher levels of circulating MTg for several days. This interval appears sufficient to heighten suppressor function. Studies are in progress to determine if Ts are involved in TSH-induced suppression as seen after the administration of exogenous MTg[48]. The possibility that endogenously released Tg somehow down-regulates Tg-reactive cells has not been excluded.

**Table 1.15** Resistance to induction of autoimmune thyroiditis following chronic thyroid stimulation

| Exp. | Treatment* | MTg antibody titre† (Mean log$_2$ ± SE) | Thyroiditis† (Mean index ± SE) |
|---|---|---|---|
| 1 | TSH pump (0.25 U/day) | 11.2 ± 1.6 | 0.5 ± 0.2 |
| | Saline pump | 19.8 ± 1.5 | 1.8 ± 0.3 |
| 2 | TSH pump (0.25 U/day) | 15.5 ± 0.6 | 0.9 ± 0.2 |
| | Sham operation | 16.4 ± 0.9 | 1.7 ± 0.2 |

Modified from Lewis et al.[50].
*Osmotic pump released thyroid-stimulating hormone (TSH) for 7 days (0.25 U/day); mice were immunized 10 days after pump implantation with mouse thyroglobulin (MTg) and lipopolysaccharide.
†Data from day 28.

## SUMMARY

Several working hypotheses dealing with recognitory, regulatory and pathogenic mechanisms in autoimmune thyroid disease have been presented in this chapter. The possible interactions of T- and B-cells and the role T-cell subsets may play *in vivo* have been integrated into a diagrammatic summary (Figure 1.3). In genetically susceptible individuals possessing the MHC-linked immune response gene (Ir-Tg), there normally exist clones of Tg-specific suppressor and inducer T-cells, providing clonal balance[49] (Ts:Ti) in homoeostasis. Each set of clones can be selectively activated with Tg. It is possible to override initial suppressor influences by multiple exposures to Tg alone, or after the combined stimulation of Tg and adjuvant-like signals from the natural environment. Expansion and differentiation of T-cell subsets then promote lymphokine production, Ia (DR-like) expression, autoantibody formation and thyroid damage. One prime pathogenic mechanism may be the destruction of thyroid epithelial cells by cytotoxic T-cells. Autoantibodies may aggravate thyroiditis in EAT by yet unknown mechanisms; definite roles have not been described for the various human antibodies to thyroid antigens. Thus, if idiotypic regulation has a role in controlling autoimmunity[52], the T-cell idiotypes should receive major attention.

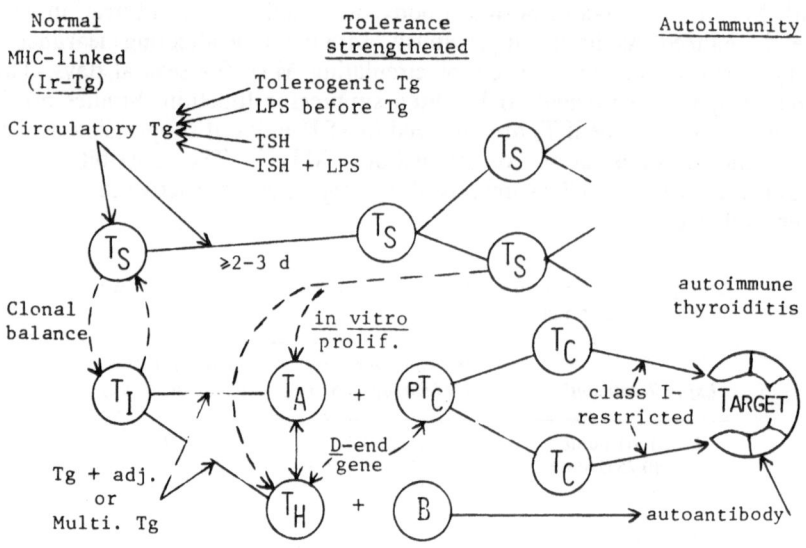

**Figure 1.3** Schematic diagram illustrating the current working hypotheses of the interactions of T-cells involved in suppressor and pathogenic mechanisms of experimental autoimmune thyroiditis. Abbreviations: Tg, thyroglobulin; LPS, lipopolysaccharide; Adj., adjuvant; TSH, thyroid-stimulating hormone; B, B-lymphocyte; T-cell subsets: S, suppressor; I, inducer; H, helper; A, amplifier; C, cytotoxic; pTc, precursor of Tc

As depicted in Figure 1.3, suppressor influences can be bolstered to withstand strong autoantigenic and adjuvant stimuli by the increase in circulatory Tg several fold above baseline levels. Both exogenous Tg and endogenous Tg, released by TSH infusion, can sustain elevated levels for 2–3 days; the former has been shown to expand the suppressor T-cell population. In addition, as yet unknown polygenic influences at different steps will contribute to the outcome of autoantigenic stimulation. As indicated in the introduction, many correlates between the human and mouse immune networks have been found. Recently, human Tg-reactive T-cells with proliferating and cytotoxic potentials have been described in Hashimoto's patients[34,53]. The numerous correlations instil confidence that the approaches taken in the mouse model will someday aid our understanding of mechanisms in autoimmune disease and provide a rationale for preventive as well as therapeutic measures.

## ACKNOWLEDGEMENTS

Space does not permit the mention of each co-worker whose diligence and fresh outlook have contributed to the concepts presented here. However, three colleagues of long duration deserve special thanks for the continually stimulating discussions: in particular, Noel R. Rose for his unique background and insight in autoimmune disease; Chella S. David for his expert analyses of immunogenetic interactions; and Alvaro A. Giraldo for his expertise in immunopathology.

This work was supported by US Public Health Service grants AM 30975 and AM 31827 from the National Institute of Arthritis, Diabetes, and Digestive and Kidney Diseases. Chuty Erves provided the unfailing secretarial help.

### References

1a. Roitt, I. M., Doniach, D., Campbell, P. N. and Hudson, R. V. (1956). Autoantibodies in Hashimoto's disease (lymphadenoid goitre). *Lancet*, **2**, 820–1
1b. Witebsky, E., Rose, N. R., Terplan, K., Paine, J. R. and Egan, R. W. (1957). Chronic thyroiditis and autoimmunization. *J. Am. Med. Assoc.*, **164**, 1439–47
2. Rose, N. R., Bacon, L. D., Sundick, R. S., Kong, Y. M., Esquivel, P. and Bigazzi, P. E. (1977). Genetic regulation in autoimmune thyroiditis. In Talal, N. (ed.) *Autoimmunity: Genetic, Immunologic and Clinical Aspects.* pp. 63–87. (New York: Academic Press)
3. Weetman, A. P. and McGregor, A. M. (1984). Autoimmune thyroid disease: developments in our understanding. *Endocrine Rev.*, **5**, 309–55
4. Lewis, M. and Rose, N. R. (1985). Experimental models in autoimmune endocrine disease. In Volpé, R. (ed.) *Autoimmunity and Endocrine Disease.* pp. 33–91. (New York: Marcel Dekker)
5. Rose, N. R., Twarog, F. J. and Crowle, A. J. (1971). Murine thyroiditis: importance of adjuvants and mouse strain for the induction of thyroid lesions. *J. Immunol.*, **106**, 698–704
6. Vladutiu, A. O. and Rose, N. R. (1971). Autoimmune murine thyroiditis: relation to histocompatibility (H-2) type. *Science*, **174**, 1137–9
7. Farid, N. R. and Bear, J. C. (1983). Autoimmune endocrine disorders and major histocompatibility complex. In Davis, T. F. (ed.) *Autoimmune Endocrine Disease.* pp. 59–91. (New York: Wiley)
8. Tomazic, V., Rose, N. R. and Shreffler, D. C. (1974). Autoimmune thyroiditis. IV.

Localization of genetic control of the immune response. *J. Immunol.*, **112**, 965–9

9. Esquivel, P. S., Rose, N. R. and Kong, Y. M. (1977). Induction of autoimmunity in good and poor responder mice with mouse thyroglobulin and lipopolysaccharide. *J. Exp. Med.*, **145**, 1250–63

10. Rose, N. R. and Kong, Y. M. (1983). T-cell regulation of experimental autoimmune thyroiditis in the mouse. *Life Sci.*, **32**, 85–95

11. Beisel, K. W., Kong, Y. M., Babu, K. S. J., David, C. S. and Rose, N. R. (1982). Regulation of experimental autoimmune thyroiditis: influence of non-*H-2* genes. *J. Immunogenetics*, **9**, 257–65

12. Esquivel, P. S., Kong, Y. M. and Rose, N. R. (1978). Evidence for thyroglobulin-reactive T-cells in good responder mice. *Cell. Immunol.*, **37**, 14–19

13. Kong, Y. M., Audibert, F., Giraldo, A. A., Rose, N. R. and Chedid, L. (1985). Effects of natural or synthetic microbial adjuvants on induction of autoimmune thyroiditis. *Infect. Immun.*, **49**, 40–5

14. Beisel, K. W., David, C. S., Giraldo, A. A., Kong, Y. M. and Rose, N. R. (1982). Regulation of experimental autoimmune thyroiditis: mapping of susceptibility to the *I-A* subregion of the mouse *H-2*. *Immunogenetics*, **15**, 427–30

15. Salamero, J. and Charreire, J. (1983). Syngeneic sensitization of mouse lymphocytes on monolayers of thyroid epithelial cells. V. The primary syngeneic sensitization is under *I-A* subregion control. *Eur. J. Immunol.*, **13**, 948–51

16. Pujol-Borrel, R., Hanafusa, T., Chiovato, L. and Bottazzo, G. F. (1983). Lectin-induced expression of DR antigens on human cultured follicular thyroid cells. *Nature (London)*, **304**, 71–3

17. Vladutiu, A. O. and Rose, N. R. (1975). Cellular basis of the genetic control of immune responsiveness to murine thyroglobulin in mice. *Cell. Immunol.*, **17**, 106–13

18. Kong, Y. M., David, C. S., Giraldo, A. A., ElRehewy, M. and Rose, N. R. (1979). Regulation of autoimmune response to mouse thyroglobulin: influence of *H-2D*-end genes. *J. Immunol.*, **123**, 15–18

19. Kong, Y. M., David, C. S., Giraldo, A. A., ElRehewy, M. and Rose, N. R. (1978). Fine structure of genetic control of autoimmune response to mouse thyroglobulin. In Rose, N. R., Bigazzi, P. E. and Warner, N. L. (eds.) *Genetic Control of Autoimmune Disease*. pp. 433–44. (New York: Elsevier/North Holland)

20. Creemers, P., Rose, N. R. and Kong, Y. M. (1983). Experimental autoimmune thyroiditis: *in vitro* cytotoxic effects of T lymphocytes on thyroid monolayers. *J. Exp. Med.*, **157**, 559–71

21. Womack, J. E. and David, C. S. (1982). Mouse gene for neuraminidase activity (Neu-1) maps to the *D* end of *H-2*. *Immunogenetics*, **16**, 177–80

22. Maron, R. and Cohen, I. R. (1979). Mutation of H-2K locus influences susceptibility to autoimmune thyroiditis. *Nature (London)*, **279**, 715–6

23. Ben-Nun, A., Maron, R., Ron, Y. and Cohen, I. R. (1980). *H-2* gene products influence susceptibility of target thyroid gland to damage in experimental autoimmune thyroiditis. *Eur. J. Immunol.*, **10**, 156–9

24. Beisel, K. W. and Rose, N. R. (1983). Genetics of the autoimmune endocrinopathies: animal models. In Davis, T. F. (ed.) *Autoimmune Endocrine Disease*, pp. 49–58. (New York: Wiley)

25. Roubinian, J. R., Talal, N., Greenspan, J. S., Goodman, J. R. and Siiteri, P. K. (1978). Effect of castration and sex hormone treatment on survival, anti-nucleic acid antibodies, and glomerulonephritis. *J. Exp. Med.*, **147**, 1568–83

26. Penhale, W. J. and Ansar Ahmed, S. (1981). The effect of gonadectomy on the sex-related expression of autoimmune thyroiditis in thymectomized and irradiated rats. *Am. J. Reprod. Immunol.*, **1**, 326–30

27. Okayasu, I., Kong, Y. M. and Rose, N. R. (1981). Effect of castration and sex hormones on experimental autoimmune thyroiditis. *Clin. Immunol. Immunopathol.*, **20**, 240–5

28. ElRehewy, M., Kong, Y. M., Giraldo, A. A. and Rose, N. R. (1981). Syngeneic thyroglobulin is immunogenic in good responder mice. *Eur. J. Immunol.*, **11**, 146–51

29. Pontes de Carvalho, L. C. and Roitt, I. M. (1982). The nature of the autoantibody response to thyroglobulin in murine strains with high or low susceptibility to the experimental induction of autoimmune thyroiditis. *Clin. Exp. Immunol.*, **48**, 519–26

30. Christadoss, P., Kong, Y. M., ElRehewy, M., Rose, N. R. and David, C. S. (1978). Genetic control of T-lymphocyte proliferative autoimmune response to thyroglobulin in mice. In Rose, N. R., Bigazzi, P. E. and Warner, N. L. (eds.) *Genetic Control of Autoimmune Disease*. pp. 445–54. (New York: Elsevier/North Holland)

31. Okayasu, I., Kong, Y. M., David, C. S. and Rose, N. R. (1981). *In vitro* T-lymphocyte proliferative response to mouse thyroglobulin in experimental autoimmune thyroiditis. *Cell. Immunol.*, **61**, 32–9

32. Simon, L. L., Krco, C. J., David, C. S. and Kong, Y. M. (1985). Characterization of the *in vitro* murine T-cell proliferative responses to murine and human thyroglobulins in thyroiditis-susceptible and -resistant mice. *Cell. Immunol.*, **94**, 243–53

33. Kong, Y. M., Simon, L. L., Creemers, P. and Rose, N. R. (1986). *In vitro* T-cell proliferation and cytotoxicity in murine autoimmune thyroiditis. *Mt. Sinai J. Med.*, **53**, 46–52

34. Canonica, G. W., Consulich, M. E., Croci, R., Ferrini, S., Bagnasco, M., Dirienzo, W., Ferrini, O., Bargellesi, A. and Giordano, G. (1984). Thyroglobulin-induced T-cell *in vitro* proliferation in Hashimoto's thyroiditis: identification of the responsive subset and effect of monoclonal antibodies directed to Ia antigens. *Clin. Immunol. Immunopathol.*, **32**, 132–41

35. Maron, R., Zerubavel, R., Friedman, A. and Cohen, I. R. (1983). T lymphocyte line specific for thyroglobulin produces or vaccinates against autoimmune thyroiditis in mice. *J. Immunol.*, **131**, 2316–22

36. Champion, B. R., Varey, A. M., Katz, D., Cooke, A. and Roitt, I. M. (1985). Autoreactive T-cell lines specific for mouse thyroglobulin. *Immunology*, **54**, 513–9

37. Braley-Mullen, H., Johnson, M., Sharp, G. C. and Kyriakos, M. (1985). Induction of experimental autoimmune thyroiditis in mice with *in vitro* activated splenic T-cells. *Cell. Immunol.*, **93**, 132–43

38. Okayasu, I. (1985). Transfer of experimental autoimmune thyroiditis to normal syngeneic mice by injection of mouse thyroglobulin-sensitized T lymphocytes after activation with concanavalin A. *Clin. Immunol. Immunopathol.*, **36**, 101–9

39. Simon, L. L., Justen, J. M., Giraldo, A. A., Krco, C. J. and Kong, Y. M. (1986). Activation of cytotoxic T cells and effector cells in experimental autoimmune thyroiditis by shared determinants of mouse and human thyroglobulins. *Clin. Immunol. Immunopathol.* **39**, 345–56

40. Nye, L., Pontes de Carvalho, L. C. and Roitt, I. M. (1980). Restrictions in the response to autologous thyroglobulin in the human. *Clin. Exp. Immunol.*, **41**, 252–63

41. Romball, C. G. and Weigle, W. O. (1984). T cell competence to heterologous and homologous thyroglobulins during the induction of experimental autoimmune thyroiditis. *Eur. J. Immunol.*, **14**, 887–93

42. Kong, Y. M., Rose, N. R., ElRehewy, M., Michaels, R., Giraldo, A. A., Accavitti, M. A. and Leon, M. A. (1980). Thyroid alloantigens in autoimmunity. *Transpl. Proc.*, **12** (Suppl. 1), 129–34

43. Salamero, J. and Charreire, J. (1985). Syngeneic sensitization of mouse lymphocytes on monolayers of thyroid epithelial cells. VII. Generation of thyroid-specific cytotoxic effector cells. *Cell. Immunol.*, **91**, 111–8

44. Creemers, P., Giraldo, A. A., Rose, N. R. and Kong, Y. M. (1984). T-cell subsets in the thyroids of mice developing autoimmune thyroiditis. *Cell. Immunol.*, **87**, 692–7

45. Kojima, A., Tanaka-Kojima, Y., Sakahura, T. and Nishizuka, Y. (1976). Spontaneous development of autoimmune thyroiditis in neonatally thymectomized mice. *Lab. Invest.*, **34**, 550–7

46. Penhale, W. J., Farmer, A. and Irvine, W. J. (1975). Thyroiditis in T cell-depleted rats. *Clin. Exp. Immunol.*, **21**, 362–75

47. Fessia, S. L. and Kong, Y. M. (1977). Studies on interference with tolerance induction in T cells. *Scand. J. Immunol.*, **6**, 1209–16

48. Kong, Y. M., Okayasu, I., Giraldo, A. A., Beisel, K. W., Sundick, R. S., Rose, N. R., David, C. S., Audibert, F. and Chedid, L. (1982). Tolerance to thyroglobulin by activating suppressor mechanisms. *Ann. N.Y. Acad. Sci.*, **392**, 191–209

49. Rose, N. R., Kong, Y. M., Okayasu, I., Giraldo, A. A., Beisel, K. and Sundick, R. S. (1981). T-cell regulation in autoimmune thyroiditis. *Immunol. Rev.*, **55**, 299–314

50. Lewis, M., Giraldo, A. A. and Kong, Y. M. (1986). Resistance to experimental autoimmune

thyroiditis induced by physiologic manipulation of thyroglobulin level. (Submitted)

51. Lewis, M., Giraldo, A. A. and Kong, Y. M. (1984). The crucial role of circulatory thyroglobulin in activation of suppressor mechanisms. *Immunobiology*, **167**, 44–5

52. Zanetti, M. (1985). The idiotype network in autoimmune processes. *Immunol. Today*, **6**, 299–302

53. Canonica, G. W., Caria, M., Bagnasco, M., Cosulich, M. E., Giordano, G. and Moretta, L. (1985). Proliferation of T8-positive cytolytic T lymphocytes in response to thyroglobulin in human autoimmune thyroiditis: analysis of cell interactions and culture requirements. *Clin. Immunol. Immunopathol.*, **36**, 40–8

# 2
# Recent Developments in the *in vitro* Bioassay of TSH and Thyroid-Stimulating Antibodies

**N. J. MARSHALL AND P. A. EALEY**

## INTRODUCTION

Circulating immunoglobulins with thyroid-stimulating activity were origin-ally discovered 30 years ago[1]. These thyroid-stimulating antibodies (TSAb) are now established as important pathogenetic factors in the hyperthyroidism of Graves' disease. They appear to interact with a site on or close to the TSH receptor and generally mimic the bioactivity of TSH. It has now become apparent that another group of related antibodies may specifically or preferentially stimulate thyroid growth as opposed to differentiated function, and these are discussed in Chapter 3. Such antibodies are now referred to as thyroid growth-stimulating antibodies, or TGAb. In the present chapter we will largely be concerned with recent developments in techniques to measure antibodies which hitherto have been regarded as stimulators of differentiated function leading to the excess production of thyroid hormones. These continue to be referred to as TSAb as opposed to TGAb.

It is generally anticipated that reliable TSAb assays have potential value in the clinical management of patients with Graves' disease in the areas listed in Table 2.1. Given the widespread availability of well-established thyroid function tests and the recent emergence of sensitive immunoradiometric assays for TSH, TSAb assays are not necessary for the initial diagnosis of Graves' disease, except perhaps for a clearer definition of occasional preclinical presentation. However, it is considered likely that spontaneous remission, which is a characteristic of this disease and occurs in a high proportion of patients, may well be correlated with a decrease in circulating TSAb. Alternatively, persistently high TSAb levels, for example during an initial period of antithyroid drug therapy, might indicate that remission is unlikely and that more drastic treatment such as thyroid ablation is necessary. Moreover, since neonatal Graves' disease involves the transplacental transfer of TSAb from the mother to the fetus[2,3], high maternal TSAb in the last months of pregnancy might well justify unusually close observation of the infant. In addition, measurement of TSAb is of potential value in the diagnostic evaluation of selected patients with exophthalmos in whom underlying Graves' disease is suspected.

**Table 2.1** The potential clinical value of TSAb assays in Graves' disease

(1) Prediction of relapse or remission of hyperthyroidism after a limited period of antithyroid drug therapy.

(2) Indication of a need for more drastic treatment after antithyroid drug therapy, e.g. thyroid ablation by surgery or [131]I.

(3) Prediction of relapse after a period of remission.

(4) Prediction of neonatal Graves' disease.

(5) Confirmation that ophthalmopathy is related to autoimmune thyroid disease.

TSAb not only bind to a site on the cell surface TSH receptor but also stimulate the activity of membrane-bound adenylate cyclase (Figure 2.1). This leads to increased production of the intracellular hormone mediator cAMP and is followed by general activation of the follicular cell. This includes the stimulation of iodine metabolism which is characteristic of differentiated thyroid cells, relating to increased synthesis and release of thyroid hormones. As such TSAb are the prime example of antibodies which not only interact with cell-surface receptors, but also stimulate post-receptor events related to an autoimmune disease state.

Bioassays to measure the activity of TSAb in patient sera have been designed around many different metabolic responses of the thyroid follicular cell (Figure 2.1), some of which are listed in Table 2.2. However, the achievement of robust, precise and reproducible bioassays for the measurement of TSAb in clinical medicine, which also have the appropriate sensitivity and can be conveniently run in a well-controlled manner, has long proved elusive. The inability to obtain such assays to date may be understood since we are aiming to develop functional bioassay systems for thyroid stimulators. These can be more experimentally demanding than those which rely upon the recognition and detection of a specific structure (e.g. the radioimmunoassay for TSH) rather than the expression of bioactivity.

The difficulties encountered in the different bioassay systems have largely been due to the variability of the starting thyroid tissue and its preparation, and/or the insensitivity of the response systems. The latter is revealed by the doses of TSH required to elicit a response (e.g. >50 mU TSH/l) which are far higher than the normal circulating levels of TSH (0.5–5 mU TSH/l). Most of these assays are unable to detect TSAb in all patients with Graves' disease. In addition these features inevitably lead to poor within assay precision and between assay reproducibility.

Recently, major advances have been made in the technology of thyroid cell culture, which as described below holds promise of a new era of TSAb assays. It is appropriate, however, to first consider the *in vivo* bioassay system

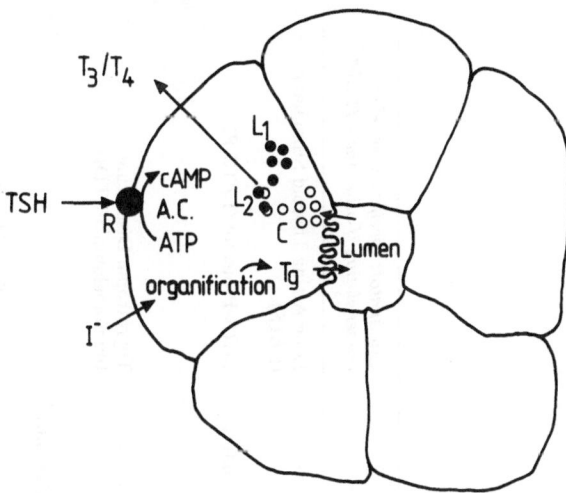

**Figure 2.1** Diagram of a thyroid follicle, which is the functional unit of the thyroid gland. The major metabolic responses of the thyroid epithelial cell when stimulated by TSH and TSAb are represented; these are utilized in the different *in vitro* bioassays listed in Table 2.2. Key: R = TSH receptor, A.C. = adenylate cyclase, Tg = thyroglobulin, C = colloid droplet, $L_1$ = primary lysosome with associated $\beta$-naphthylamidase activity, $L_2$ = secondary lysosome formed by fusion of a colloid droplet and a primary lysosome. Iodide influx is stimulated in a cAMP dependent manner, and the iodide is then organified by incorporation into thyroglobulin, which is stored in the lumen of the follicle as colloid. Iodinated thyroglobulin is reintroduced into the cell as colloid droplets, and the acid hydrolases of the lysosomes degrade the thyroglobulin, leading eventually to the release of thyroid hormones ($T_3/T_4$) into the local capillaries which surround each follicle

available for the measurement of TSAb in serum, and briefly review the alternative *in vitro* bioassays.

## *IN VIVO* BIOASSAY OF TSAb AND THE LATS-PROTECTOR ASSAY

TSAb were first detected following experiments designed to develop an *in vivo* bioassay for TSH[1]. The endogenous secretion of TSH of guinea pigs was first suppressed by thyroxine injection and their thyroid gland was preloaded with radioactive iodine. Sera from thyrotoxic patients were then injected intravenously and stimulated the release of the radioactivity in a concentration dependent manner. This was detected by monitoring blood sampled from the animals at specific time intervals after the original injection of serum. The bioactivity in the thyrotoxic sera, although originally thought to be due to TSH, was soon shown to be located in the immunoglobulin G (IgG) fraction of serum proteins[57,58]. Stimulation by the IgG was slower in onset and more prolonged than that due to equivalent doses of TSH. This characteristic gave rise to the early name of TSAb, namely Long Acting Thyroid Stimulator (LATS).

This *in vivo* bioassay was made technically easier when mice were

**Table 2.2** Examples of assay systems for TSAb and related stimulators

| Assay system | Target tissue preparation | Response system | Stimulator: specific assay related nomenclature if other than TSAb* |
|---|---|---|---|
| In vivo bioassay† | Guinea-pig or mouse thyroid in vivo preloaded with $^{125}$I (endogenous TSH suppressed) | radioactivity released in vivo from guinea pig[1] or mouse[6] thyroid | Long Acting Thyroid Stimulator (LATS) |
| In vitro assays (non-functional) | Solubilized fraction of thyroid homogenate obtained by freezing and thawing (LATS absorbing activity (LAA)) | LATS-Protector activity; binding of the antibody to LAA[7,8] | LATS-Protector (LATS-P) |
| | Membrane-bound or solubilized TSH receptors | inhibition of [$^{125}$I]TSH binding to receptor preparations[9,10] | Thyrotropin Displacing Immunoglobulins (TDI) |
| | Membrane-bound TSH receptors | direct binding of receptor purified Graves' immunoglobulins[11] | — |
| In vitro bioassays (functional) | Subcellular fraction of thyroid tissue enriched with plasma membranes | adenylate cyclase activity[12-14] | Human Thyroid Adenylate Cyclase Stimulator (HTACS) |
| | Thyroid slices (generally human) | cAMP[15,16] colloid droplets[17,18] T$_3$,T$_4$ release[19,20] | — Human Thyroid Stimulator (HTS) |

| Response system | Response measured | Thyroid Growth | Stimulating Antibodies (TGAb) |
|---|---|---|---|
| Segments of guinea-pig thyroid lobes (Cytochemical bioassay) | (i) β-Naphthylamidase Activity[21] | — | |
| | (ii) Feulgen Reaction[22] | | |
| | NADPH (i)[23] | — | — |
| | NADPH (ii)[24] | | |
| Thyroid tissue sections (12 μm) (Cytochemical bioassay) | β-Naphthylamidase Activity[25] | — | — |
| Follicle suspensions | [³H]thymidine incorporation[26,27] | | TGAb |
| Isolated cell suspension | I⁻ uptake[28,29] | — | |
| Cultures of thyroid cells (generally human) (generally porcine) | ↑cAMP (cells/medium)[30-44] | — | |
| | I⁻uptake[30,45-48] | | |
| FRTL-5 cell line | ↑cAMP[49-52] | | TGAb |
| | I⁻ uptake[53,54] | — | TGAb |
| | [³H]thymidine incorporation[49,55] | | |
| | number of metaphases[56] (Metaphase Index Assay) | | |

*Descriptions of some assay systems include the expression of the stimulator by a name derived from the specific response system utilized in the assay.

†There is also an *in vivo*, but non-serum based bioassay for TSAb, which utilizes $^{99}TcO_4$ trapping by the patient's thyroid[4,5].

substituted for guinea pigs[6], and in this form is frequently referred to as the 'McKenzie Assay'. Much valuable work has been carried out with this system, including the establishment of an international reference preparation for TSAb bioactivity, LATS-B. However, numerous studies have consistently found that a large proportion of the sera from thyrotoxic patients fail to produce any response in this assay and that LATS-levels do not often correlate well with the degre of hyperthyroidism[59,60]. This has frequently been attributed to a species specificity of TSAb, such that although the immunoglobulin in the patient serum is able to stimulate the human thyroid, it cannot cross-react with the mouse or guinea-pig gland. Such species specificity has yet to be established, since for example in the ultrasensitive Cytochemical Bioassay[21,24,25] which uses guinea-pig thyroid tissue virtually all sera from untreated thyrotoxics have been reported to stimulate.

Using the LATS *in vivo* bioassay, it was shown that bioactivity could be absorbed out of a given serum by incubating it with a soluble fraction prepared by freeze-thawing a crude homogenate of human thyroid tissue[7]. However, this abolition of the bioactivity could be prevented by the addition of LATS-negative sera from other thyrotoxic patients. Immunoglobulins in the latter were seen to 'protect' the LATS activity from absorption and were termed LATS-protectors (LATS-P). A quantitative assay based upon this interaction and known as the LATS-P assay, was established by careful manipulation of the experimental conditions. LATS-protectors were detected in almost 90% of sera from patients with untreated Graves' disease[8]. These findings have frequently been interpreted to indicate that LATS-P is a human specific TSAb which is unable to stimulate the mouse thyroid. However, it binds to TSH receptors solubilized from the human thyroid homogenate and thereby can prevent the absorption of LATS activity. As such the LATS-P assay would appear to be a non-functional ligand assay (see Table 2.2) since it primarily measures the interaction of the immunoglobulins at the TSH receptor level. It may not be possible to relate this activity to bioactivity, although a direct relationship has been claimed[61].

The *in vivo* bioassay is currently expertly carried out in only a few specialized centres worldwide, since it is labour intensive and requires the maintenance and careful control of large colonies of laboratory animals. In addition, this experimental system is inherently difficult to standardize, and assay precision difficult to achieve. Due to these problems much effort has been expended in many laboratories to develop simpler systems which we will now describe. These are based either upon the binding characteristics of the immunoglobulins of Graves' disease or on their stimulating effects on thyroid preparations *in vitro*.

## *IN VITRO* RECEPTOR ASSAYS

The binding of TSH to its receptor was characterized subsequent to the improved techniques of iodination of TSH and the preparation of subcellular fractions of thyroid tissue enriched with TSH receptors[62]. It was found that IgG preparations from a large number of Graves' sera inhibited TSH binding to its receptor[9,10], and this system was quickly exploited in numerous studies to detect what are now termed 'thyroid receptor antibodies' (Table 2.2). The receptor assay system that emerged measured the competition between the [125I]TSH and the TSAbs to bind to a preparation of TSH receptors associated with plasma membranes subfractionated from thyroid homogenates. The results were expressed directly as a function of the response parameter. This was usually a 'Displacement Index', which was the ratio of the [125I]TSH bound in the presence of the test IgG: the [125I]TSH bound in the presence of IgG from controls, (or some slight transformation of this ratio). In its earliest forms, this assay proved tantalizingly difficult to standardize in different laboratories. The routine technical procedures of the assay are as straightforward as those for radioimmunoassays, but despite this undoubted convenience, problems associated with reagent preparations proved difficult to resolve. These included control and reproducibility of the preparation of labelled TSH and TSH-receptor enriched subcellular fractions[63] and also the variable effects of 'control' IgG preparations from euthyroid individuals[64]. Another major problem was the reluctance to express the results in terms of a reference standard as opposed to the response parameter, i.e. the displacement of [125I]TSH. However, a recently modified system which uses solubilized receptors has probably overcome these problems. Solubilized receptors do not seem to be as susceptible to the non-specific effects of control IgG and components in unextracted serum[65-67] and the use of a reference material will reduce interassay variation.

An alternative approach has been to 'receptor-purify' anti-TSH receptor immunoglobulins by preincubation with fat cell membranes which are rich in TSH receptors, and subsequently to study the direct binding of the purified immunoglobulins to TSH receptors on human thyroid membranes[11]. Clearly, however, both forms of receptor assays are based upon recognition of *structures* by a TSH binding site on the TSH receptor, and do not measure TSAb bioactivity *per se*. Such structural as opposed to functional assays may not be directly related to TSAb bioactivity.

## *IN VITRO* BIOASSAYS FOR TSAb

The maintenance of a wide variety of thyroid tissue preparations *in vitro*, under conditions which allow the expression of the stimulation of post-TSH receptor events, has generated a large number of *in vitro* bioassay systems for TSH and TSAb (Table 2.2).

Three main factors have governed the extent to which they have been exploited, i.e. their convenience, technical difficulty and their response characteristics. Each system with its own particular advantages has contributed to long-term *in vitro* bioassay developments. They form a wide range of assays, any one of which might prove especially suitable for investigating new concepts relating to TSAb in the future. We will now discuss several recent developments which appear to be leading directly to the achievement of convenient, rugged, sensitive and precise *in vitro* bioassays which look promising for general clinical application. These assays are a consequence of advancements in the technology of thyroid cell culture, and the realization that culture systems offer the basis of superior assays.

## THE MERITS OF CELL CULTURE SYSTEMS

A major group of *in vitro* bioassays for both TSH and TSAb has been established using the stimulation of adenylate cyclase as the basic response system. These bioassays can be designed using a variety of thyroid tissue preparations ranging from subcellular fractions through to immortalized cell cultures (Table 2.2). The response characteristics of these different systems are summarized in Figure 2.2, which is based upon the experiences of several laboratories, including our own[16,35,43]. These characteristics illustrate the particular advantages of cell culture systems.

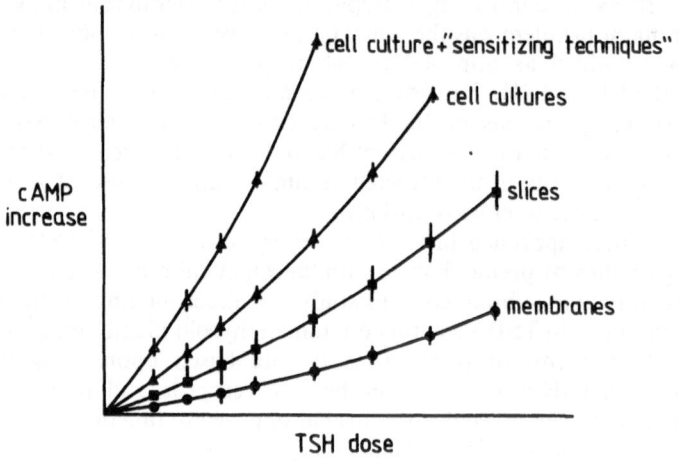

**Figure 2.2** Diagrammatic comparison between the response characteristics of the three thyroid tissue preparations most commonly used for *in vitro* bioassays measuring increased production of cAMP. It is based upon the results of several comparative studies such as those described in references 16, 34, 37, 38. Error bars indicate magnitudes of errors in response as estimated by standard deviations

The magnitude of response to a given dose of TSH, when using membranes, i.e. the most disrupted of the tissue preparations, has often been found to be relatively low. Larger responses are observed when the cellular integrity is retained, as for example with slices of thyroid tissue. However, with slices the errors in the responses can be disappointingly large, presumably because of the inherent heterogeneity of thyroid tissue slices. This necessitates the use of many replicates (e.g. $n = 6$–8) per experimental variable to observe statistically significant TSAb stimulation. With cell cultures, however, there is a larger magnitude of response and within assay errors are reduced. The plating of cells in multiwell plates with a similar number of cells from a common pool results in homogeneous cultures which minimizes within assay errors and accounts for the excellent precision which can be attained with this system (Figure 2.2). Moreover the general reproducibility of different subcultures has led to systematic work which has resulted in progressive increases in bioassay sensitivity. These modifications are referred to in Figure 2.2 as 'sensitizing techniques' and are discussed in more detail later.

Many laboratories have accordingly accepted the challenge of the demanding techniques of cell culture and exploited thyroid cell monolayers for the *in vitro* bioassay of TSH and TSAb. Although cells from the thyroids of several species have been successfully maintained in culture, much recent work on the development of new TSAb bioassays has centred upon the use of two systems, namely the culture of human thyroid cells and FRTL-5 cells, and is described below.

## Human thyroid cell culture systems

In view of the suspected human specificity of a proportion of TSAb, it has clearly been appropriate to investigate intensively the use of monolayer cultures prepared from human thyroids for TSAb bioassay. The basic flow diagram of the procedures involved is shown in Figure 2.3. These TSAb *in vitro* bioassays have almost exclusively utilized the measurement of cAMP as their end-point.

Encouraging results were obtained with this system at an early stage, and the anticipated merits, which have been discussed above, were confirmed. Apart from the obvious problem of obtaining adequate and consistent supplies of human thyroid tissue, the difficulties encountered largely derived from the inherent instability of the thyroid cells when maintained as monolayers. In our experience[38] a decrease in the magnitude of response occurred by about 21 days, which was presumed to be due to extensive dedifferentiation of the thyroid follicular cells or overgrowth by fibroblasts. As a consequence the frequent preparation of new cultures from fresh thyroids became an unavoidable necessity. Working with many different thyroid cultures, two subsequent problems were revealed. Firstly, the magnitudes of response observed with different cultures can be very variable. This is presumably largely due to inherent variations between the human thyroids used to prepare each culture. Secondly, there is evidence that the relative potencies of different TSAbs can change when tested on cultures obtained from different thyroids[38,68]. This phenomenon, which could be of considerable significance, has yet to be rigorously investigated.

### The use of cryopreserved human thyroid cells

The first of these problems, i.e. the variation of the starting tissue, has now been largely circumvented by cryopreservation of dispersed human thyroid cells. They can be cryopreserved over a period of years without detriment to their viability and response characteristics[39,42,43], and aliquots taken for successive bioassays. In addition, the availability of sensitized radioim-

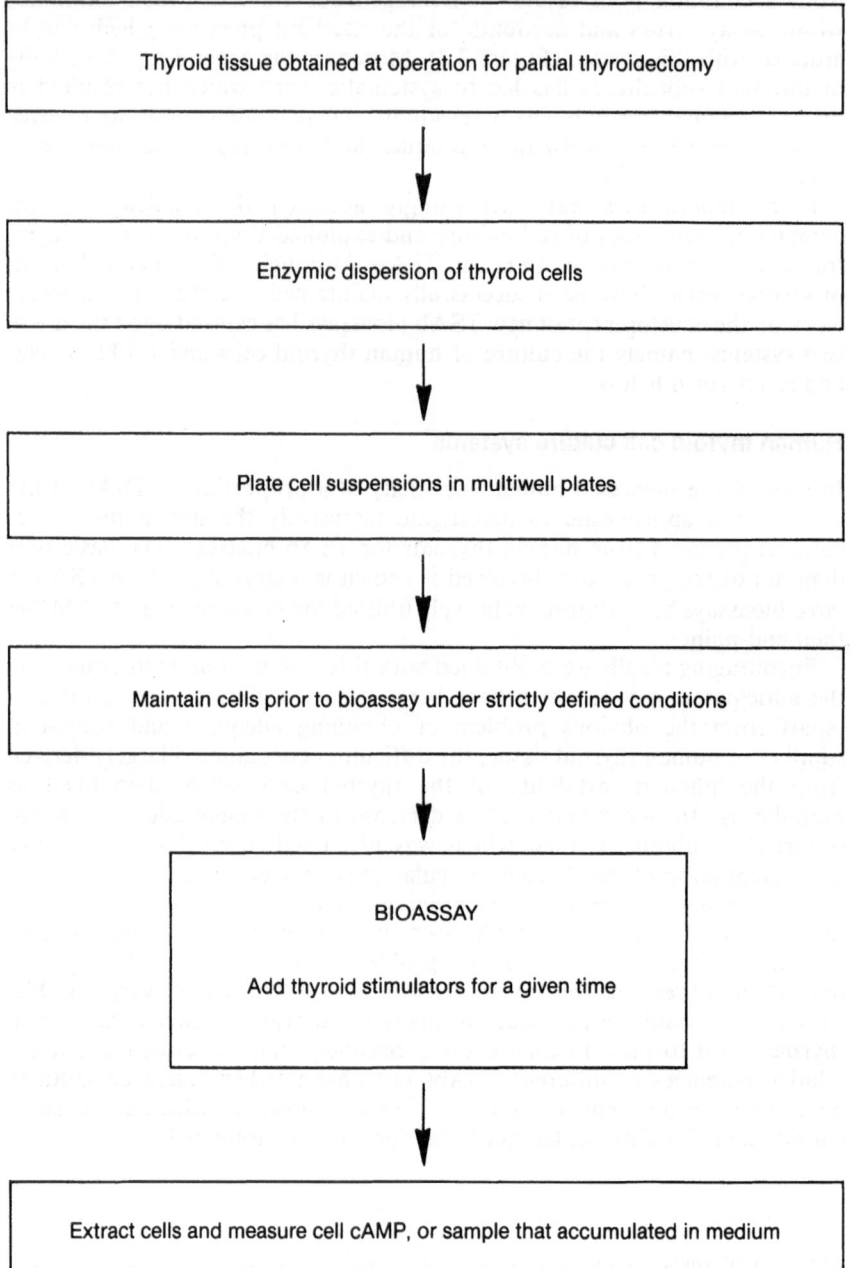

**Figure 2.3** An outline of the procedures involved in the preparation of monolayer cultures from human thyroids, and their use for the bioassay of TSH and TSAb based upon increases in cAMP[33–43]

munoassays for cAMP, with detection limits of the order of 50 fmoles/ml, has allowed much smaller numbers of cells to be used per bioassay, making it possible to use one cell-preparation for many months rather than a few days. For example, sufficient cells for 10 successive assays, each with 25 samples and a standard curve can be prepared from one gram of starting thyroid tissue[43].

Freezing the cells in liquid nitrogen allows one to use them at convenient times for a routine assay, and reduces the frequency of establishing primary cultures. Moreover, the sensitivity of a given culture to TSH and TSAb can be tested in advance prior to commitment for bioassay; clearly the use of a batch of cells of known sensitivity increases confidence that the bioassay can be performed on a regular basis.

Recently, one particularly interesting modification of this system has been the use of hypotonic incubation conditions during the exposure of the cells to the stimulators in the bioassay. Kasagi *et al.*[40] showed that a low sodium chloride concentration in the incubation medium had two advantages. Firstly, the swollen cells release a larger proportion of the total cAMP accumulated in response to the stimulators into the incubation medium. Consequently the extraction step (Figure 2.3), which is both laborious and responsible for a large error component in the assay, can be avoided. Thus the assays are made more precise by simply sampling the incubation medium. Secondly, the 'low-salt' conditions enhance the magnitude of response of the cells to thyroid stimulators such as TSH and TSAb. Intriguingly, sensitivity to TSAb is increased by a far greater extent than that to TSH[40,42]. This differential effect of NaCl on TSAb and TSH activity has yet to be explained, but one is tempted to speculate that it is related to the long-standing controversy concerning the effects of NaCl on TSH binding to its receptors[69].

Combining the use of cryopreserved human thyroid cells, and hypotonic 'sensitizing' conditions, a promising *in vitro* bioassay for TSH and TSAb has been described by Rapoport and co-workers[43]. This is relatively sensitive, technically straightforward and has a high sample capacity. Using this, TSAb were detected in 93% of a total of 61 patients with untreated hyperthyroidism due to Graves' disease, and the specificity of the assay as an indication of Graves' disease was 100% with no false positives. However, about 40% of those which were positive were giving a response equal to or less than that observed with 10 mU bTSH/l, which emphasizes the necessity for sensitive bioassays. After treatment, the prevalence of detectable TSAb decreased and was lowest during antithyroid drug therapy, when after a mean period of ~2 years only 44% remained positive. In addition, TSAb levels correlated well with relapse or remission after antithyroid drug therapy. This assay is now being evaluated on a long-term basis in several different laboratories.

At present there have been no reports that this system suffers from the changes in relative potencies of different TSAbs when tested on cultures derived from different thyroids, as found previously with human thyroid cell monolayers[38,68].

## FRTL-5 cell cultures

An alternative approach to solving the problems encountered with *in vitro* bioassays based upon thyroid cell monolayers, has been provided by the development of a continually proliferating substrain of an epithelial thyroid cell line, the FRTL-5 cells. These cells were obtained by Ambesi-Impiombato and co-workers[70,71], and are the first example of such a strain. In principle they can be maintained indefinitely in culture, and since they are responsive to TSH and TSAb, they clearly present us with new opportunities for designing *in vitro* bioassays based upon a continuous stable cell-culture system.

The parent cell-line, FRTL (Fisher Rat Thyroid Line) was initially obtained by selection in medium with a low serum concentration, but the cells grow and remain differentiated in 5% serum. The FRTL-5 cells have a doubling time of about 30 h in the presence of TSH, which is much faster than the FRTL cells from which they were cloned[70,71]. FRTL-5 cells have maintained their rapid growth and response characteristics over a few years. Cell stocks can be cryopreserved providing an assured indefinite source even in the eventuality of deleterious mutations.

The major advantages of using FRTL-5 cells for TSH and TSAb *in vitro* bioassays are summarized in Table 2.3. They clearly provide a standardized bioassay tissue which can be used in a highly controlled manner within one laboratory, allowing investigators to run rigorous quality control procedures. Moreover, for the first time they provide a bioassay tissue which can be distributed between many different laboratories. This will inevitably reduce between-laboratory bioassay variation and allow a more realistic comparison of results from different centres.

**Table 2.3** The use of FRTL-5 cells in *in vitro* bioassays

---

*Advantages*

(1)  They provide continuous, convenient and stable systems which can be used for different laboratories.

(2)  They can be manipulated prior to use in the bioassay to 'sensitize' cells to the subsequent addition of thyroid stimulators.

(3)  Unlike human thyroid cells in culture, FRTL-5 cells are acutely responsive to TSH in terms of growth.

(4)  Parallel bioassays using different response systems (e.g. ↑cAMP, ↑iodide uptake, ↑[³H]thymidine uptake, ↑cell number, ↑metaphases) can be carried out on replicate cultures.

*Disadvantages*

(1)  Derived from rat, not human thyroid; might be inappropriate for the measurement of human specific TSAb.

(2)  They are obviously not 'normal' thyroid cells; caution required before extrapolating results concerning the control systems of the FRTL-5 cells to thyroid cells *in vivo*.

---

The typical regime for the routine growth of the FRTL-5 cells in the laboratory, and their use in the bioassay based upon stimulation of cAMP accumulation, is shown in Figure 2.4. The cells are manipulated prior to use

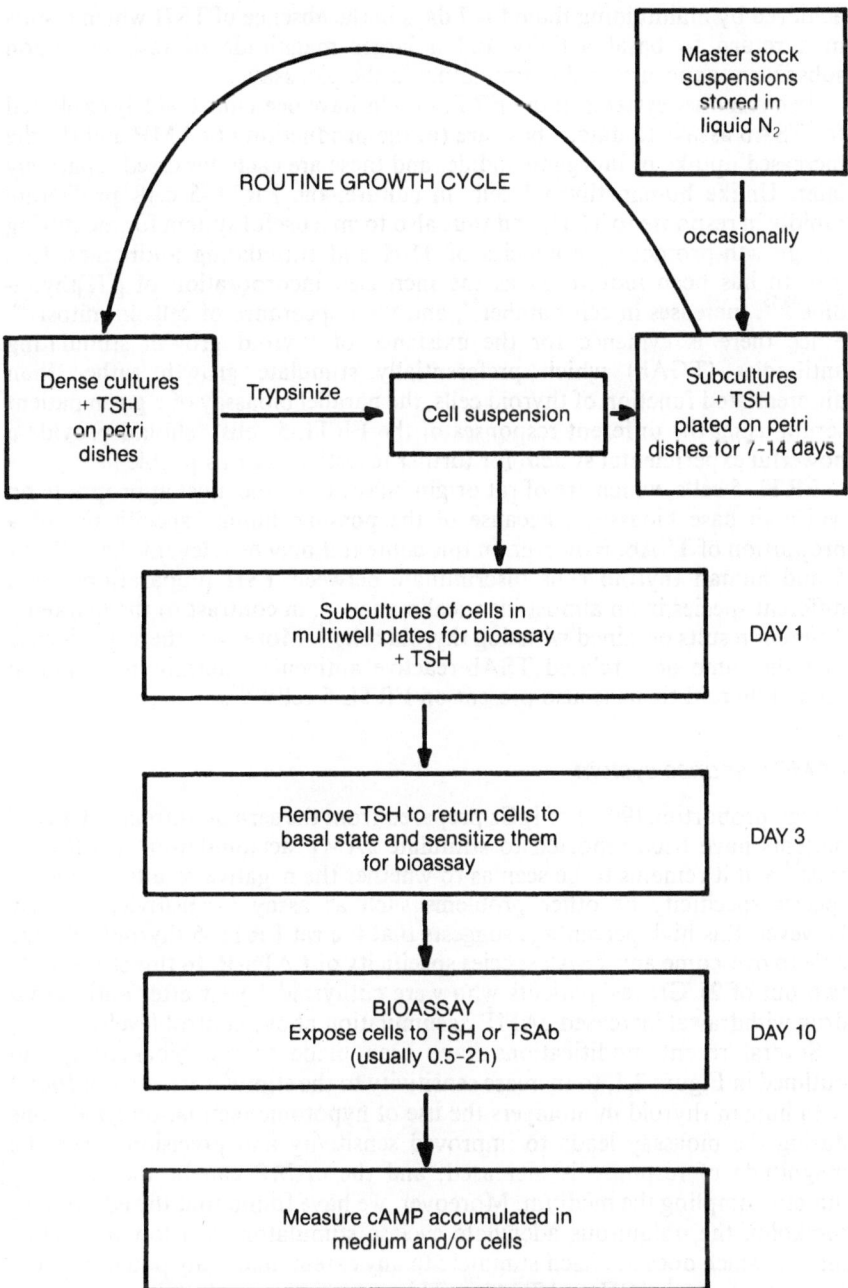

**Figure 2.4** An outline of the procedures involved in the maintenance of FRTL-5 cells, and the preparation and use of monolayers in bioassays for TSH and TSAb based upon increases in cAMP[49–52]

in the bioassay to increase their sensitivity to TSH and TSAb[52]. This is achieved by maintaining them for 7 days in the absence of TSH which results in a return to basal activity and a larger magnitude of response upon subsequent exposure to the stimulators in the bioassay.

Two response systems of the FRTL-5 cells have been most widely exploited for TSAb assays to date. These are (a) the production of cAMP and (b) the increased uptake of inorganic iodide, and these are each discussed separately later. Unlike human thyroid cells in culture, the FRTL-5 cells proliferate rapidly in response to TSH, and thus also form a useful system for measuring the growth-promoting potencies of TSH and stimulating antibodies. Cell growth has been monitored as the increased incorporation of [$^3$H]thymidine[49,55], increases in cell number[49], and the appearance of cells in mitosis[56]. Since there is evidence for the existence of thyroid growth stimulating antibodies (TGAb) which preferentially stimulate growth rather than differentiated function of thyroid cells, the parallel bioassay of a given patient serum using the different responses of the FRTL-5 cells[55] should provide a powerful experimental system for further investigating this problem.

FRTL-5 cells, which are of rat origin, may not be the most appropriate on which to base bioassays, because of the possible human specificities of a proportion of TSAb. However, in this context it may be relevant that FRTL-5 and human thyroid cells discriminate between TSH preparations from different species in an almost identical manner[72], in contrast to the markedly different results obtained with dog thyroid cells[73]. Moreover, there is evidence that the same or a related TSAb-reactive antigenic determinant found in human thyroid tissue is also present on FRTL-5 cells[52,74].

## cAMP response system

A high proportion (90%) of IgGs prepared from the sera of untreated Graves' patients have been reported to stimulate cAMP accumulation in FRTL-5 cells[52] and it remains to be seen as to whether the negative results are due to species specificity or other problems such as assay insensitivity. Clearly however, this high percentage suggests that the rat FRTL-5 thyroid cells are able to overcome any TSAb species specificity of LATS-P. In this study, only two out of 21 Graves' patients who were euthyroid 1 year after antithyroid drug withdrawal increased cAMP accumulation above control levels.

Several recent modifications have been made to the bioassay system outlined in Figure 2.4, to increase sensitivity to the stimulators. As was found with human thyroid monolayers the use of hypotonic incubation conditions during the bioassay leads to improved sensitivity and precision, since the magnitude of response is increased, and the cAMP can be measured by directly sampling the medium. Moreover, we have found that the addition of forskolin, the ubiquitous adenylate cyclase stimulator, at a low dose ($10^{-7}$ mol/l), which does not itself stimulate to any extent, markedly potentiates the responses to both TSH and TSAb[75]. This potentiation is also observed under the 'low-salt' conditions, leading to yet further sensitization with a bioassay sensitivity of about 1 mU TSH/l (Ealey, Mitchell and Marshall, unpublished results).

## *Iodide uptake response system*

The ability of thyroid cell cultures to concentrate inorganic iodide in response to TSH, has formed the basis of *in vitro* bioassay systems using cells derived from several species (Table 2.2). The sensitivity to TSH has frequently been reported to be impressive, with responses detected to <1 mU/l, making it more sensitive than the cAMP system. However, iodide uptake has yet to be exploited as extensively for the bioassay of TSH and TSAb.

The use of FRTL-5 cells for an *in vitro* bioassay based upon the stimulation of iodide uptake is illustrated in Figure 2.5, and follows the procedure recently described by Marcocci *et al.*[53]. The unstimulated control levels of iodide uptake may be reduced by depriving the cells of TSH for about 7 days as with the cAMP-based system. After readdition of the stimulators, iodide uptake is measured 48 h later, when a pulse of $^{125}$I is added for 40 min. Intracellular uptake can then be measured in ethanol extracts of the cells. Alternatively, since the cells do not organify iodide to an appreciable extent, accumulated $^{125}$I may be discharged into fresh medium containing $10^{-4}$ mol/l sodium perchlorate, and the medium can then be sampled[54].

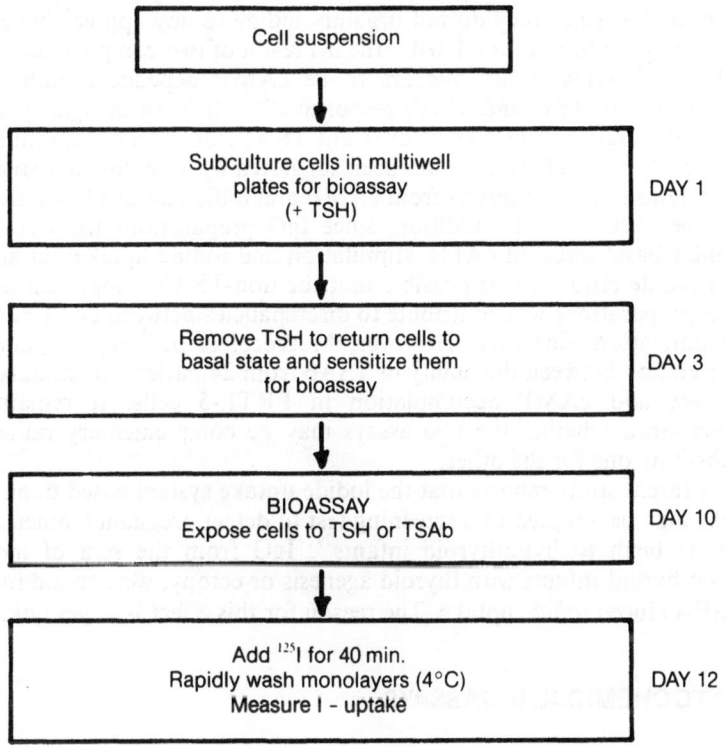

**Figure 2.5** A flow diagram of the preparation and utilization of monolayers of FRTL-5 cells in bioassays for TSH and TSAb based upon increased uptake of iodide, as first described by Marcocci *et al.*[53]

It is estimated that TSAb stimulation can result in iodide being concentrated 30-fold in the cells compared with the medium[53]. IgG from the sera of about 80% of untreated Graves' patients showed significant stimulation above control values observed in the presence of IgG prepared from euthyroid individuals, using this system[53,54]. In these limited studies, 15 of the 16 patients in clinical and biochemical remission after a course of thionamide drug treatment, were inactive with respect to iodide accumulation.

It is possible that bioassays based upon intracellular accumulation of iodide will form an alternative to those based on stimulation of cAMP production. They eliminate the time-consuming and expensive cAMP radioimmunoassay, which must decrease overall bioassay errors. Direct comparison of dose–response curves to TSH[53], LATS-B[54] and patient TSAb[54] in the two systems, showed that iodide uptake was the more sensitive, responding to 10-fold lower doses than the cAMP system. However, in these studies, comparable bioassay incubation conditions were used for the two bioassays, and as discussed above, 'sensitizing techniques' can improve the potential sensitivity of cAMP bioassays.

The use of FRTL-5 cells for iodide uptake bioassays is complicated by the finding that since they do not organify iodide to any appreciable extent the amount of iodide accumulated is the net result of two components, influx and efflux[76–78]. Only influx appears to be cAMP dependent, although both processes are TSH and TSAb responsive[54,76]. It is an intriguing possibility that the relative potencies of different TSABs on influx and efflux may be different, in which case, as has been suggested by a preliminary study, direct correlation between results from cAMP and iodide uptake based assays may not be observed[54]. In addition, since IgG preparations from control sera inhibit basal levels of cAMP stimulation and iodide uptake but apparently not iodide efflux[54], it is possible that the non-TSAb component of Graves' IgG preparations will contribute to discrepancies between cAMP and iodide accumulation bioassays. However, Marcocci et al.[53] report good overall correlation between the ability of TSAb from 24 patients to stimulate iodide uptake and cAMP accumulation in FRTL-5 cells. It remains to be determined whether the two assays may be complementary rather than a substitute one for the other.

A recent study reports that the iodide uptake system based upon FRTL-5 cells may be adapted as a screening test to detect pregnant women at risk of giving birth to hypothyroid infants[79]. IgG from the sera of mothers of hypothyroid infants with thyroid agenesis or ectopy, were found to enhance TSH-induced iodide uptake. The reason for this effect is as yet unknown.

## CYTOCHEMICAL BIOASSAYS

Since we have placed much emphasis on the necessity to attain sensitive bioassays for TSAb, it is appropriate to comment upon the cytochemical bioassay (CBA) for TSAb, which exhibits exceptional sensitivity. The development of cytochemical bioassay systems was pioneered by Chayen,

Bitensky and co-workers[21], who have recently developed new CBAs for detecting TGAb[22,23], which are discussed in detail in Chapter 3.

The most frequently used CBA for the detection of TSAb is that based upon the stimulation of $\beta$-naphthylamidase in the thyroid follicular cells in sections of guinea-pig thyroid tissue[2]. An outline of the procedures involved is shown in Figure 2.6. The sections are exposed to TSH or TSAb for a brief and carefully timed period. This exposure time is predetermined and is generally between 90 and 180 seconds, with the longer times giving the more sensitive assays (e.g. detection limit of about $10^{-5}$ mU TSH/l)[80,81]. The sections are then reacted for $\beta$-naphthylamidase activity using a chromogenic substrate ($\beta$-leucine naphthylamide). Finally, the intensity of the cytochemical reaction product is quantified with a scanning and integrating microdensitometer, utilizing a wavelength of 550 nm. Readings are taken from ten follicular cells for each section and the results are expressed as the mean integrated extinction obtained from these.

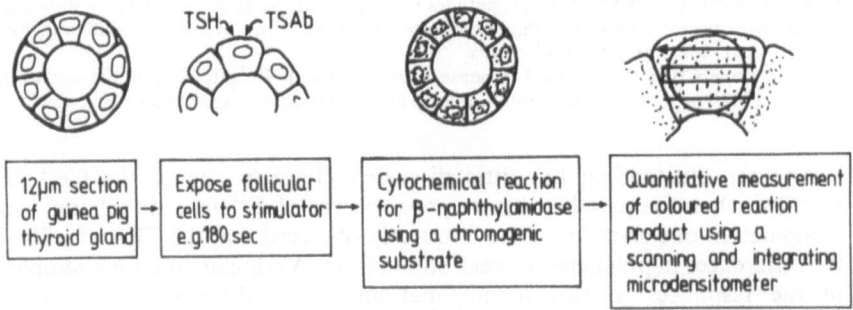

**Figure 2.6** An outline of the procedures involved in the Cytochemical Bioassay for TSH and TSAb based upon the stimulation of $\beta$-naphthylamidase activity in sections of guinea-pig thyroid tissue

Some of the outstanding features of the CBA are illustrated diagrammatically in Figure 2.7. A typical dose–response curve for the CBA is compared with that obtained from one of the cell culture bioassay systems based upon the stimulation of cAMP production which we discussed previously. Selecting a bioassay exposure time of 180 seconds, the maximum response of the CBA usually occurs at $10^{-3}$ mU TSH/l[81] and higher doses give a lower response. The CBA is capable of detecting concentrations of TSH which are several orders of magnitude below normal circulating levels. In contrast, sensitivities approaching normal physiological levels of TSH can only be achieved with the bioassay based upon the cultured cells using the 'sensitizing techniques' (Figure 2.7). The latter systems however, though less sensitive, are capable of greater within assay precision[38,42,50-52,72]. The ultrasensitivity of the CBA is seen with all thyroid stimulators which we have tested (TSH[81], TSAb[81], forskolin[82] and VIP[83]). This sensitivity of the CBA may account for its ability to detect TSAb in virtually all sera of untreated Graves' patients, overcoming any human specificity attributed to some TSAb.

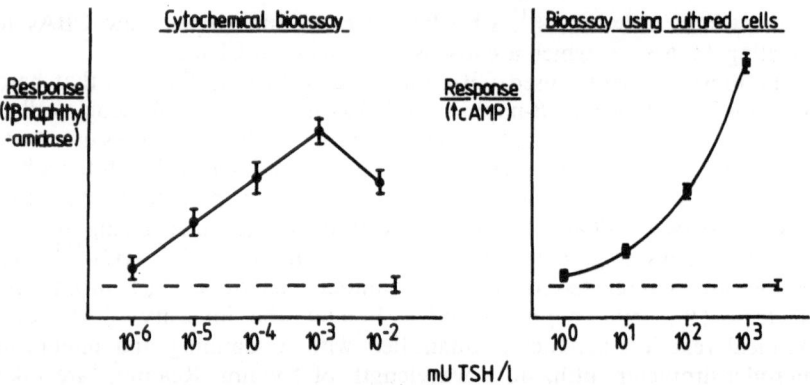

**Figure 2.7** A diagrammatic representation of typical dose-response curves to TSH as observed by the authors when using (a) the cytochemical bioassay ($\uparrow\beta$-naphthylamidase activity; tissue exposure time 180s) and (b) *in vitro* bioassays based upon monolayers of thyroid epithelial cells ($\uparrow$cAMP). Error bars indicate the magnitudes of errors in response as estimated by standard deviations with $n = 3$ or 4. The figure has been constructed from results obtained with the CBA[80–83] and monolayers of FRTL-5 cells[51,72].

Note: in some CBAs the maximal response is observed with $10^{-2}$ mU TSH/l, and not with $10^{-3}$ mU TSH/l as shown. This is presumed to be due to between-thyroid variation

Another outstanding but little discussed characteristic of the CBA is revealed when the parallel dose–response curves of different stimulators are compared in one assay. We have frequently observed that the CBA amplifies the differences in potencies between stimulators. A comparison, for example, of the responses to two monoclonal antibodies derived from Graves' lymphocytes, one of which was about 3 times more potent when assessed in a cell-culture *in vitro* bioassay, showed the relative potencies to be $10^7$: 1 in the CBA[84].

We have also observed this phenomenon when comparing the potencies of different TSAb derived directly from patient sera[85] and also different preparations of TSH[86]. The potency ranking is retained but the differences in potencies are magnified. Clearly the relative potencies markedly depend upon the response systems employed in the different bioassays but we cannot at present explain the enhanced discrimination observed with the CBA.

Because of the high level of technical expertise required to conduct cytochemical bioassays, and their inability to accommodate more than a small number of samples per assay, their use has been restricted to a few centres. However, despite their impracticability, they remain powerful assay systems which will continue to be exploited in specialized studies such as those relating to TGAb (see Chapter 3).

## FUTURE DEVELOPMENTS

The motivation behind the efforts to achieve improved measurement systems for TSAb is the widely held conviction that TSAb are important pathological factors in Graves' disease. Consequently reliable assessments of TSAb activity in serum should become an essential adjunct to the established thyroid function tests used for the evaluation of several aspects of autoimmune thyroid disease. In this chapter we have described recent developments which have improved the techniques for the measurement of TSAb bioactivity.

Inevitably work is in progress to gain from the advantages of cell culture systems which are already apparent. Several centres are investigating the development of human thyroid cell lines[87], to avoid problems due to the possible human species specificity of some TSAbs. Should a responsive human thyroid cell line be established, the experience gained from work with the currently available cell culture systems, including the primary cultures of human thyroid cells and the FRTL-5 cells, will doubtless be rapidly applied to the new cell line. This will include the manipulation of the cell-cultures to reduce basal levels of activity prior to use in the bioassay and the careful selection of incubation medium to optimize sensitivity. Work with any of these 'immortalized' cell culture systems will, however, require vigilance against long-term culture instability. Clearly a programme of periodic recloning should be established, which will both obviate problems due to deleterious mutations and also yield useful new cell lines with advantageous characteristics. It is not inconceivable that cells will be 'designed' for bioassays rather than *vice versa* as at present.

Undoubtedly, new assays using alternative response systems will be set up based upon thyroid cell-cultures. The iodide uptake response, which appears to be significantly more sensitive to TSH than the adenylate cyclase based systems[48], has to date been little exploited for TSAb *in vitro* bioassay. Moreover, it may be possible to circumvent many technical difficulties of the CBA, by redesigning the assay using cell monolayers as opposed to tissue sections.

One pragmatic problem, which has only been briefly discussed, is the question of the most appropriate and helpful method of expressing the results obtained with a TSAb bioassay. It has been common practice to express TSAb bioactivity as a ratio of the response observed with the given TSAb to that obtained in the presence of a control from euthyroid individuals. In a few recent studies results are compared with a TSH dose–response curve and expressed as 'TSH-equivalents'[40,42,43]. This has an appealing directness, and facilitates the comparison of results from different assays using one technique but may unfortunately be misleading. These results may alter markedly by merely changing any assay conditions which have differential effects upon TSH compared with TSAb. This was demonstrated by Kasagi *et al.*[40] who showed that TSAb activity expressed as $\mu$U TSH/ml could increase between 3 and 100-fold, by reducing the ionic strength of the incubation medium. Moreover, to derive the 'TSH equivalents' one has to implicitly assume that the response curves to TSH and the given TSAb are parallel. For practical reasons this is infrequently checked. We have observed parallelism between LATS-B and TSH when tested in both the 'forskolin sensitized' FRTL-5 system[75], and the CBA[81]. However, using the latter assay system we have also observed responses to TSAb from patients with euthyroid goitres which were not parallel to that of TSH (Ealey and Marshall, unpublished). Given the widespread speculation that TSAb activity in a given serum is the net result of the combined effects of a number of polyclonal anti-TSH receptor antibodies, some of which might block rather than stimulate post-receptor events, one might anticipate that parallelism with TSH would not be a consistent feature. It is not inconceivable that different monoclonal antibodies directed against sites on the TSH-receptor complex[88,89] which are associated with specific biological activities[84,90], might prove to be more appropriate reference preparations.

As discussed recently by Kohn and co-workers[88], such monoclonal antibodies may lead to a new generation of binding assays. This could be achieved by raising an anti-idiotype against an individual monoclonal antibody which had previously been shown to express a specific action at the TSH receptor. The anti-idiotype would then bind to antibodies present in patient serum which shared the idiotype of the original monoclonal. Clearly by labelling the anti-idiotype this system would yield ligand binding assays designed to recognize idiotypes associated with activation of specific functions.

Characterization of the monoclonals raised against the TSH receptor has emphasized the existence of antibodies which bind strongly to the TSH receptor and block TSH action, but which do not stimulate of their own accord[88-92]. These findings have direct relevance to the few clinical studies to date, which link the action of blocking antibodies to adult and infant hypothyroidism[93-97]. The *in vitro* bioassays based on cell monolayers, which have highly reproducible TSH dose–response characteristics, should be readily adaptable to quantify such 'blocking' antibodies, by directly testing for inhibition of TSH stimulation. Some blocking antibodies, e.g. monoclonal 11E8, discriminate between stimulation by TSH and TSAb[92] and in future may be used as subtle probes of the bioactivities of different stimulatory autoantibodies.

Probably the most challenging area for the immediate future will be to utilize the new systems to derive multi-assay strategies to identify the separate and integrated effects of the 'spectrum' of anti-TSH receptor antibodies which may be present in a patient. One test alone may not be of absolute predictive value to determine the future course of an autoimmune thyroid condition such as Graves' disease[55]. Such an approach will require a critical examination of the specificity of the different response parameters employed in each bioassay. This is only now possible due to the improved reliability, precision and sensitivity of these systems.

## ACKNOWLEDGEMENTS

The authors are grateful to the Sir Jules Thorn Charitable Trust and the Locally Organized Research Scheme for financial support.

### References

1. Adams, D. D. and Purves, H. D. (1956). Abnormal responses in the assay of thyrotropin.

*Proc. Univ. Otago Med. Sch.*, **34**, 11–12

2. McKenzie, J. M. (1964). Neonatal Graves' disease. *J. Clin. Endocrinol. Metab.*, **24**, 660–5
3. Munro, D. S., Dirmikis, S. M., Humphries, H. and Smith, T. (1978). The role of thyroid stimulating immunoglobulins of Graves' disease in neonatal thyrotoxicosis. *Br. J. Obstet. Gynaecol.*, **85**, 837–42
4. Alexander, W. D., McLarty, D. G., Horton, P. and Pharmakiotis, A. D. (1973). Sequential assessment during drug treatment of thyrotoxicosis. *Clin. Endocrinol.*, **2**, 803–10
5. Wilson, R., McKillop, J. H., Pearson, D. W. M., Cuthbert, G. F. and Thomson, J. A. (1985). Relapse of Graves' Disease after medical therapy: predictive value of thyroidal technetium-99m uptake and serum thyroid stimulating hormone receptor antibody levels. *J. Nucl. Med.*, **26**, 1024–8
6. McKenzie, J. M. (1958). The bioassay of thyrotropin in serum. *Endocrinology*, **63**, 372–82
7. Adams, D. D. and Kennedy, T. H. (1967). Occurrence in thyrotoxicosis of a gamma globulin which protects LATS from neutralization by an extract of thyroid gland. *J. Clin. Endocrinol. Metab.*, **27**, 173–7
8. Dirmikis, S., Kendall-Taylor, P. and Munro, D. S. (1976). The nature and significance of LATS-protector. In Robbins, J. and Braverman, L. E. (eds). *Thyroid Research*. pp. 403–6. (Amsterdam: Excerpta Medica American Elsevier)
9. Rees Smith, B. and Hall, R. (1974) Thyroid-stimulating immunoglobulins in Graves' disease. *Lancet*, **2**, 427–30
10. Mehdi, S. Q. and Nussey, S. S. (1975). A radio-ligand receptor assay for long-acting thyroid stimulator. *Biochem. J.*, **145**, 105–11
11. Endo, K., Borges, M., Amir, S. and Ingbar, S. (1982). Preparation of [125]I-labelled receptor purified Graves' immunoglobulins: properties of their binding to human thyroid membranes. *J. Clin. Endocrinol. Metab.*, **55**, 566–76
12. Kaneko, T., Zor, U. and Field, J. B. (1970). Stimulation of thyroid adenyl cyclase activity and cyclic adenosine 3′, 5′-monophosphate by long-acting thyroid stimulator. *Metabolism*, **19**, 430–8
13. Orgiazzi, J., Chopra, I. J., Williams, D. E. and Solomon, D. H. (1976). Human thyroid adenylate cyclase-stimulating activity in immunoglobulin G of patients with Graves' disease. *J. Clin. Endocrinol. Metab.*, **42**, 341–54
14. Bech, K. and Madsen, S. N. (1979). Thyroid adenylate cyclase stimulating immunoglobulins in thyroid disease. *Clin. Endocrinol.*, **11**, 47–58
15. McKenzie, J. M., Zakarija, M. and Sato, A. (1978). Humoral immunity in Graves' disease. *Clin. Endocrinol. Metab.*, **7**, 31–45
16. Bidey, S. P., Marshall, N. J. and Ekins, R. P. (1981). Adenylate cyclase activity and the accumulation and release of adenosine 3′, 5′-monophosphate in normal human thyroid tissue slice preparations: responses to thyrotropin and thyroid-stimulating antibodies. *J. Clin. Endocrinol. Metab.*, **53**, 246–53
17. Shishiba, Y., Shimizu, T., Yoshimura, S. and Shizume, K. (1973). Direct evidence for human thyroidal stimulation by LATS-protector. *J. Clin. Endocrinol. Metab.*, **36**, 517–21
18. Onaya, T., Kotani, M., Yamada, T. and Ochi, Y. (1973). New *in vitro* tests to detect the thyroid stimulator in sera from hyperthyroid patients by measuring colloid droplet formation and cyclic AMP in human thyroid slices. *J. Clin. Endocrinol. Metab.*, **36**, 859–66
19. Laurberg, P. and Weeke, J. (1975). T3 release from thyroid slices as an assay for thyroid stimulators. *Scand. J. Clin. Lab. Invest.*, **35**, 723–7
20. Atkinson, S. and Kendall-Taylor, P. (1981). The stimulation of thyroid hormone secretion *in vitro* by thyroid-stimulating antibodies. *J. Clin. Endocrinol. Metab.*, **53**, 1263–6
21. Bitensky, L., Alaghband-Zadeh, J. and Chayen, J. (1974). Studies on thyroid stimulating hormone and the long-acting thyroid stimulator. *Clin. Endocrinol.*, **3**, 363–74
22. Drexhage, H. A., Bottazzo, G. F., Doniach, D., Bitensky, L. and Chayen, J. (1980). Evidence for thyroid growth stimulating immunoglobulins in some goitrous thyroid diseases. *Lancet*, **2**, 287–92
23. Drexhage, H. A., Hammond, L. J., Bitensky, L., Chayen, J., Bottazzo, G. F. and Doniach, D. (1982). The involvement of the pentose shunt in thyroid metabolism after stimulation with TSH or with immunoglobulins from patients with thyroid disease. I. The generation of NADPH in relation to stimulation of thyroid growth. *Clin. Endocrinol*, **16**, 49–56
24. Drexhage, H. A., Hammond, L. J., Bitensky, L., Chayen, J., Bottazzo, G. F. and Doniach,

D. (1982). The involvement of the pentose shunt in thyroid metabolism after stimulation with TSH or with immunoglobulins from patients with thyroid disease. II. The reoxidation of NADPH and stimulation of hormone synthesis. *Clin. Endocrinol.*, **16**, 57–63

25. Chayen, J., Gilbert, D. M., Robertson, W. R., Bitensky, L. and Besser, G. M. (1980). A cytochemical section bioassay for thyrotropin. *J. Immunoassay*, **1**, 1–13

26. Chiovato, L., Hammond, L. J., Hanafusa, T., Pujol-Borrell, R., Doniach, D. and Bottazzo, G. F. (1984). Detection of thyroid growth immunoglobulins (TGI) by [$^3$H]-thymidine incorporation in cultured rat thyroid follicles. *Clin. Endocrinol.*, **19**, 581–90

27. Schatz, H., Beckmann, F. H. and Floren, M. (1983). Radioassay for thyroid growth stimulating immunoglobulins (TGI) with cultivated porcine thyroid follicles. *Hormone Metab. Res.*, **15**, 627–8

28. Edmonds, M. W., Row, V. V. and Volpe, R. (1970). Action of globulin and lymphocytes from peripheral blood of patients with Graves' disease on isolated bovine thyroid cells. *J. Clin. Endocrinol. Metab.*, **31**, 180–5

29. Burke, G. and Kowalski, K. (1971). Comparative effects of thyrotrophin and long acting thyroid stimulator on iodide trapping in isolated thyroid cells. *Acta Endocrinol. (Kbh)*, **68**, 675–80

30. Povey, P. M., Rees Smith, B., Davies, T. F. and Hall, R. (1976). Thyrotrophin receptor binding, intracellular cyclic AMP levels and iodine release in isolated thyroid cells. *FEBS Letts.*, **72**, 251–5

31. Takasu, N., Charrier, B., Mauchamp, J. and Lissitzky, S. (1978). Modulation of adenylate cyclase/cAMP response by TSH and $PGE_2$ in cultured thyroid cells: positive regulation and negative regulation. *Eur. J. Biochem.*, **90**, 131–8

32. Rapoport, B. (1976). Dog thyroid cells in monolayer tissue culture: adenosine 3′, 5′-cyclic monophosphate response to thyrotrophic hormone. *Endocrinology*, **98**, 1189–97

33. Kaneko, Y. (1976). Cyclic AMP level of human thyroid cells in monolayer culture: TSH induced refractoriness to TSH action. *Hormone Metab. Res.*, **8**, 202–6

34. Bidey, S. P., Marshall, N. J. and Ekins, R. P. (1981). Characterisation of the cyclic AMP response to thyrotrophin in monolayer cultures of normal human thyroid cells. *Acta Endocrinol. (Kbh).*, **98**, 370–8

35. Ollis, C. A., Munro, D. S. and Tomlinson, S. (1982). Characteristics of TSH stimulated cyclic AMP production in cultured human thyroid cells from thyrotoxic tissue and non-toxic goitres. *J. Endocrinol.*, **95**, 237–44

36. Toccafondi, R. S., Aterinin, S., Medicin, M. A., Rotella, C. M., Tanini, A. and Zonefrati, R. (1980). Thyroid stimulating antibody (TSAb) detected in sera of Graves' patients using human thyroid cell cultures. *Clin. Exp. Immunol.*, **40**, 532–9

37. Hinds, W. E., Takai, N., Rapoport, B., Filleti, S. and Clark, O. H. (1981). Thyroid-stimulating immunoglobulin bioassay using cultured human thyroid cells. *J. Clin. Endocrinol. Metab.*, **52**, 1204–10

38. Bidey, S. P., Marshall, N. J. and Ekins, R. P. (1983). Bioassay of thyroid stimulating immunoglobulins using human thyroid cell cultures: optimization and clinical assessment. *Clin. Endocrinol.*, **18**, 193–206

39. Davies, T. F., Platzer, M., Schwartz, A. and Friedman, E. (1983). Functionality of thyroid-stimulating antibodies assessed by cryopreserved human thyroid cell bioassay. *J. Clin. Endocrinol. Metab.*, **57**, 1021–7

40. Kasagi, K., Konishi, J., Iida, Y., Ikekubo, K., Mori, T., Kuma, K. and Torizuka, K. (1982). A new *in vitro* assay for human thyroid stimulator using cultured thyroid cells: effect of sodium chloride on adenosine 3′, 5′-monophosphate increase. *J. Clin. Endocrinol. Metab.*, **54**, 108–14

41. Etienne-Decerf, J. and Winand, R. J. (1981). A sensitive technique for determination of thyroid-stimulating immunoglobulin (TSI) in unfractionated serum. *Clin. Endocrinol.*, **14**, 83–91

42. Rapoport, B., Filetti, S., Takai, N., Seto, P. and Halverson, G. (1982). Studies on the cyclic AMP response to thyroid stimulating immunoglobulins (TSI) and thyrotrophin (TSH) in human thyroid cell monolayers. *Metabolism*, **31**, 1159–67

43. Rapoport, B., Greenspan, F. S., Filetti, S. and Pepitone, M. (1984). Clinical experience with a human thyroid cell bioassay for thyroid stimulating immunoglobulins. *J. Clin. Endocrinol. Metab.*, **58**, 332–8

44. Creagh, F., Teece, M., Williams, S., Didcote, S., Perkins, W., Hashim, F. and Rees Smith, B. (1985). An analysis of thyrotrophin receptor binding and thyroid stimulating activities in a series of Graves' sera. *Clin. Endocrinol.*, **23**, 395–404
45. Dickson, J. G., Hovsepian, S., Fayet, G. and Lissitzky, S. (1981). Follicle formation and iodide metabolism in cultures of human thyroid cells. *J. Endocrinol.*, **90**, 113–24
46. Bourke, J. R., Carseldine, K. L., Ferris, S. H., Huxham, G. J. and Manley, S. W. (1981). Changes in membrane potential of cultured porcine and human thyroid cells in response to thyrotrophin and other agents. *J. Endocrinol.*, **88**, 187–196
47. Ginsberg, J., Shewring, G., Howells, R., Rees-Smith, B. and Hall, R. (1983). Stimulation of iodide organification in porcine thyroid cells by thyroid stimulators. *Life Sci.*, **32**, 153–60
48. Reader, S. C. J., Davison, B., Ratcliffe, J. G. and Robertson, W. R. (1985). Measurement of low concentrations of bovine thyrotrophin by iodide uptake and organification in porcine thyrocytes. *J. Endocrinol.*, **106**, 13–20
49. Valente, W. A., Vitti, P., Kohn, L. D., Brandi, M. L., Rotella, C. M., Toccafondi, R., Tramontano, D., Aloj, S. M. and Ambesi-Impiombato, S. (1983). The relationship of growth and adenylate cyclase activity in cultured, thyroid cells: separate bioeffects of thyrotrophin. *Endocrinology*, **112**, 71–9
50. Vitti, P., Valente, W. A., Ambesi-Impiombato, F. S., Fenzi, G. F., Pinchera, A. and Kohn, L. D. (1982). Graves' IgG stimulation of continuously cultured rat thyroid cells: a sensitive and potentially useful clinical assay. *J. Endocrinol. Invest.*, **5**, 179–82
51. Bidey, S. P., Chiovato, L., Day, A., Turmaine, M., Gould, P., Ekins, R. P. and Marshall, N. J. (1984). Evaluation of the rat thyroid cell strain FRTL-5 as an *in vitro* bioassay system for thyrotrophin. *J. Endocrinol.*, **101**, 269–76
52. Vitti, P., Rotella, C. M., Valente, W. A., Cohen, J., Aloj, S. M., Lacetti, P., Ambesi-Impiombato, F. S., Grollman, E. F., Pinchera, A., Toccafondi, R. and Kohn, L. D. (1983). Characterization of the optimal stimulatory effects of Graves' monoclonal and serum immunoglobulin G on adenosine 3′, 5′-monophosphate production in FRTL-5 thyroid cells: a potential clinical assay. *J. Clin. Endocrinol. Metab.*, **57**, 782–91
53. Marcocci, C., Valente, W. A., Pinchera, A., Aloj, S. M., Kohn, L. D. and Grollman, E. F. (1983). Graves' IgG stimulation of iodide uptake in FRTL-5 rat thyroid cells: a clinical assay complementing FRTL-5 assays measuring adenylate cyclase and growth stimulating antibodies in autoimmune thyroid disease. *J. Endocrinol. Invest.*, **6**, 463–71
54. Bidey, S. P. and Ekins, R. P. (1986). Comparative evaluation of cyclic AMP and iodide accumulation responses to thyroid-stimulating immunoglobulins using cultured FRTL-5 cells. *J. Endocrinol.* (in press)
55. Valente, W., Vitti, P., Rotella, C. M., Aloj, S. M., Ambesi-Impiombato, F. S. and Kohn, L. D. (1983). Growth-promoting antibodies in autoimmune thyroid disease: a population of thyroid stimulating antibodies measurable using rat FRTL-5 cells. *N. Engl. J. Med.*, **309**, 1028–34
56. Ealey, P. A., Emmerson, J. M., Bidey, S. P. and Marshall, N. J. (1985). Thyrotrophin stimulation of mitogenesis of the rat thyroid cell strain FRTL-5: a metaphase index assay for the detection of thyroid growth stimulators. *J. Endocrinol.*, **106**, 203–10
57. Kriss, J. P., Pleshakov, V. and Chien, J. R. (1964). Isolation and identification of the long-acting thyroid stimulator and its relation to hyperthyroidism and circumscribed pretibial myxoedema. *J. Clin. Endocrinol.*, **24**, 1005–28
58. Meek, J. C., Jones, A. E., Lewis, U. J. and Vanderlaan, W. P. (1964). Characterization of the long-acting thyroid stimulator of Graves' disease. *Proc. Natl. Acad. Sci., USA.*, **52**, 342–9
59. Chopra, I. J., Solomon, D. H., Johnson, D. E. and Chopra, U. (1970). Thyroid gland in Graves' disease: victim or culprit? *Metabolism*, **19**, 760–72
60. Henneman, G., Dolman, A., Docter, R., De Reus, A. and Van Zijl, J. (1975). Dissociation of serum LATS activity and hyperfunction and autonomy of the thyroid gland in Graves' disease. *J. Clin. Endocrinol. Metab.*, **40**, 935–41
61. Adams, D. D., Kennedy, T. H. and Stewart, R. D. H. (1974). Correlation between long-acting thyroid stimulator protector level and thyroid [131]I uptake in thyrotoxicosis. *Br. Med. J.*, **2**, 199–201
62. Manley, S. W., Bourke, J. R. and Hawker, R. W. (1974). The thyrotrophin receptor in guinea pig thyroid homogenate: interaction with long-acting thyroid stimulator. *J.*

*Endocrinol.*, **61**, 437–45

63. Gossage, A. A. R., Byfield, P. G. H., Copping, S. and Himsworth, R. L. (1981). A comparative study of the binding of Graves' immunoglobulins by the patient's own and other thyroid membranes. *Clin. Endocrinol.*, **14**, 301–10

64. Sato, A., Zakarija, M. and McKenzie, J. M. (1978). The influence of normal human IgG and of thyroid-stimulating antibody (TSAb) on the binding of thyrotrophin to thyroid plasma membranes. *Endocrinol. Res. Commun.*, **5**, 259–69

65. Kotulla, P. and Schleusener, H. (1978). Improvement of the radioligand receptor assay (RRA) for thyroid stimulators by using solubilized receptors. *Ann. d'Endocrinol.*, **39**, 2

66. Shewring, G. and Rees Smith, B. (1982). An improved radioreceptor assay for TSH receptor antibodies. *Clin. Endocrinol.*, **17**, 409–17

67. Southgate, K., Creagh, F., Teece, M., Kingswood, C. and Rees Smith, B. (1984). A receptor assay for the measurement of TSH receptor antibodies in unextracted serum. *Clin. Endocrinol.*, **20**, 539–48

68. Stockle, G., Wahl, R. and Seif, F. J. (1981). Micromethod of human thyrocyte cultures for detection of thyroid-stimulating antibodies and thyrotropin. *Acta Endocrinol. (Kbh)*, **97**, 369–74

69. Pekonen, F. and Weintraub, B. D. (1980). Salt-induced exposure of high affinity thyrotropin receptors in human and porcine thyroid membranes. *J. Biol. Chem.*, **255**, 8121–6

70. Ambesi-Impiombato, F. S., Parks, L. A. M. and Coon, H. G. (1980). Culture of hormone-dependent epithelial cells from rat thyroids. *Proc. Natl. Acad. Sci., USA*, **77**, 3455–9

71. Ambesi-Impiombato, F. S., Tramontano, D. and Coon, H. G. (1980). Hormones, cell growth and differentiation in *vitro*: the thyroid system. In Jimenez de Asua, L. (ed.) *Control Mechanisms in Animal Cells.* pp. 7–14. (New York: Raven Press)

72. Bidey, S. P., Ryder, K., Gaines-Das, R., Marshall, N. J. and Ekins, R. P. (1984). A comparison of the bioactivity of human and bovine thyrotrophin preparations as determined by intracellular cyclic AMP responses of cultured FRTL-5 cells and human thyroid cell monolayers. *Acta Endocrinol., (Kbh)*, **106**, 482–9

73. Rapoport, B., Takai, N. A. and Filetti, S. (1982). Evidence for species specificity in the interaction between thyrotropin and thyroid stimulating immunoglobulin and their receptor in thyroid tissue. *J. Clin. Endocrinol. Metab.*, **54**, 1059–62

74. Kohn, L. D., Yavin, E., Yavin, Z., Lacetti, P., Vitti, P., Grollman, E. F. and Valente, W. (1984). Autoimmune thyroid disease studied with monoclonal antibodies to the thyrotrophin receptor. In Haynes, B. F. and Eisenbarth, G. S. (eds.) *Monoclonal Antibodies: Probes for the Study of Autoimmunity and Immunodeficiency.* (New York: Academic Press)

75. Bidey, S. P., Emmerson, J. M., Marshall, N. J. and Ekins, R. P. (1985). Characterization of thyroid-stimulating immunoglobulin-induced cyclic AMP accumulation in the rat thyroid cell strain FRTL-5: potentiation by forskolin and calibration against reference preparations of thyrotrophin. *J. Endocrinol.*, **105**, 7–15

76. Weiss, S. J., Philp, N. J. and Grollman, E. F. (1984). Iodide transport in a continuous line of cultured cells from rat thyroid. *Endocrinology*, **114**, 1090–8

77. Weiss, S. J., Philp, N. J. and Grollman, E. F. (1984). Effect of thyrotropin on iodide efflux in FRTL-5 cells mediated by $Ca^{2+}$. *Endocrinology*, **114**, 1108–13

78. Corda, D., Marcocci, C., Kohn, L. D., Axelrod, J. and Luini, A. (1985). Association of the changes in cytosolic $Ca^{2+}$ and iodide efflux induced by thyrotropin and by the stimulation of $\alpha_1$-adrenergic receptors in cultured rat thyroid cells. *J. Biol. Chem.*, **260**, 9230–6

79. Dussault, J. H. and Bernier, D. (1985). $^{125}$I-uptake by FRTL-5 cells: a screening test to detect pregnant women at risk of giving birth to hypothyroid infants. *Lancet*, **2**, 1029–31

80. Ealey, P. A., Marshall, N. J. and Ekins, R. P. (1981). Time-related thyroid stimulation by thyrotropin and thyroid-stimulating antibodies, as measured by the cytochemical section bioassay. *J. Clin. Endocrinol. Metab.*, **52**, 483–7

81. Ealey, P. A., Marshall, N. J. and Ekins, R. P. (1984). Further studies on the response of a cytochemical bioassay to thyroid stimulators, using reference preparations of thyrotropin and long acting thyroid stimulator. *J. Endocrinol. Invest.*, **7**, 25–8

82. Ealey, P. A., Kohn, L. D., Marshall, N. J. and Ekins, R. P. (1985). Forkolin stimulation of naphthylamidase in guinea pig thyroid sections detected with a cytochemical bioassay.

*Acta Endocrinol., (Kbh),* **108**, 367–71

83. Ealy, P. A., Marshall, N. J. and Ekins, R. P. (1985). VIP stimulation of β-naphthylamidase activity in guinea-pig thyroid sections. *Acta Endocrinol., (Kbh),* **109**, 505–10

84. Ealey, P., Kohn, L. D., Ekins, R. P. and Marshall, N. J. (1984). Characterization of monoclonal antibodies derived from lymphocytes from Graves' disease patients in a cytochemical bioassay for thyroid stimulators. *J. Clin. Endocrinol. Metab.*, **58**, 909–14

85. Ealey, P. A., Marshall, N. J., Lawton, N., Dandona, P., Lightman, S. and Ekins, R. P., (1984). The application of a cytochemical bioassay to measure thyroid stimulating antibodies; a study of patients with euthyroid Graves' ophthalmopathy. *J. Endocrinol. Invest.*, **7**, 597–602

86. Gaines Das, R. E. and Bristow, A. F. (1985). The Second International Preparation of Thyroid-Stimulating Hormone, Human, for Immunoassay: calibration by bioassay and immunoassay in an international collaborative study. *J. Endocrinol.*, **104**, 367–79

87. Karsenty, G., Michel-Bechet, M. and Charreire, J. (1985). Monoclonal human thyroid cell line GEJ expressing human thyrotropin receptors. *Proc. Natl. Acad. Sci., USA*, **82**, 2120–4

88. Kohn, L. D., Alvarez, F., Marcocci, C., Kohn, A. D., Corda, D., Hoffman, W. E., Tombaccini, D., Valente, W., Deluca, N., Santisteban, T. and Grollman, E. F. (1985). Monoclonal antibody studies defining the origin and properties of autoantibodies. In Rose, N. and Schwartz, R. S. (eds.) *Autoimmunity–Experimental and Clinical Aspects.* (New York: Ann. N.Y. Acad. Med.)

89. Yavin, E., Yavin, Z., Schneider, M. D. and Kohn, L. D. (1981). Monoclonal antibodies to the thyrotrophin receptor: implications for receptor structure and the action of autoantibodies in Graves' disease. *Proc. Natl. Acad. Sci., USA*, **78**, 3180–4

90. Kohn, L. D., Valente, W., Laccetti, P., Marcocci, C., De Luca, M., Ealey, P. A., Marshall, N. J. and Grollman, E. F. (1984). Monoclonal antibodies as probes of thyrotropin receptor structure. In Venter, J. C., Fraser, C. M. and Lindstrom, J. M. (eds.) *Receptors Biochemistry and Methodology: 'Monoclonal and antiidiotype antibodies as probes for receptor structure and function.* Vol. 4, pp. 85–116. (New York: Alan R. Liss)

91. Valente, W. A., Vitti, P., Yavin, Z., Yavin, E., Rotella, C. M., Grollman, E. F., Toccafondi, R. S. and Kohn, L. D. (1982). Graves' monoclonal antibodies to the thyrotrophin receptor: stimulating and blocking antibodies derived from the lymphocytes of patients. *Proc. Natl. Acad. Sci., USA*, **79**, 6680–4

92. Ealey, P. A., Valente, W. A., Ekins, R. P., Kohn, L. D. and Marshall, N. J. (1984). Characterization of monoclonal antibodies raised against solubilized thyrotropin receptors in a cytochemical bioassay for thyroid stimulators. *Endocrinology*, **116**, 124–31

93. Matsuura, N., Yamada, Y., Nohara, Y., Konishi, J., Kasagi, K., Endo, K., Kojima, H. and Wataya, K. (1980). Familial neonatal transient hypothyroidism due to maternal TSH-binding inhibitor immunoglobulins. *N. Engl. J. Med.*, **303**, 738–41

94. Konishi, J., Iida, Y., Endo, K., Misaki, T., Nohara, Y., Matsuura, N., Mori, T. and Torizuka, K. (1983). Inhibition of thyrotropin-induced adenosine 3′ 3′-monophosphate increase by immunoglobulins from patients with primary myxedema. *J. Clin. Endocrinol. Metab.*, **57**, 544–9

95. Steel, N. R., Weightman, D. R., Taylor, J. J. and Kendall-Taylor, P. (1984). Blocking activity to action of thyroid stimulating hormone in serum from patients with primary hypothyroidism. *Br. Med. J.*, **288**, 1559–62

96. Arikawa, K., Ichikawa, Y., Yoshida, T., Shinozawa, T., Homma, M., Momotani, N. and Ito, K. (1985). Blocking type antithyrotropin receptor antibody in patients with non-goitrous hypothyroidism: its incidence and characteristics of action. *J. Clin. Endocrinol. Metab.*, **60**, 953–9

97. Takasu, N., Naka, M., Mori, T. and Yamada, T. (1984). Two types of thyroid-function blocking antibodies in autoimmune atrophic thyroiditis and transient neonatal hypothyroidism due to maternal IgG. *Clin. Endocrinol.*, **21**, 345–55

# 3
# Immunoglobulins Affecting Thyroid Growth

## H. A. DREXHAGE AND R. D. VAN DER GAAG

## INTRODUCTION

The first impetus for our study on immunoglobulins (Igs) stimulating the growth of the thyroid gland (thyroid growth stimulating Igs – TGI) was given by observations on a selective series of ten patients with euthyroid 'colloid' goitres[1]. The patients had been collected over a period of 20 years because they had some features resembling thyrotoxicosis including raised iodine-uptake values, partially suppressible with $T_3$ and flat or absent TRH responses. Several authors have reported similar abnormalities of thyroid function in euthyroid colloid goitre disease[2,3]. The ten patients were suspected of having TGI. Only in 1980 were we able to prove this, using an assay system in which patient immunoglobulin stimulated the growth of guinea-pig thyroid explants in organ culture. The observations were taken as evidence that at least some sporadic colloid goitres were related to Graves' disease and Hashimoto goitre, both well-known thyroid autoimmune diseases.

Immunoglobulins stimulating thyroid growth were reported as early as 1970 by Garry and Hall[4], using a mitotic-arrest assay on rat thyroid tissue in culture. They interpreted their findings in the view that the autoreactive immunoglobulins represented antagonists to the thyroid 'chalone'. Such a mitotic inhibitor has not yet been demonstrated.

In 1978 Brown et al.[5] developed an ultrasensitive assay for measuring immunoglobulins competing with TSH for its receptor (TBII). They were able to show that TBII levels were elevated in patients with sporadic non-toxic and toxic multinodular goitres. It was postulated that these goitres – like Graves' disease – resulted from increased circulating TGIs, which in some cases were present in sufficient concentration to cause thyrotoxicosis (Plummer's disease).

We favour a concept that TGI is involved in the pathogenesis of sporadic goitre and that it represents an antibody activity to a cell-membrane receptor for growth. This might be – but is not necessarily – the TSH receptor. Stimulation of the TSH receptor by the hormone results in both stimulation of function and growth[6]. Two types of biochemical pathways have been discovered for these effects; one is linked to cAMP stimulation and the other to the phosphatidyl-inositol turnover cycle[7].

Since 1980 several authors have provided further evidence on the existence of at least two varieties of Igs with separate specificities for either hormone production or growth[8-11]. Whether these two Ig varieties indeed reflect antibody activities to one single or a variety of receptors, or whether these antibodies trigger separate biochemical pathways resulting in either growth or hormone synthesis is still a matter of debate.

## METHODOLOGY FOR THE DETECTION OF TGI

### Cytochemical bioassays

Bitensky et al.[12] developed the initial cytochemical bioassay for thyroid-stimulating Igs and this test probably still remains the most sensitive method available. It is based on the labilization of thyroid lysosomes by TSH or by TSI. This is one of the rapid effects of TSH and one that is related to hormone synthesis and secretion. To assay the effects of various agents on cell growth, which involves the slower actions of TSH, we focused on different cellular events. Two quantitative cytochemical techniques have been applied to this detection. One is based on nucleic acid cytophotometry (Feulgen CBA) and the other on the measurement of glucose-6-phosphate dehydrogenase (G6PD) activity (G6PD-CBA).

Nucleic acid cytophotometry involves the measurement of the amount of DNA in individual follicle-cell nuclei of a guinea-pig thyroid segment kept in organ culture. The DNA is visualized by the Feulgen reaction and is quantified in individual nuclei (in arbitrary units) by means of a microdensitometer or cytophotometer (Figure 3.1). Many nuclei are measured, and the results are expressed by a computer connected to the microdensitometer as population histograms. The DNA content is plotted along the horizontal axis and the number of nuclei showing a particular content of DNA on the vertical axis (Figure 3.2).

The cell-cycle forms the basis of the assessments. In differentiated tissues we will find cells with only the diploid (2c) content of DNA, but in proliferating tissues some nuclei will be in S-phase and these nuclei will have DNA content values intermediate between the 2c and 4c amounts. From the population histograms the percentage of cells in S-phase ($>2.8c$) can easily be computed and these high values are taken as evidence for proliferation. A detailed description of the methodology has been given elsewhere[13].

The optimal concentration of immunoglobulin for the Feulgen CBA was defined by dose–response curves, using immunoglobulins obtained from patients with non-toxic goitres and untreated thyrotoxic Graves' disease patients with large goitres. The dose–response data of these immunoglobulins were compared with those of the human TSH-standard MRC 63–14 (Figure 3.3). In all instances bell-shaped curves were observed. The optimal amount for the TSH standard ranged from 0.01 to $1 \mu U/ml$ culture fluid. For immunoglobulins from patients with untreated goitrous Graves' disease the

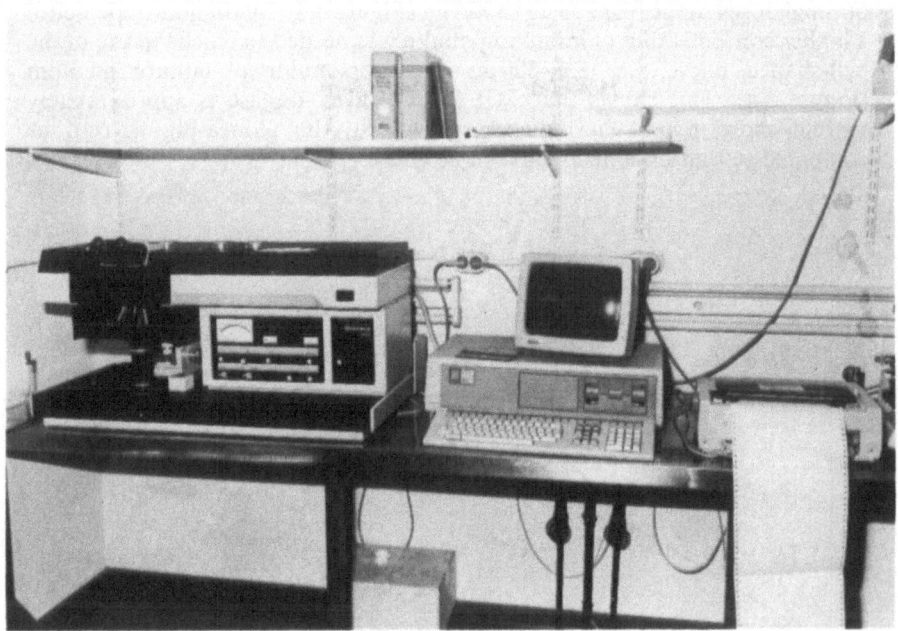

**Figure 3.1** A scanning and integrating microdensitometer (Vickers M85a) connected to a Personal Computer (Digital)

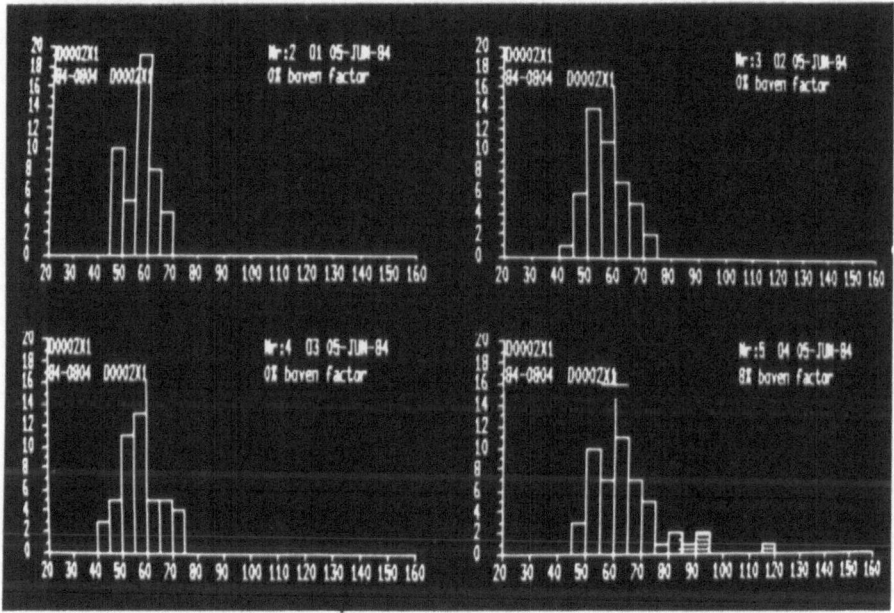

**Figure 3.2** Histograms of DNA values as plotted by the personal computer. No. 5 represents a histogram of proliferating thyroid tissue

optimal doses range from 15 μg to 125 μg (Figure 3.4), but in non-toxic goitre a higher concentration of immunoglobulin was needed to reach the top of the bell-shaped curve, i.e. 125–500 μg immunoglobulin/ml culture medium (Figure 3.4). This shows that TGI from Graves' disease is approximately tenfold more potent in inducing growth in the guinea-pig thyroid as compared to that obtained from simple goitre.

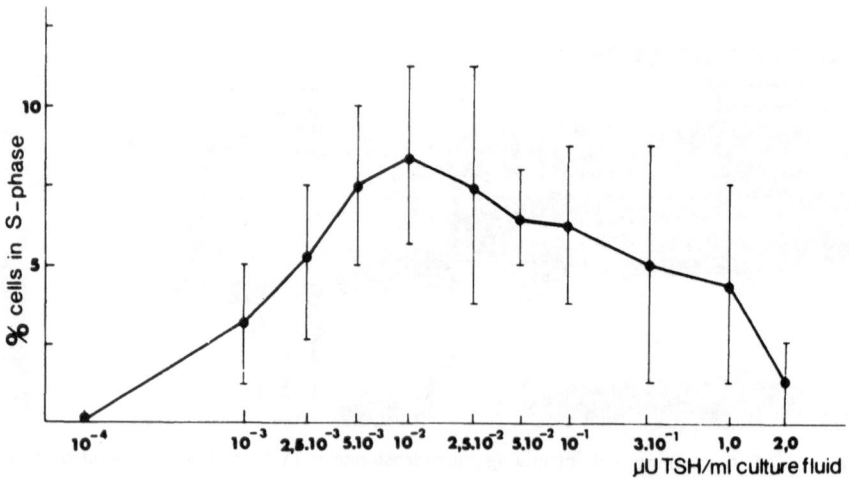

**Figure 3.3** Dose–response curve for thyroid growth obtained in Feulgen CBA with hTSH (MRC-A standard 63–14), showing mean values (*n* = 15)

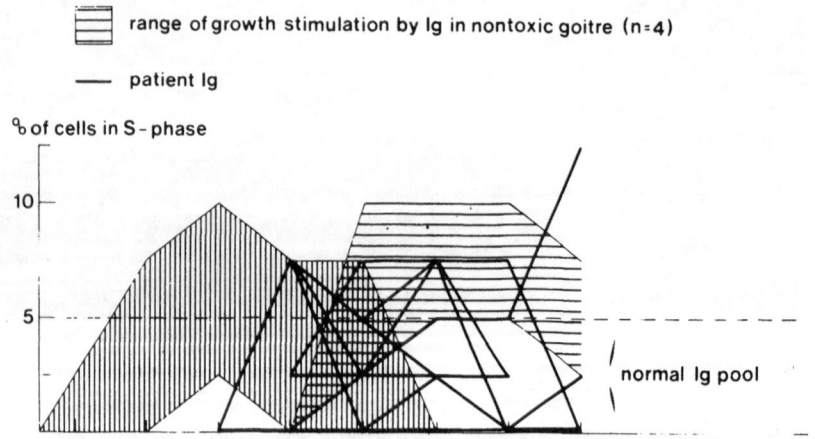

**Figure 3.4** Dose–response curves for thyroid growth obtained in Feulgen CBA with immunoglobulins from patients with goitrous Graves' disease, sporadic non-toxic goitre and Plummer's disease (solid lines)

TGI can also be assayed with another quantitative cytochemical method that measures activity of glucose-6-phosphatase dehydrogenase (G6PD-CBA). G6PD is the first and rate-controlling enzymatic step of the pentose shunt, which is the major source of ribose sugars needed for the synthesis of DNA[14]. It also provides much of the NADPH of the cytosol, which is essential for many biosynthetic steps required for cellular growth ($E_0$ at – 320 mV) (Figure 3.5). NADPH is also used by the microsomal respiratory pathway (with an $E_0$ at +170 mV) in many hydroxylation and mixed-function oxidation processes, as well as being involved in the generation of $H_2O_2$, important for iodination in the synthesis of thyroid hormones (Figure 3.5).

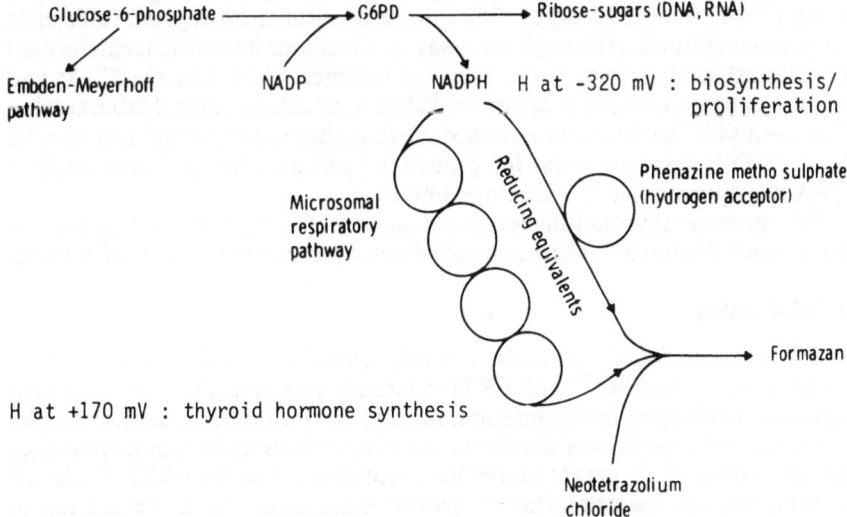

**Figure 3.5** Pentose shunt. Energy transfers measured in the glucose-6-phosphate dehydrogenase (G6PD) cytochemical bioassay for both thyroid growth-stimulating and thyroid function-stimulating immunoglobulins

The total generation of NADPH by G6PD in a particular thyroid cell can be measured by reacting tissue sections with G6P and NADPH in the presence of the intermediate hydrogen carrier, phenazine methosulphate (PMS), which transfers reducing equivalent quantitatively from NADPH to the final acceptor, neotetrazolium chloride, which on reduction precipitates as a formazan (Figure 3.5). The amount of formazan per follicle cell is again measured by microdensitometry.

The advantage of this type of quantitative cytochemical study on the pentose shunt is that it permits an analysis of how reducing equivalents from NADPH are apportioned between growth activities ($E_0$ of –320 mV) and hormone-production activities ($E_0$ of +170 mV) involving the microsomal pathway[15].

A detailed description of the methodology is given in references 13, 16 and 17.

McMullan and Smyth[10] adapted our methods for the G6PD-CBA, since they found that the reaction media described by us did not result in their laboratory in a separation of NADPH generation between TSH-treated and control thyroid segments. They optimized the reaction conditions at section thicknesses of $10\,\mu m$, coenzyme NADP concentrations of $0.3\,mmol/l$ and a reaction time of $10-12\,min$.

### Rat thyroid follicle assay

Efforts have also been directed at developing other more simplified methods for measuring TGI levels.

Chiovato et al.[8] described an assay for measuring thyroid growth effects using [³H]thymidine incorporation into reconstituted rat thyroid follicles in suspension cultures. Although the assay is still labour intensive, it can be used for clinical studies since it requires less technical skill than the CBA; and isotope culture techniques are more widely available in clinical laboratories. The method is, however, far less sensitive than the cytochemical bioassays. Its limit of TSH responsiveness for growth is $1\,\mu U/ml$ whereas in the Feulgen CBA it is approximately 1000 times lower.

For the assay thyroid follicles are prepared from rat glands as described by Nitsch and Wollman[18]. Further detailed descriptions are given in reference 8.

### FRTL-5 assay

A differentiated functional strain of rat thyroid cells in continuous culture has recently been described[19] (the FRTL-5 strain). The cells allow measurement of cyclic AMP-stimulating autoimmune thyroid antibodies in serum samples from patients with Graves' disease nearly as effectively as human thyroid-slice and cell systems[20]. Separate studies have also shown that the FRTL-5 cells are suitable for the measurement of growth stimulation, with the uptake of radiolabelled thymidine as a simple parameter.

The cell line has an absolute requirement of thyrotropin for growth and they are grown in Coon's modified Ham's F-12 medium supplemented with 5% fetal calf serum and a six-hormone mixture[19]. Detailed descriptions for the methodology of TGI detection in this system are given in reference 9.

## TGI IN GRAVES' DISEASE

Most cases of Graves' disease have some enlargement of their thyroid gland, but the size of the goitre bears little relation to the amounts of thyroid hormone generated: about 10% of thyrotoxic patients have no goitre, yet the overproduction of thyroid hormones is such that they often present with clinically overt hyperthyroidism. For our initial studies on Graves' goitre we selected the two extremes of the spectrum and compared cases having large or moderate goitres, with patients with a just palpable or impalpable thyroid gland but proven elevations of serum $T_3$ and $T_4$ and an absent response of serum TSH to intravenous TRH. The Ig preparations from 17 out of 18 of such goitrous thyrotoxic cases stimulated DNA synthesis in the Feulgen CBA when added in a fixed concentration of 125 $\mu$g Ig/ml to the culture system. By contrast the Igs from six non-goitrous thyrotoxics lacked such effects and were comparable to Igs from normal individuals. Though the assay system was not accurate enough to establish individual potencies of TGI (dose–response studies are a prerequisite for that, see earlier) we nevertheless found that the growth stimulus, expressed as the percentage of cells in S-phase, correlated fairly well with goitre size ($r = 0.76$). On the other hand, when we tried to match the severity of hyperthyroidism (pretreatment $T_3$ levels), with *in vitro* DNA synthesis, the relationship was negative ($r = 0.01$).

The growth stimulus was organ-specific since a TGI-positive Ig preparation from a thyrotoxic patient failed to increase the DNA synthesis in segments of stomach and parathyroid.

Although LATS responses are not always proportional to clinical toxicity owing to coexisting lymphoid thyroiditis in some Graves' glands or to the use of mice as test animals, it does nevertheless measure hormone production in these animals. Therefore it was of interest that the height of the LATS response found positive in half our Graves' patients tested for TGI did not correlate at all ($r = 0.16$) with the growth stimulus present in the sera. Another interesting negative correlation was obtained when comparing TGI results with TBII data obtained with the radioligand test of Smith and Hall[21]. This test is positive in about 60–80% of Graves' patients and correlates in general with the cAMP stimulation test[22,23].

With regard to the G6PD-CBA Ig preparations from 12 out of 14 Graves' disease patients with goitres stimulated the generation of NADPH. The Ig from five patients with Graves' disease but with minimal enlargement of the thyroid gland behaved like normal Ig and gave negative responses. In all specimens tested there was good correlation between the amount of DNA synthesis, measured by Feulgen CBA, and the generation of NADPH measured by G6PD-CBA ($r = 0.71$, $p<0.01$).

McMullan and Smyth confirmed this presence of Igs stimulating NADPH generation in goitrous Graves' disease[10]. These authors additionally showed that antisera to human IgG significantly diminished the NADPH generating capacity of Graves' immunoglobulin while antisera to human TSH had no such effect. They also found in analogy to our previous mentioned studies that a positive response largely depended on the concentration of immunoglobulin used in the culture system: bell-shaped dose–response curves were obtained reaching maximal values at different concentrations; and TGI of goitrous Graves' disease was 10 times more potent than that of non-toxic goitre. In the isolated rat thyroid follicle assay of Chiovato, 68% of patients with goitrous Graves' disease were positive. Positivity was found in proportion with goitre size, but again showed no correlation with serum $T_3$ levels, or three accepted methods for measuring TSI, e.g. cAMP stimulation, LATS activity and the TBII assay[8].

Using the FRTL-5 assay, Valente *et al.*[9] found that IgG preparations from 117 of 156 patients (75%) with active Graves' disease could augment thyroid-cell growth. Performed in parallel with TSI assays (measuring cAMP levels), their occurrence was unrelated to this activity. The presumption of the authors was that the growth promoting activity was in some manner linked to goitrogenesis, and in a preliminary series they found indeed a gross correlation between goitre sizes and TGI activity.

All these data make it clear that distinct classes of Igs participate in the pathogenesis of Graves' disease. TSIs stimulate thyroid follicle cells to produce excessive amounts of $T_3$ and $T_4$, whereas TGI stimulates follicle cells to grow.

TGI activity appeared in general independent of the action of TSI. There is even evidence that TSI and TGI react with different domains of the TSH receptor. Valente et al.[24] generated human monoclonal antibodies from heterohybridomas obtained by fusing mouse myeloma cells with peripheral lymphocytes from patients with active Graves' disease. Four antibodies were characterized as presumptive thyrotropin receptor antibodies, since TSH specifically inhibited their binding to human thyroid membranes. Two of these antibodies were representative of autoimmune stimulators in Graves' disease, since they could stimulate thyroid function in several assays, including the mouse bioassay. These stimulating antibodies interacted strongly with ganglioside preparations but were poor inhibitors of TSH binding to the glycoprotein receptor component embedded in liposomes. One of the monoclonal antibodies stimulated thymidine incorporation in the FRTL-5 cell line and also showed positive results in the Feulgen CBA. This monoclonal TGI had no intrinsic stimulatory action in assays of thyroid function but rather inhibited thyrotropin activity in the assays. Although this antibody did not react with human thyroid gangliosides it inhibited the binding of TSH to the glycoprotein part of the receptor. This indicates that TGI may interact with domains on the TSH receptor differently from those reacting with TSI.

The surface of cells is known to expose receptors for a wide variety of intercellular messages, including neurotransmitters, hormones, growth factors and lectins. The cellular responses to such chemical messages (increased function and proliferation) occur via and at intracellular sites. The adenylate cyclase system is one such site translating messages. However, it is confusing how one signalling system can serve multiple functions and other second messengers must be involved. Such new second messengers are now identified but knowledge is still scanty, and interactions between the systems have not fully been elucidated. The phosphatidyl–inositol turnover pathway is one such newly identified second messenger system. Protein kinase C plays a crucial role in this system in signal transduction for a variety of biologically active substances which activate cellular function and proliferation. When cells are stimulated, protein kinase C is transiently activated by diacylglycerol, which is produced in the membrane during the turnover of inositol phopholipids[7,25,26].

The phosphatidyl–inositol turnover cycle is present in a variety of tissues – including the thyroid[27] – and is activated by numerous substances of different origin, most notably growth factors.

We favour a hypothesis that there may be several TGIs in Graves' disease and non-toxic goitre with specificities for more than one receptor, not only stimulating cAMP but also systems such as the phosphatidyl–inositol pathway. Such a concept is illustrated by our recent findings in a collaborative double-blind study with Bliddal *et al.* (in preparation) on autoreactive thyroid antibodies in Graves' disease. This study focused on the mutual relationships between TBII, Igs stimulating cAMP and TGI, the latter quantitatively measured in dose–response. The correlation of these Igs with circulating thyroid hormones and the size of the goitre measured by an ultrasound technique was studied as well. The study confirmed that TGI correlates to thyroid volume (Figure 3.6). However, exceptions were noted in two patients with large goitres without TGI, and one patient having a very large gland with only intermediate TGI activity. These results indicate the complexity of goitrogenesis and underline the possibility suggested by Studer *et al.*[28] of large variations in the individual response to a goitrogen.

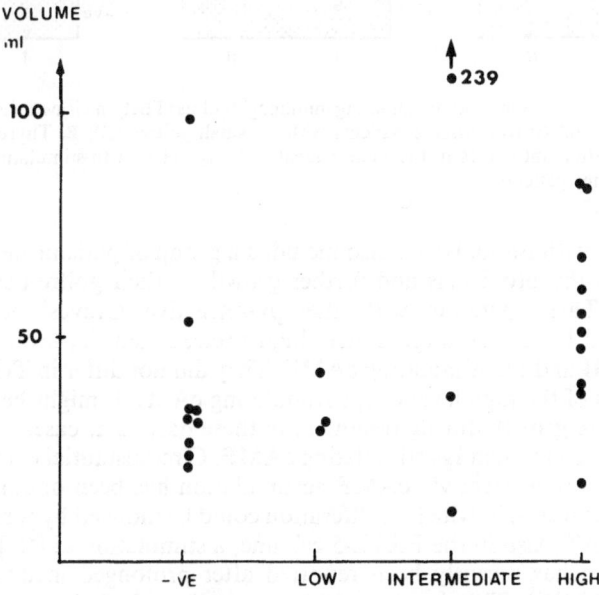

**Figure 3.6** The correlation between thyroid volume determined by ultrasound and TGI in patients with untreated Graves' disease, $n = 25$, $Rs = 0.54$, $p < 0.03$

The correlation found in this study between TBII and Igs stimulating cAMP, though weak, is in agreement with previous studies[22,23]. The correlation between TBII and Igs stimulating cAMP with thyroid function has also been observed before[29,30]; other studies have, however, been negative in this respect[31]. Ig stimulating cAMP did not correlate with goitre size, underlining the notion that cAMP is, in general, not involved in the pathway leading to proliferation. Previous attempts to correlate TGI to TBII in Graves' disease had been negative (see before). The results of the present double-blind study indicate, however, that the TBII assay probably measures both some TGI as well as some TSI (Figure 3.7). This is supported by the aforementioned experiments of Valente *et al.* on the monoclonal TBIIs of which some were TGIs, while others were TSIs.

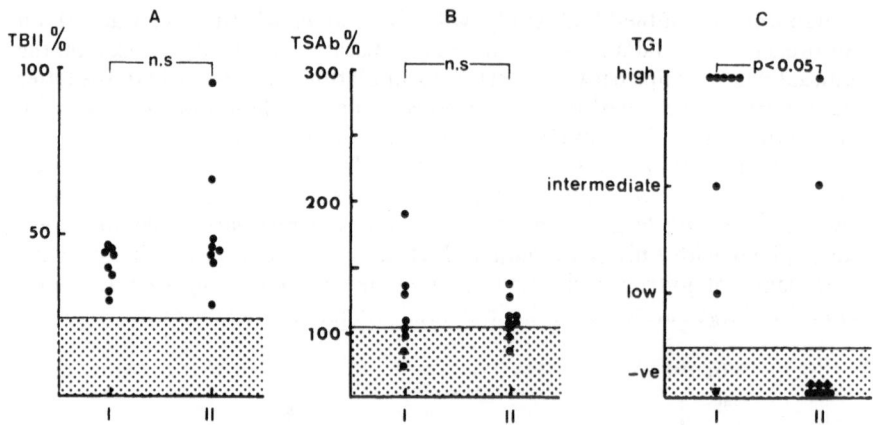

**Figure 3.7 A.** Thyrotropin-binding inhibiting immunoglobulins (TBII) in Graves' disease patients with goitre (I) and Graves' disease patients with no/small goitres (II); **B.** Thyroid adenylate cyclase stimulating antibodies in the same patients; **C.** thyroid growth-stimulating antibodies (TGI) in the same patients

The study with Bliddal *et al.* also included a group of patients developing a recurrent $T_3$ thyrotoxicosis and further growth of their goitre despite PTU treatment. These patients with therapy-refractive Graves' goitre were characterized by a very large goitre, high pretreatment $T_3$ levels and high levels of TBII and Igs stimulating cAMP. They did not differ in TGI activity. On the basis of the high level of Igs stimulating cAMP it might be suggested that the goitre growth during treatment in these particular cases is caused in addition to TGI by such Igs stimulating cAMP. Circumstantial evidence for a growth-promoting effect via cAMP-accumulation has been obtained in dog thyroid cell cultures, in which proliferation could be induced by forskolin and cholera toxin[32]. Also in the FRTL-5 cell line, a stimulation of [$^3$H]thymidine incorporation has recently been reported after prolonged incubation with dibutyryl cAMP[33]. This is in contrast to studies which have indicated a separation of TSH effects on adenylate cyclase and growth[20].

The findings of the collaborative study with Bliddal *et al.* highlight the complexity of the growth stimuli exerted by Graves' Igs and the pathways involved.

## TGI IN SPORADIC DIFFUSE AND NODULAR GOITRES

The TGI results of the ten cases of euthyroid colloid goitres selected for our initial studies are shown in Figure 3.8. In these investigations we tested the Igs at fixed concentrations of $125\,\mu g$ Ig/ml culture fluid.

The highest TGI values were seen in patients who had undergone subtotal thyroidectomies in the past and whose goitres had regrown after 1–5 years. All patients had been given prolonged therapy with thyroxine but their goitres had failed to shrink. There was no difference in TGI positivity between

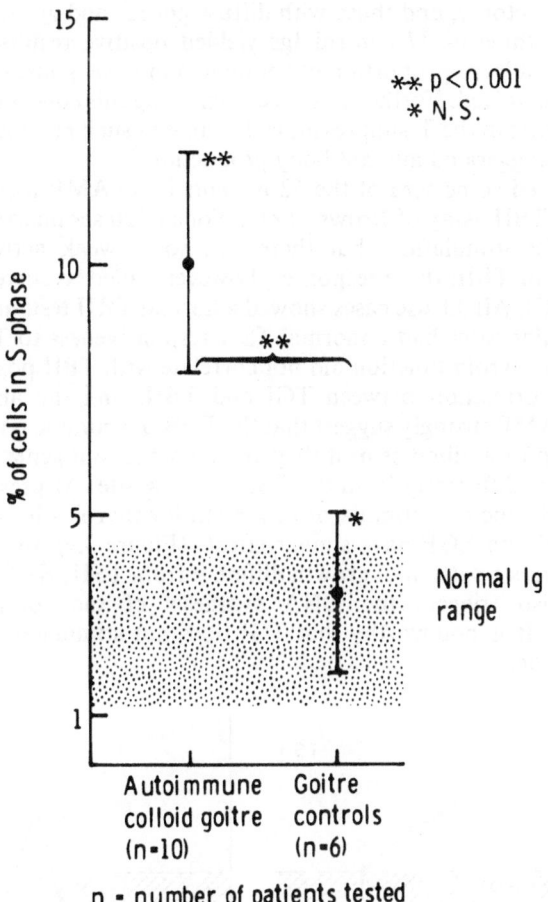

**Figure 3.8** Thyroid growth-stimulating immunoglobulins (TGI) in sporadic non-toxic goitres. Goitre controls: dyshormonogenic goitre patients, and patients with 'single hot adenomas'

patients who had normal TRH responses and those with flat or absent responses. Unresponsiveness to TRH appears to depend on the amount of circulating $T_3$ in the patient, and in some of the non-toxic goitre cases this hormone was at the upper part of the normal range or even slightly above it. There were also cases amongst the ten patients where the TRH response returned to normal after being flat, yet at no time were there any clinical signs of hyperthyroidism.

Recently we extended the studies on non-toxic goitre by testing 62 consecutive cases (57 females, 5 males, living in London or Amsterdam, both non-iodine-deficient areas)[34]. Of these, 15 were classified as diffuse, 39 as multinodular and 8 as single nodules. Sera from these patients were tested for the presence of TGI by the Feulgen CBA. Forty-three (67%) were positive. Titres of TGI tended again to be high in nodular goitres that recurred after partial thyroidectomy, and those with diffuse goitres and goitres with recent growth. Only three of 37 control Igs yielded positive results. These data suggest that in a large proportion of sporadic non-toxic goitres autoimmune processes are involved. Further evidence supporting this concept is our recent finding of defects in the T-suppressor cell system in such patients, which may underlie the exaggerated autoantibody production[35].

We also tested some sera of the 62 patients in a cAMP assay and in the ultrasensitive TBII assay of Brown *et al.*[5]. None of 20 serum samples studied showed cAMP stimulation, but there was some weak activity of some preparations for TBII; these responses, however, failed to correlate with the presence of TGI. All diffuse cases showed a normal TRH test; around 40% of the multinodular cases had abnormal TSH responsiveness to TRH but this disturbance in thyroid function did not correlate with TBII positivity either. The lack of correlation between TGI and TBII, and the absence of Igs stimulating cAMP strongly suggest that the TGIs of sporadic goitre are either not TSH receptor antibodies or if they are, recognize antigenic determinants on the receptor differently from the TSH binding site. At present we know that TSH is not the sole stimulator of growth for thyroids in organ culture. HCG, α-MSH and EGF have similar effects (Figure 3.9); the latter factor, however, induces a pattern of growth different from TSH, HCG and α-MSH in that it also triggers the DNA synthesis of the connective tissue compartment. It is noteworthy that TGI does not stimulate the growth of connective tissue.

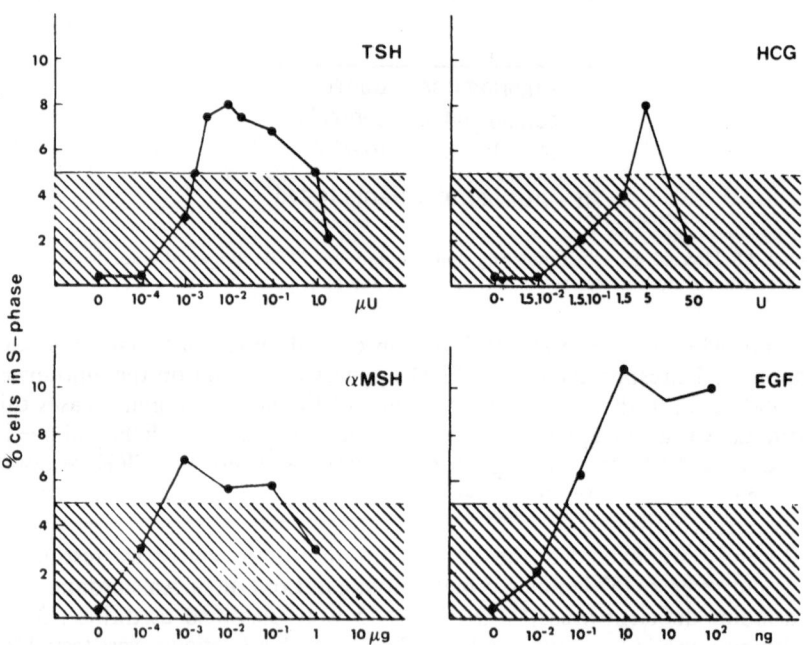

**Figure 3.9** Dose–response curves for thyroid growth obtained in Feulgen CBA with hTSH, HCG, αMSH and EGF

Regarding the presence of TGI in non-toxic goitre, similar findings have been reported by Smyth et al.[10], testing Igs in their G6PD-CBA. TGI was found to be present in 68% of cases. Their finding, that TGI, when present in non-toxic goitre, caused only a maximum increase in G6PD activity at a relatively high IgG concentration of $500 \mu g/ml$ culture fluid in the vast majority of their patients, confirms that TGI of sporadic goitre is about 10 times less potent than that of goitrous Graves' disease (see before). Measurements of goitre size were not available in their studies, but a few non-toxic euthyroid patients whose Igs caused maximal increases in G6PD activity at relatively low IgG concentration of $50 \mu g/ml$ had very large goitres.

The presence of relatively low activities of sporadic goitre TGI – as found by us and the group of Smyth – supports the concept of Studer et al. on the development of this thyroid anomaly. These investigators view the normal thyroid gland as composed of follicular cells that differ in their ability to synthesize thyroid hormones, to respond to TSH, and to replicate[28]. If a relatively potent goitrogen acts upon such a normal heterogeneous gland, a diffuse enlargement will result showing both hypertrophy and hyperplasia in most acini (Graves' disease and diffuse non-toxic goitre). Conversely, multinodular goitres would develop when a relatively mild goitrogenic stimulus exerts its influence over a longer period, stimulating only those follicles with a relatively low threshold for growth. Such follicles may intrinsically possess a high or low basal metabolism for hormone production. Consequently, multinodular goitres will show wide differences in function between one follicle and the next, and differences in sizes, thyroglobulin content and other biochemical parameters.

In this view mild stimulation of growth rather than of function is at the basis of the development of subclinical and clinically overt toxic multinodular goitre (Plummer's disease). Toxicity in these disorders will supervene only when the mass of intrinsically hyperactive cells with TSH-independent function surpasses certain limits. Indeed, Plummer in 1913[36] already noted that 'the onset of disease is usually insidious' and that the average interval between the detection of a goitre and 'the evidence of intoxication' was 14.5 years in his patients with 'non-hyperplastic toxic goitre'. Recently we tested nine cases of Plummer's disease for the presence of TGI in the Feulgen CBA[37]; seven were found positive, TGI activities ranging from low to intermediate activity (Figure 3.4). Smyth et al. (personal communication) found similar data showing four of eight cases of toxic nodular goitres positive in the G6PD-CBA. They have argued on earlier occasions for Plummer's disease being related to autoimmune phenomena and based their assumption on the detection of low levels of TSI in six out of six cases, as detected by the ultrasensitive LNA-se CBA. They found similar TSIs in non-toxic multinodular cases with a flat TSH responsiveness to TRH. The significance of such TSIs in Plummer's disease and subclinical hyperthyroid multinodular goitres is unknown. It is possible that these TSIs when arising in relatively longstanding non-toxic goitres, may contribute to the development of hyperthyroidism by a functional stimulation of the nodules grown under the influence of TGI. Some of these nodules may already function independently from the action of TSH due to a relatively high intrinsic metabolism. A concept that some TSI is involved in subclinical hyperthyroidism in some of the sporadic goitres may explain cases where TRH responsiveness returned to normal after being flat since levels of TSI may fluctuate (see for further illustration Table 3.1).

**Table 3.1** TRH responsiveness and TGI

| Goitre<br>TRH test | Euthyroid | | | Hyperthyroid |
|---|---|---|---|---|
| | Diffuse<br>Normal (n = 9) | Multinodular<br>Normal (n = 14) | Flat (n = 10) | Multinodular<br>Flat (n = 7) |
| Age<br>(median, years) | 29 | 48 | 60 | 67 |
| Goitre duration<br>(median, years) | 5 | 15 | 19 | Not known |
| Serum $T_3$ (nmol/l)<br>Serum $T_4$ (nmol/l) | 2.1 ± 0.2<br>121 ± 24 | 1.8 ± 0.8<br>110 ± 24 | 3.3 ± 0.8<br>129 ± 29 | 3.5 ± 0.3<br>213 ± 40 |
| TGI<br>(Feulgen and<br>G6PD-CBA) | Clearly positive<br>in practically all<br>patients | Positive in 60–70%<br>of patients | | Positive in 60–70%<br>of patients |
| TSI<br>(LNA'se and type 1<br>hydrogen CBA) | Trace amounts in<br>half the patients | Trace amounts in half<br>the patients | | Some weak activity<br>in all patients |
| Genetic trait | z ax (g) | Km (1) | | Not done |

Recent reports have suggested that not only patients with sporadic but also those with endemic goitres may have growth-promoting antibodies. Schatz *et al.* found 14% of such cases positive in the Giessen area, using an isolated porcine thyroid follicle assay[11], whereas a 50–60% positivity was reported in cases from Tuscany and Brazil by Kohn *et al.*[38], using the FRTL-5 assay. The antibody profile of these latter endemic goitre cases is, however, different from that observed in sporadic goitre cases, since around 60% were additionally positive for Igs stimulating cAMP synthesis. Iodized oil treatment resulted in a disappearance of TGI and TSI from the circulation of almost every patient initially positive. The possibility thus exists, that the thyroid autosensitization in this syndrome might earlier be the consequence rather than the cause of the thyroid enlargement. Nevertheless, these findings highlight what appears to be a potentially fascinating relationship between intrathyroidal metabolism and thyroid autoimmunity.

## Igs BLOCKING THYROID GROWTH IN THYROID ATROPHY

Autoantibodies capable of blocking the cAMP stimulation produced by TSH (TSI block) were described in sera from thyrotoxic patients[31] and later in patients with primary myxoedema[39–41]. Blocking antibodies for the growth pathway (TGI block) are also present in sera of patients with thyroid atrophy[42]: when Igs from these patients are incubated together with TSH in Feulgen CBA, they depress the cell division stimulated by the hormone.

Mothers with thyroid atrophy occasionally give birth to babies with a familial form of congenital athyreotic cretinism. Goldsmith et al.[43] were the first to study such a family in detail. Thyroid suppression was present in all six offspring of a myxoedematous mother showing positive thyroid microsomal antibodies. Two of the siblings died in the neonatal period. Although hypothyroidism was transient in two of the remaining offspring, all were mentally and physically retarded at a later age, despite full $T_4$ replacement therapy. To account for the familial clustering of this form of cretinism, the authors postulated the transplacental passage of a 'thyrocytosuppressive' factor in addition to thyroid microsomal antibodies.

More recently, Japanese investigators provided the evidence for the transplacental passage of a TBII capable of blocking TSH-induced adenylate cyclase stimulation and interfering with thyroid hormone synthesis[39,40]. The maternal antibody was present in high titre in the siblings at 2 months of age. The levels decreased at 3 months and tests were negative at approximately 10 months of age. These children had only mild transient forms of congenital hypothyroidism.

We have studied a Turkish family in which four members (two sisters, an aunt and an uncle) were affected by more persistent forms of congenital hypothyroidism[44]. In three, the thyroid gland could not be seen by radioactive thyroid imaging. The mother of the two sisters was clinically euthyroid throughout the period of observation, but showed high levels of microsomal antibodies in addition to Igs that blocked the trophic action of TSH. The serum of the father was weakly positive for microsomal antibodies. The maternal growth-blocking antibodies underwent transplacental transfer in the younger child. The older sibling, the aunt and the uncle produced growth-blocking antibodies themselves and may thus represent forms of thyroid autoimmunity with a very early onset.

The Turkish family appeared to have many features in common with the earlier reported Cincinatti family, the Japanese family and a Swedish family[45] (see Table 3.2), but differed, however, also in several aspects. Though positive for microsomal antibodies and TGI-block the Turkish mother never showed any clinical or biochemical signs of primary myxoedema, except for a raised TSH during her second pregnancy. This is puzzling: the data may speak for a subclinical symptomless thyroiditis that may later progress to hypothyroidism. Furthermore, the cause of the disease of the two Turkish siblings differed from that of the siblings of the Japanese families, who had only transient forms of hypothyroidism. The cretinism of the Turkish infants was persistent and more or less similar to the disease form observed in the Cincinatti family where the first two infants died, and the remaining four siblings were still clearly disturbed at later ages. They are also comparable to the majority of sporadic CHT-cases (vide infra).

Furthermore, it is important to note that the Turkish sera containing the growth blockers of immune origin did not compete with hTSH for its receptor.

The family studies indicate that familial forms of congenital hypo-

**Table 3.2** Data of familial CHT in relation to sporadic CHT

| | Persistence of CHT | Thyroid status of the mother | M-AAbs | | TBII | | TGI block | |
|---|---|---|---|---|---|---|---|---|
| | | | Mother | Child at birth | Mother | Child at birth | Mother | Child at birth |
| The Cincinatti family (Goldsmith et al., 1973)[43] | persistent | hypothyroid/at first thyroxine treatment | + | + | not done | | not done | |
| Two Japanese families (Matsuura et al., 1980)[39] | transient | thyroxine treatment | + | + | + | + | not done | |
| Iseki et al., 1983[40] | transient | thyroxine treatment | + | + | + | + | not done | |
| The Swedish family (Ritzen et al., 1981)[45] | transient | thyroxine treatment | + | + | not done | | not done | |
| The Turkish family[44] | persistent | euthyroid | + | + | − | − | + | + |
| Sporadic CHT (Van der Gaag et al., 1986)[46] | almost all persistent (32/34) | euthyroid | 5/34 + | − | − | − | 16/34 + | 8/16 + |

thyroidism are complex and, at least in some cases, may be brought about by transplacental passage of thyroid receptor antibodies, whereas others may be associated with the inheritance of a trait for thyroid autoimmunity.

Intriguing are recent data on TGI-block in sporadic forms of congenital hypothyroidism[46]. This disorder has a prevalence of about 1 to 4000 live births in iodine-replete areas. Most industrialized countries screen all newborns for the presence of this disease in an attempt to eradicate the permanent neurological sequelae of delayed T4 replacement therapy. The pathogenesis of sporadic congenital hypothyroidism is largely unknown.

Of 34 mothers of infants detected in the Quebec screening programme (1979–1983) 15 serum samples were positive for TGI block when tested in the ultrasensitive Feulgen CBA. At childbirth, all mothers were clinically and biochemically euthyroid. In general, the blocking Igs were found in the absence of thyroid microsomal antibodies. Two mothers, however, had significant titres of antimicrosomal antibodies and thus had an autoantibody profile similar to that which characterizes adult thyroid atrophy. They were the only two mothers who became hypothyroid in a follow-up of 1–3 years, and their infants can be considered to be affected by familial congenital hypothyroidism. Sixteen postpartum infant blood samples from the Quebec programme were also available for study; eight were positive for Igs that blocked TSH-induced thyroid growth. There was a generally good correlation in the positivity for these Igs between mothers and their own children.

Seven mothers with positive sera were tested up to 3 years after childbirth, when the results for four of the seven were negative. This suggests that blocking Igs may disappear from the maternal circulation in the course of time.

The data from the Quebec series raise the possibility that a transplacental passage of maternal Igs influencing processes of thyroid growth may play a role in the pathogenesis of a substantial proportion of cases of sporadic congenital hypothyroidism.

After our initial report Drs Dussault and Bernier described another variety of thyroid-reactive Igs, present in mothers of children with thyroid agenesis or ectopy[47]. It is confusing that these Igs acted as stimulators of TSH-mediated $^{125}I$ uptake in cells of the rat thyroid cell-line FRTL-5. Since the $^{125}I$ uptake assay is relatively simple and all of 20 mothers tested positive, the authors proposed to investigate the use of the test in a prenatal screening of pregnant women to predict birth of CHT infants.

Also to devise a practical method for prenatal screening, we have recently looked into the presence of yet another variety of thyroid reactive antibodies in CHT mothers, e.g. antibodies to second colloid antigen (CA2). Such antibodies have been reported as early as 1961 in CHT[48]. CA2 antibodies are detected by way of indirect immunofluorescence on methanol-fixed human thyroid sections. Around 40% of our earlier reported Canadian series of mothers (e.g. 14 in 35) were positive, versus a positivity of 8% (1 in 12) in normal pregnancies. The presence of CA2 antibodies showed a positive correlation to the presence of thyroid growth-blocking Igs (Table 3.3, $\chi^2 =$ 9.32; $p < 0.01$).

**Table 3.3** Contingency table between presence of CA2 antibodies and the presence of thyroid growth-blocking Igs

|  | TGI block + ve | TIG block – ve |
|---|---|---|
| CA2 antibodies + ve | 9 | 5 |
| CA2 antibodies – ve | 3 | 18 |

Regarding a more precise prevalence of the Feulgen CBA growth-blocking antibodies in CHT we have found uptil now 9 in 11 (80%) of Dutch cases positive when employing the sensitive, but time-consuming cytochemical bioassay in dose–response.

The way we view these findings on the separate thyroid reactive Igs in CHT is that the maternal autosensitization apparently affects several thyroid functions. There is (a) stimulation of TSH-mediated $^{125}$I uptake in all or almost all of the cases; (b) blockade of TSH-induced thyroid growth in around 80%; and (c) sensitization to a colloid component in 40%. The possibility thus exists that the immune reaction is polyclonal, as in Graves'

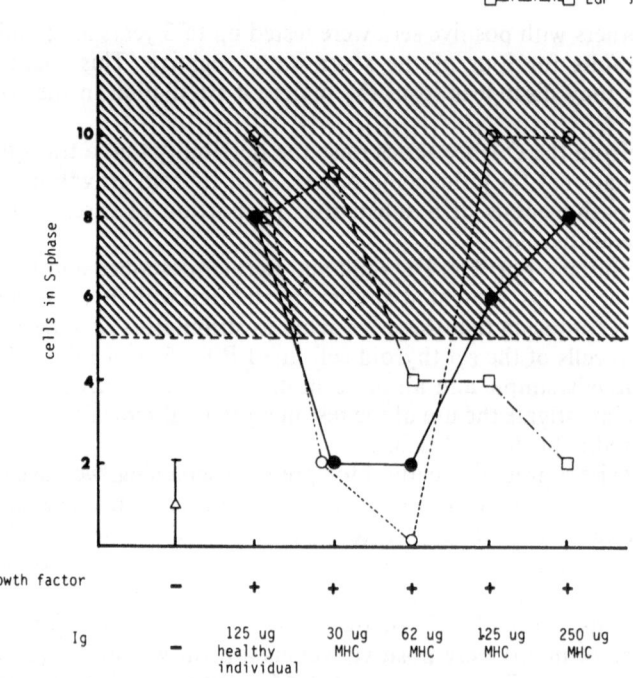

**Figure 3.10** Dose–response curves for the blockade by an Ig preparation from a mother of a congenital hypothyroid child of thyroid growth induced by hTSH, HCG and EGF

disease[24], and directed to a variety of epitopes.

The thyroid-reactive immunoglobulins need not necessarily be directed to the TSH receptor itself but may change the function and conformation of the receptor by reacting with a close domain or membrane component. Such a mechanism of action has been proposed earlier for Igs blocking TSH-mediated cAMP stimulation in primary myxoedema[49]. It is indeed a fact that antibodies competing for radiolabelled TSH with its receptor are absent or very rare in primary myxoedema and sporadic CHT (in our series, none). These notions may imply that not only TSH-mediated growth will be affected by the maternal antibodies but also growth induced by other hormones. This has prompted us to a further investigation on growth-blockade potential of the Igs and we have found that they also abolish growth of thyroid cells induced by stimulators such as EGF, HCG and $\alpha$-MSH (Figure 3.10). Thus it is likely that Igs present in mothers giving birth to CHT babies are not primarily directed to the TSH receptor, but to other membrane components. The triggering of such 'receptors' apparently exerts negative influences on thyroid growth in general, whereas at the same time positive effects are evident on iodine accumulation. Further studies will elucidate whether a prenatal screening for CHT is within reach, employing assays for the detection of such maternal thyroid-reactive immunoglobulins.

## References

1. Drexhage, H. A., Bottazzo, G. F., Doniach, D., Bitensky, L. and Chayen, J. (1980). Evidence for thyroid-growth-stimulating immunoglobulins in some goitrous thyroid diseases. *Lancet*, **2**, 287–92
2. Emrich, D. and Bahre, M. (1978). Autonomy in euthyroid goitre: maladaptation to iodine deficiency. *Clin. Endocrinol. (Oxf.)*, **8**, 257–65
3. Morgans, H. E., Thomson, B. S. and Whitehouse, S. A. (1978). Sporadic non-toxic goitre: an investigation of the hypothalamic-pituitary axis. *Clin. Endocrinol. (Oxf.)*, **8**, 101–8
4. Garry, R. and Hall, R. (1970). Stimulation of mitosis in rat thyroid by long-acting thyroid stimulator. *Lancet*, **1**, 693–5
5. Brown, R. S., Jackson, I. M. D., Pohl, S. L. and Reichlin, S. (1978). Do thyroid-stimulating immunoglobulins cause non-toxic and toxic multinodular goitre? *Lancet*, **1**, 904–6
6. Dumont, J. E., Takeuchi, A., Lamy, F., Gervy-Decoster, C., Cochaux, P., Roger, P., Van Sande, J., Lecocq, R. and Mochel, J. (1981). Thyroid control: an example of complex cell regulation network. *Adv. Cyclic Nucleotide Res.*, **14**, 479–89
7. Berridge, M. J. (1984). Inositol triphosphate and diacylglycerol as second messengers. (Review). *Biochem. J.*, **220**, 345–60
8. Chiovato, L., Hammond, L. J., Hanafusa, T., Pujol-Borell, B., Doniach, D. and Bottazzo, G. F. (1983). Detection of thyroid growth immunoglobulins (TGI) by 3H-thymidine incorporation in cultured rat thyroid follicles. *Clin. Endocrinol. (Oxf.)*, **19**, 581–90
9. Valente, W. A., Vitti, P., Rotella, C. M., Vaughan, M. M., Aloj, S. M., Grollman, E. F., Ambesi-Impiombato, F. S. and Kohn, L. D. (1983). Antibodies that promote thyroid growth: a distinct population of thyroid stimulating autoantibodies. *N. Engl. J. Med.*, **309**, 1028–34
10. McMullan, N. M. and Smyth, P. P. A. (1984). *In vitro* generation of NADPH as an index of thyroid stimulating immunoglobulins (TGI) in goitrous disease. *Clin. Endocrinol. (Oxf.)*, **20**, 269–80
11. Schatz, H., Beckman, F. H. and Floren, M. (1983). Radioassay for thyroid growth stimulating immunoglobulins (TGI) with cultivated porcine thyroid follicles. *Horm. Metab. Res.*, **15**, 626–7
12. Bitensky, L., Alaghband-Zadeh, J. and Chayen, J. (1974). Studies on thyroid stimulating

hormone and the long-acting thyroid stimulating hormone. *Clin. Endocrinol. (Oxf.)*, **3**, 363–74

13. Drexhage, H. A., Bottazzo, G. F. and Doniach, D. (1983). Thyroid growth stimulating and blocking immunoglobulins. In Chayen, J. and Bitensky, L. (eds.) *Cytochemical Bioassays*, pp. 153–72 (New York: Marcel Dekker, Inc. and Butterworths)

14. Eggleston, L. V. and Krebs, H. A. (1974). Regulation of the pentose phosphate cycle. *Biochem. J.*, **138**, 425–35

15. Gillette, J. R., Conney, A. H., Cosmides, G. J., Estabrook, R. W., Fouts, J. R. and Mannering, G. J. (eds.) (1969). *Microsomes and Drug Oxidations.* (New York, London: Academic Press)

16. Drexhage, H. A., Hammond, L. J., Bitensky, L., Chayen, J., Bottazzo, G. F. and Doniach, D. (1982). The involvement of the pentose shunt in thyroid metabolism after stimulation with TSH or with immunoglobulins from patients with thyroid disease. I. The generation of NADPH in relation to stimulation of thyroid growth. *Clin. Endocrinol. (Oxf.)*, **16**, 49–56

17. Drexhage, H. A., Hammond, L. J., Bitensky, L., Chayen, J., Bottazzo, G. F. and Doniach, D. (1982). The involvement of the pentose shunt in thyroid metabolism after stimulation with TSH or with immunoglobulins from patients with thyroid disease. II. The reoxidation of NADPH and stimulation of hormone synthesis. *Clin. Endocrinol. (Oxf.)*, **16**, 57–63

18. Nitsch, L. and Wollman, S. H. (1980). Suspension culture of separated follicles consisting of differentiated thyroid epithelial cells. *Proc. Natl. Acad. Sci. USA*, **77**, 472–6

19. Ambesi-Impiombato, F. S., Parks, L. A. M. and Coon, H. G. (1980). Culture of hormone-dependent functional epithelial cells from rat thyroids. *Proc. Natl., Acad. Sci. USA*, **77**, 3455–9

20. Valente, W. A., Vitti, P., Kohn, L. D., Brandi, M. L., Rotella, C. M., Toccafondi, R. S., Tramontano, D., Aloj, S. M and Ambesi-Impiombato, F. S. (1983). The relationship of growth and adenylate cyclase activity in cultured thyroid cells: separate bioeffects of thyrotropin. *Endocrinology*, **112**, 71–9

21. Rees Smith, B. and Hall, R. (1974). Thyroid-stimulating immunoglobulins in Graves' disease. *Lancet*, **2**, 427–31

22. Bliddal, H., Bech, K., Petersen, P. H., Siersback-Nielsen, K. and Friis, T. (1982). Evidence for a correlation between thyrotropin receptor binding inhibition and thyroid adenylate cyclase activation by immunoglobulins in Graves' disease before and during long-term anti-thyroid treatment. *Acta Endocrinol. (Copenh.)*, **101**, 35–40

23. Hensen, J., Kotulla, P., Finke, R., Bogner, U., Badenhoop, K., Meinhold, H. and Schleusener, H. (1984). Methodological aspects and clinical results of an assay for thyroid-stimulating antibodies: correlation with thyrotropin binding-inhibiting antibodies. *J. Clin. Endocrinol. Metab.*, **58**, 980–7

24. Valente, W. A., Vitti, P., Yavin, E., Rotella, C. M., Grollman, E. F., Toccafondi, R. S. and Kohn, L. D. (1982). Monoclonal antibodies to the thyrotropin receptor; stimulating and blocking antibodies derived from the lymphocytes of patients with Graves' disease. *Proc. Natl. Acad. Sci. USA*, **79**, 6680–4

25. Marx, J. L. (1984). A new view of receptor action. Research on the calcium ion-linked receptors features the identification of a new second messenger and a possible connection to oncogene action. *Science*, **224**, 271–4

26. Nishizuka, Y. (1984). The role of protein kinase C in cell surface signal transduction and tumour promotion. *Nature (London)*, **308**, 693–8

27. Michel, R. H. and Kirk, C. J. (1981). Why is phosphatidyl inositol degraded in response to stimulation of certain receptors. *TIPS Reviews*

28. Studer, H. and Ramelli, F. (1982). Simple goiter and its variants: euthyroid and hyperthyroid multinodular goiters. *Endocr. Rev.*, **3**, 40–61

29. Bech, K. and Madsen, S. N. (1979). Thyroid adenylate cyclase stimulating immunoglobulins in thyroid diseases. *Clin. Endocrinol. (Oxf.)*, **11**, 47–58

30. McGregor, A. M., Peterson, M. M., Capiferri, R., Evered, D. C., Rees Smith, B. and Hall, R. (1979). Effects of radioiodine on thyrotrophin binding inhibiting immunoglobulins in Graves' disease. *Clin. Endocrinol. (Oxf.)*, **11**, 437–44

31. Orgiazzi, J., Williams, D. E., Chopra, I. J. and Solomon, D. H. (1976). Human thyroid adenyl cyclase-stimulating activity in immunoglobulins G of patients with Graves' disease. *J. Clin. Endocrinol. Metab.*, **42**, 341–54

32. Roger, P. P., Servais, P. and Dumont, J. E. (1983). Stimulation by thyrotropin and cyclic AMP of the proliferation of quiscent canine thyroid cells cultured in a defined medium containing insulin. *FEBS Lett.*, **157**, 323-9

33. Neylan, D., Zakarija, M., Claflin, A. and McKenzie, J. M. (1985). Evidence that stimulation of thyroid growth is mediated by cyclic AMP (cAMP). Presented at the *9th International Thyroid Congress*, September 1-6, Sao Paulo, Brazil

34. Van der Gaag, R. D., Drexhage, H. A., Wiersinga, W. M., Brown, R. S., Docter, R., Bottazzo, G. F. and Doniach, D. (1985). Further studies on thyroid growth-stimulating immunoglobulins in euthyroid nonendemic goiter *J. Clin. Endocrinol. Metab.*, **60**, 972-9

35. Van der Gaag, R. D., Von Blomberg-van der Flier, M., Van de Plassche-Boers, E., Kokjé-Kleingeld, M. and Drexhage, H. A. (1986). T suppressor cell defects in euthyroid nonendemic goitre. *Acta Endocrinol. (Copenh.)* (In press)

36. Plummer, H. S. (1913). The clinical and pathological relationship of simple and exophthalmic goiter. *Am. J. Med. Sci.*, **146**, 790

37. Wiener, J. D. and Van der Gaag, R. D. (1986). Autoimmunity and the pathogenesis of localized thyroid autonomy (Plummer's disease). *Clin. Endocrinol. (Oxf.)*, (In press)

38. Kohn, L. D., Valente, W. A., Alvarez, F. Z., Rotella, C. M., Marcocci, C., Toccafondi, R. S. and Grollman, E. F. (1985). New procedures for detecting Graves' immunoglobulins. In Walfish, P. G., Wall, J. R. and Volpé, R. (eds.). *Autoimmunity and the Thyroid*. pp. 217-48. (New York: Academic Press)

39. Matsuura, M., Yamada, Y., Nohara, Y., Konishi, I., Kasagi, K., Endo, K., Kojima, H. and Wataya, K. (1980). Familial neonatal transient hypothyroidism due to maternal TSH-binding inhibitor immunoglobulins. *N. Engl. J. Med.*, **303**, 738-41

40. Iseki, M., Shimizu, U., Oikawa, T., Hojo, H., Arikawa, K., Ichikawa, Y., Momotani, N. and Ito, K. (1983). Sequential serum measurements of thyrotropin binding inhibitor Ig in transient familial neonatal hypothyroidism. *J. Clin. Endocrinol. Metab.*, **57**, 384-9

41. Steel, N. R., Weightman, D. R., Taylor, R. R. and Kendall-Taylor, P. (1984). Blocking activity to action of thyroid stimulating hormone in serum from patients with primary hypothyroidism. *Br. Med. J.*, **288**, 1559-62

42. Drexhage, H. A., Bottazzo, G. F., Bitensky, L., Chayen, J. and Doniach, D. (1981). Thyroid growth blocking antibodies in primary myxoedema. *Nature (London)*, **289**, 594-6

43. Goldsmith, R. E., McAdams, A. G., Larsen, P. R., McKenzie, J. M. and Hess, V. E. (1973). Familial autoimmune thyroiditis: maternal-fetal relationship and the role of generalized autoimmunity. *J. Clin. Endocrinol. Metab.*, **37**, 265-75

44. Van der Gaag, R. D., Frisch, H., Weissel, M., Wick, G. and Drexhage, H. A. (1986). Congenital hypothyroidism in a Turkish family: the role of immunoglobulins blocking the trophic effects of TSH and maternal-fetal relationship. *Acta Endocrinol. (Copenh.)* (In press)

45. Ritzen, E. M., Mahler, H. and Alveryd, A. (1981). Transitory congenital hypothyroidism and maternal thyroiditis. *Acta Paediatr. Scand.*, **70**, 765-6

46. Van der Gaag, R. D., Drexhage, H. A. and Dussault, J. H. (1985). Role of maternal immunoglobulins blocking TSH-induced thyroid growth in sporadic forms of congenital hypothyroidism. *Lancet*, **1**, 246-50

47. Dussault, J. H. and Bernier, D. (1985). [125]I-uptake by FRTL5-cells: a screening test to detect pregnant women at risk of giving birth to hypothyroid infants. *Lancet*, **2**, 1029-31

48. Balfour, B. M., Doniach, D., Roitt, I. M. and Couchman, K. G. (1961). Fluorescent antibody studies in human thyroiditis: auto-antibodies to an antigen of the thyroid colloid distinct from thyroglobulin. *Br. J. Exp. Pathol.*, **4**, 307-16

49. Konishi, J., Iida, Y., Endo, K., Misaki, T., Nohara, Y., Matsuura, N., Mori, T. and Torizuka, K. (1983). Inhibition of thyrotropin-induced adenosine 3' 5'-monophosphate increase by immunoglobulins from patients with primary myxedema. *J. Clin. Endocrinol. Metab.*, **57**, 544-9

# 4
# Islet Cell Antibodies

## S. BAEKKESKOV, M. CHRISTIE AND Å. LERNMARK

## INTRODUCTION

Over the last 30 years evidence has accumulated to suggest that autoimmune mechanisms are involved in the remarkably cell specific destruction of pancreatic $\beta$-cells preceding the clinical onset of insulin-dependent diabetes mellitus, IDDM, in man.

Small lymphocytes, inflammatory cells forming an insulitis, are present within the islets of Langerhans in IDDM patients of short duration[1-3], found preferentially in islets where $\beta$-cells still remain[4]. Cellular hypersensitivity to pancreatic antigens has been observed[5] and there is a high prevalence of islet cell autoantibodies at the time of onset[6,7] and even in the period preceding the clinical manifestations of the disease[8-11]. Furthermore, the susceptibility of developing the disease seems to be associated with certain alleles of the HLA-D/DR locus in man which frequently is associated with autoimmune disorders. In IDDM 93-98% of the patients have the HLA-DR3 and/or DR4 specificities[12,13]. These phenomena distinguish IDDM from non-insulin-dependent diabetes mellitus (NIDDM) which presents a different category of diabetes. In this chapter it is our aim to review the state of knowledge of the main immunological aberrations observed in IDDM patients (Table 4.1) and discuss which mechanisms can lead to the $\beta$-cell destruction, as well as how possible future therapies may be aimed at preventing this destruction.

## ISLET CELL ANTIBODIES

The antibodies present in serum of IDDM patients have mainly been demonstrated using indirect immunofluorescence on either frozen or fixed sections of human pancreas (from blood group O donors to prevent interference from isoagglutinins)[14] or on living islet cells in suspension[14]. The first method detects antibodies reacting with the cytoplasm of islet cells referred to as islet cell cytoplasmic antibodies (ICCA); the latter detects islet cell surface antibodies (ICSA). Furthermore, islet cell antibodies have been demonstrated by their ability to mediate complement dependent lysis of

**Table 4.1** Evidence of enhanced activity of the immune system in IDDM

|  | Reference |
|---|---|
| *Humoral immunity* |  |
| Antibodies to the $\beta$-cell surface | 27, 30, 37 |
| Antibodies to islet cell cytoplasmic components | 17 |
| Increased level of autoantibodies to other tissues | 44 |
| *Cellular immunity* |  |
| Lymphocyte infiltration (insulitis) in the islets | 1 |
| Cellular hypersensitivity to pancreatic islets | 5 |
| Signs of polyclonal activation | 45 |

viable islet cells[15] and by their ability to specifically immunoprecipitate islet cell antigens[16].

## Islet cell cytoplasmic antibodies

Islet cell cytoplasmic antibodies are the most extensively studied immunological phenomena in IDDM patients. They were first discovered in 1974[17,18] in sera from IDDM patients with polyendocrine autoimmunity and later detected in the majority (60–90%) of newly diagnosed Caucasian patients[19,20] and at a lower percentage in Japanese IDDM patients[21]. In most cases these antibodies tend to disappear with time so that only 20% of IDDM patients are still positive 3 years after onset of IDDM[14]. However, in patients with polyendocrine autoimmune disorders ICCA titres seem to sustain[22,23]. The immunofluorescence reaction, whether detected using fluorescent secondary antibodies to human IgG or using a sandwich of complement factor C3 and a fluorescent antibody to C3 (complement fixing antibodies, CF-ICCA), is positive for the cytoplasm of all endocrine cell types in the islet. It is therefore difficult to envisage that these antibodies can be responsible for the cell specific destruction of the $\beta$-cells.

It has been suggested that ICCA may be the result of a secondary immune response phenomenon initiated by the exposure of cytoplasmic components, common to all endocrine cells in islets, being released from $\beta$-cells damaged by a primary destruction mechanism. However, the antibody reaction demonstrated by this method may comprise several types of antibody molecules including some of $\beta$-cell specificity. The presence of ICCA in serum several years before clinical onset of IDDM, and at the same time as a progressive decrease of $\beta$-cell function as estimated by the intravenous glucose tolerance test (IVGTT) is observed, suggests that these antibodies are a possible indicator of ongoing or preceding $\beta$-cell destruction[11,24]. Furthermore, recent data suggest that a high ICCA titre at diagnosis or within the first 3 months of insulin therapy may be a useful predictor of a more rapid loss of residual $\beta$-cell function resulting in increased insulin dosage requirements[25]. The sensitivity of the islet cell cytoplasmic antibody assay is dependent on several non-standardized factors including the quality of the pancreas specimen, immunological reagents and inter-observer variability. An international workshop on the standardization of these antibody tests was recently held[26] with the major goal of establishing standard assay conditions for not only qualitative but also quantitative ICCA determinations using end point titres. Standardization of the assay in the future will hopefully allow reliable inter-laboratory comparisons of ICCA measurements.

## Islet cell surface antibodies

Antibodies reacting with the surface of viable dispersed mouse and rat islet cells were demonstrated in the serum of 20–30% of IDDM patients and 2–4% of control subjects in 1978[27]. Prior to that a much higher prevalence of antibodies had been demonstrated by testing binding to the surface of cultured human insulinoma cells no longer producing insulin[28]. The islet cell surface antibodies show up in the microscope as a ring of fluorescence at the cell margin. The highest prevalence (60%) was found prior to the initiation of insulin therapy and diminished thereafter with increasing duration of diabetes[29]. In young diabetics these antibodies have been shown to be $\beta$-cell specific[30]. The presence of ICSA is not always concordant with the presence of ICCA[31–33] indicating that they may recognize different antigenic epitopes.

ICSA but not ICCA can mediate a complement-dependent cellular cytotoxic reaction using rat islet cells, rat insulinoma cells or hamster islet cells as targets[34–36]. Cytotoxic antibodies were detected in 40–60% of IDDM patients[34–36] and the lysis of cells was specific for $\beta$-cells[37]. The pathogenetic importance of the ability of ICSA to confer complement-dependent lysis of $\beta$-cells was questioned on the basis of the high prevalence of the cytotoxic antibodies in non-diabetic first degree relatives of IDDM probands (25%)[34]. However, this prevalence was only 2% in a more recent study[35].

Although it has been demonstrated that ICSA are organ but not species specific[27], it is likely that the sensitivity of ICSA detection would increase if freshly isolated human islet cells were used as targets. In a study using cultured neonatal human islets nine of 11 newly diagnosed IDDM patients were found ICSA positive[31]. Thus, the prevalence of ICSA may be higher in newly diagnosed IDDM patients than measurements using non-human islet cell material indicate. The possibility also exists that IDDM patients who are ICSA negative at clinical onset may have been ICSA positive during the long period of progressive $\beta$-cell destruction which can precede the clinical onset. A period of vigorous destruction of the $\beta$-cells may be followed by a slow destruction process with a low immunoreactivity. The clinical onset is a result of destruction of $\beta$-cells to such an extent that the remaining $\beta$-cell population can no longer meet the physiological requirements for insulin. It can be suggested that the individual may stay at the lower threshold for some time until a situation which calls for a higher insulin demand (e.g. stress) arises and the symptoms of insulin deficiency appear.

Immunoglobulin fractions purified from IDDM sera have been shown to inhibit glucose-stimulated insulin release both *in vitro* and *in vivo*[38,39]. This could indicate that the antibodies interfere somehow with the glucose recognition mechanism of the cell, although that remains highly speculative.

## TARGET ANTIGENS FOR ISLET CELL ANTIBODIES

Antibodies to various non-$\beta$-cell specific molecules have been reported at an increased prevalence in IDDM patients. This includes antibodies to tubulin[40], insulin receptor[41], single stranded and double stranded DNA[42,43], intrinsic factor[44] and thyroglobulin[44]. IDDM patients have signs of polyclonal activation of B-lymphocytes[45] and the increased antibody titres to various antigens may be a result of this. Since none of these proteins are $\beta$-cell specific, the role of such antibodies in the pathogenesis of IDDM is questionable. If autoimmune reactions are responsible for a $\beta$-cell specific destruction, the immune response must be directed to a protein which, at least at the time of the immune aggression, is expressed at the surface of the $\beta$-cell and on no other cells accessible to the immune system. Furthermore, if such a protein is the target of a primary specific immune response to $\beta$-cells, the antibodies should be detectable before clinical onset of IDDM and even before the appearance of ICCA and a decrease in $\beta$-cell function as measured by IVGTT. Using detergent lysates of [$^{35}$S]methionine-labelled human islets as a source of antigen, nine out of ten newly diagnosed IDDM sera were shown[46] to recognize a human islet cell protein of $M_r$ 64000. This protein is amphiphilic[47] and therefore possibly a membrane protein, an observation supported by the fact that antibodies to it were primarily detected in sera positive for $\beta$-cell specific ICSA. This protein was neither detected in freshly isolated human peripheral lymphocytes[46] nor in 11 different endocrine and non-endocrine human cell lines indicating a cell restricted expression of the protein[47]. In a recent investigation[48], antibodies to the $M_r$ 64000 protein were studied in patients who had been followed before the clinical onset of IDDM, due to an impaired glucose tolerance test or a family history of IDDM. In eight out of 12 patients, $M_r$ 64000 antibodies were already present in the first serum sample available, 4–91 months before the clinical onset of IDDM (Figure 4.1). In some cases $M_r$ 64000 antibodies appeared before ICCA and/or abnormal glucose tolerance could be detected. One individual progressed from a $M_r$ 64000 antibody negative to a highly positive state in the period from 70 to 55 months before clinical onset of IDDM. Three patients were designated negative in the observation period. These data support the conclusion from ICCA and IVGTT studies, that the clinical onset of IDDM is preceded by a very long prodromal period of aberrant immune reaction to $\beta$-cells and a progressive decrease in $\beta$-cell function. The incidence of the $M_r$ 64000 antibodies was 86% in 28 IDDM patients, 100% in seven first degree relatives with prediabetic indications (ICCA and/or abnormal glucose tolerance) and 6% in 34 apparently healthy individuals[49]. The function of this protein in $\beta$-cells is not known.

Insulin antibodies may have been detected in newly diagnosed IDDM patients[50,51] before the initiation of insulin therapy. Whether these antibodies are the result of a polyclonal B-lymphocyte activation or structural changes in the insulin molecule is unknown. The response might also be elicited by the release of proinsulin into the circulation during destruction of $\beta$-cells. Proinsulin may be immunogenic because it is normally hidden within the cell and tolerance may not have been created during neonatal life. Its release

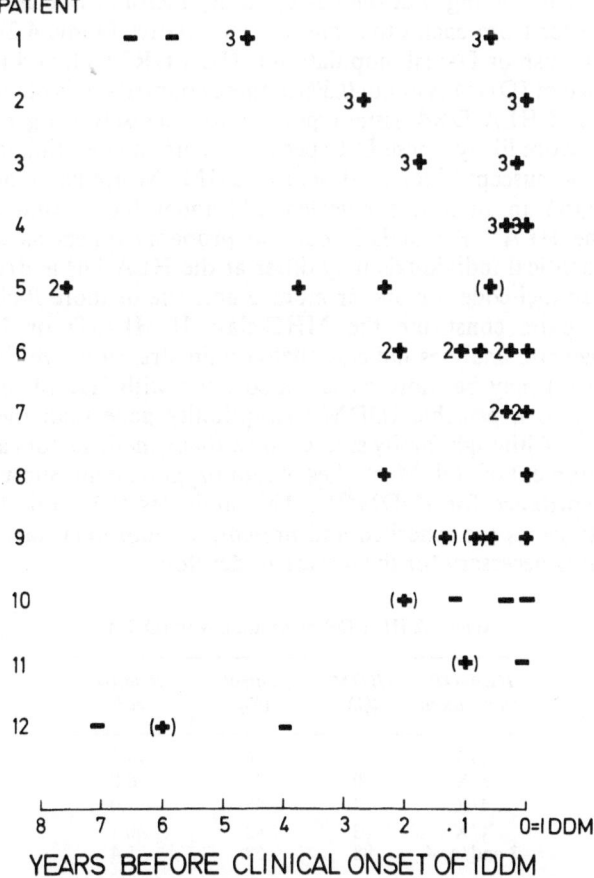

## Prospective analysis of $M_r$ 64000
## antibodies before the clinical onset of IDDM

**Figure 4.1** Immunoreactivity to a $M_r$ 64000 human islet cell antigen in sera from 12 IDDM patients followed for 4–91 months before clinical onset. Degree of $M_r$ 64000 antibody reactivity was estimated from the intensity of the [$^{35}$S]methionine-labelled $M_r$ 64000 antigen band on fluorograms of immunoprecipitates analysed by sodium dodecyl sulphate gel electrophoresis. Immunoreactivity was scored on a 0–3+ scale

could stimulate an immune response including production of antibodies which cross-react with insulin. Both the $M_r$ 64000 protein and insulin seem to satisfy the criteria of being $\beta$-cell specific and insulin may be detected in the plasma membrane of $\beta$-cells during exocytosis.

## GENETIC AND ENVIRONMENTAL FACTORS

Genetic studies have shown a strong association between IDDM and certain

MHC loci in man. The strongest association is found to the HLA DR3 and/or 4 tissue types[12,13]. The relative risk of developing IDDM is higher in HLA DR3/DR4 heterozygotes than in HLA DR3/DR3 or HLA DR4/DR4 homozygotes, indicating that the susceptibility factors associated with each haplotype differ from each other and are cumulative (Table 4.2). Since 57–58% of the British or Danish population is HLA DR3 and/or 4 positive and the prevalence of IDDM is about 0.3% in these countries, it is obvious that the HLA DR3 and HLA DR4 tissue types are not themselves a genetic marker for IDDM. More likely, these DR specificities are in close linkage to a gene conferring the susceptibility to develop IDDM. Molecular cloning of the HLA-D region in man has revealed additional loci within this region including the HLA-DP and DQ loci and probably others as well[52]. Thus HLA DR identical individuals may differ at the HLA DP and/or DQ loci. Each of these loci code for one or more $\alpha$ and one or more $\beta$-chains which together in pairs constitute the MHC-class II HLA-D or Ia antigens. Molecular genetic analyses indicate that certain structures within HLA-DQ $\beta$-chain gene(s) may be more closely associated with IDDM or in a more close linkage to a possible IDDM susceptibility gene than the HLA-DR specificity[53–55]. Although family studies show that genetic factors are involved in the development of IDDM, studies of monozygotic twins show only a 50% or less concordance for IDDM[56,57]. This indicates that, although IDDM susceptibility genes are inherited and present, an additional factor from the environment is necessary for the disease to develop.

**Table 4.2** HLA-DR association with IDDM

| HLA-DR determinant | IDDM (%) | Controls (%) | Relative risk |
|---|---|---|---|
| 3/4 | 51 | 6 | 14.3 |
| 3/X | 20 | 24 | 0.8 |
| 4/X | 27 | 28 | 1.0 |
| X/X | 3 | 42 | 0.1 |
| 3 and/or 4 | 98 | 58 | 1.4 |

Data from ref. 13. X denotes DR-types other than 3 or 4

In spite of an intensive search, a $\beta$-cell cytotoxic diabetogenic factor has not been identified. The seasonal variation in new cases of IDDM indicates that some kind of infectious agent may be involved. Twenty per cent of children exposed to congenital rubella will later develop IDDM[58] and Coxsackie B4 virus has been isolated from the pancreas of a child that died after acute onset of IDDM[59]. Several other candidates including mumps virus, reoviruses, retroviruses and encephalomyocarditis virus have been implicated in the aetiology of IDDM (see 60 for review). In animal models some viruses including encephalomyocarditis virus and Coxsackie B viruses can exert their effect by direct $\beta$-cell damage while infection with other viruses may result in the development of autoimmunity and polyendocrine disease including IDDM[61]. Furthermore, the cumulative effect of $\beta$-cell toxins like alloxan and streptozotocin and a virus infection can result in IDDM in mouse strains otherwise resistant to virally induced IDDM[62].

## MORPHOLOGY

In pancreases inspected shortly after diagnosis of IDDM, invasion by small lymphocytes is seen within the islets, primarily in association with $\beta$-cells, and $\beta$-cells are specifically lost[1-4]. In a pancreas from a patient who died at presentation, monoclonal antibodies to different lymphocyte subsets demonstrated the presence of many cytotoxic/suppressor T-cells as well as a small number of T-helper cells and natural killer/killer cells. B-lymphocytes actively synthesizing immunoglobulins were also detected. Some islets were coated with IgG on the outer membranes. Furthermore, increased expression of HLA-DR was observed on vascular endothelium. Some $\beta$-cells, but not glucagon or somatostatin cells were HLA-DR positive. In the BB-rat, which is an animal model that develops IDDM with many similarities to that of man[64], prospective immunohistological studies of pancreas using monoclonal antibodies to various lymphocyte subsets as well as MHC-class II, Ia, molecules have been performed[65]. The first change observed was an increased expression of Ia antigens on vascular endothelium. Then activated T-helper cells appeared around blood vessels in the pancreas and converged on islets. T cytotoxic/suppressor cells and B-lymphocytes in the pancreatic infiltrates increased proportionately with rat age. Macrophages were also detected. Ia expression was observed on $\beta$-cells at a late stage of destruction, while no expression was detected on glucagon or somatostatin producing cells. The BB-rat studies may provide an important indication of the sequence of events resulting in the formation of insulitis.

Before we go into details of which mechanisms may lead to an immune response to $\beta$-cells, it may be helpful to summarize concepts of an autoimmune response.

## AUTOIMMUNE RESPONSE

The major function of the immune system is to recognize and discriminate between self and non-self. When the immune system encounters a foreign antigen stimulus, the antigen is processed and presented on the surface of an antigen-presenting cell together with MHC class II antigens, the HLA-D or Ia antigen. T-helper cell clones with a T-cell receptor specific for epitopes on the foreign antigen recognize and bind the complex of Ia antigen and foreign antigen and proliferate to yield help to effector cells which can be cytotoxic T-cells and/or B-lymphocytes of the same antigen specificity. Regulatory T-cells, the T-suppressor cells, inhibit the effector arm of the immune system. These events in the immune response are schematized in Figure 4.2. Cytotoxic T-cells can mediate a killing of cells expressing the antigen, and B-lymphocytes proliferate to plasma cells producing antibodies which recognize and bind the antigen either in circulation or membrane bound. Antibodies bound to the surface of cells can mediate complement-dependent cell killing or be recognized by killer cells which mediate the killing. Several growth factors and signals participate in the different events of the immune response (see 66 for review).

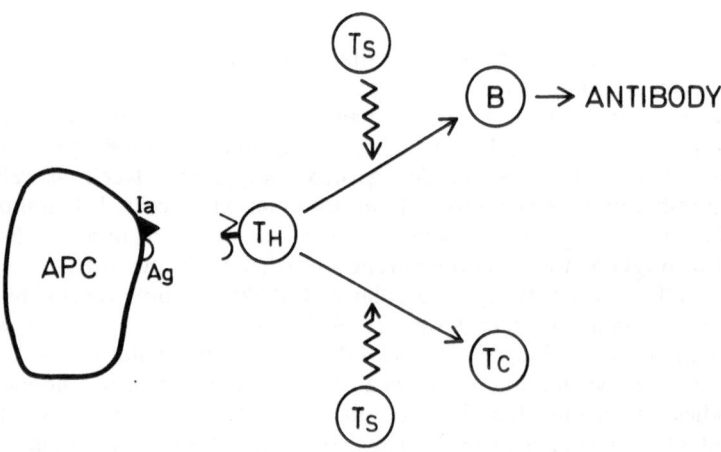

**Figure 4.2** Schematic representation of a T-cell mediated immune response. T$_H$: T-helper cells; APC: antigen presenting cells; T$_S$: T-suppressor cells; T$_C$: cytotoxic T-cells; Ia: MHC-class II antigens

During fetal and/or neonatal life the immune system becomes tolerant to self-antigens. The mechanisms by which the immune system is rendered non-reactive to self-antigens may include control by immuno-regulatory T-lymphocytes, the T-suppressor cells, and/or clonal deletion of autoreactive B- and/or T-helper cells. In neonatal life, suppressed Ia expression may be a mechanism to generate T-suppressor cells and not T-helper cells since the T-suppressor cells may recognize antigen without Ia whereas T-helper cells have to see Ia antigen on antigen-presenting cells[67]. Clones of B-lymphocytes to antigens which are present at high concentrations in the circulation are probably deleted while B-lymphocyte clones to minor antigens or antigens which are normally hidden inside cells may remain but are kept silent by regulatory means, lack of T-helper cells and/or control by T-suppressor cells. For some minimal antigens T-helper cell clones seem to be deleted[68]. Low levels of autoantibody production may be detected in apparently normal individuals[69]. Autoreactive B-cell clones may be pushed into production of antibodies by experimental methods. A classical example is the immunization with thyroglobulin, usually with an adjuvant, resulting in autoantibodies to thyroglobulin and pathological conditions which resemble chronic thyroiditis and related thyroid disorders in man[70]. An example of autoreactive B-cell clones active at low levels in a normal situation are those participating in the idiotypic network as foreseen by Jerne[71]. Immunization with a receptor ligand may result in a production of autoantibodies to the combining site of the receptor via the anti-idiotypic pathway[72].

In a healthy individual proliferation of autoreactive clones is under a tight regulatory control. The knowledge of mechanisms resulting in breakdown of control and a pathological autoimmune condition is limited but several theories have been put forward and are summarized in Table 4.3. A defect in T-suppressor cells can result in breakdown of regulation of autoreactive clones. Analysis of function and levels of circulating T-suppressor cells in IDDM patients has yielded conflicting results (see 73 for review). Analysis of β-cell autoantigen-specific T-suppressor clones has not as yet been feasible. Unresponsiveness to self can be generated by elimination of T-helper cell clones specific for self-antigens. However, T-helper cell clones generated against antigens of infectious agents may cross-react with self-antigens and activate existing autoreactive B-lymphocyte clones. For instance, cross-reactivity between antigenic determinants of *Yersinia enterocolitica* and the thyrotropin (TSH) receptor has been demonstrated. An increased frequency of new cases of Graves' disease, where the patients have antibodies against the TSH receptor, is seen after epidemics of *Yersinia*[74]. Some of the viruses which have been implicated as causative agents for IDDM (e.g. mumps virus, rubella virus and Coxsackie viruses) might sensitize T-helper cells cross-reacting with a β-cell autoantigen. A diabetogenic virus is difficult to identify since it may initiate a process of aberrant immune reaction to β-cells several years before clinical onset. Therefore, no traces of the virus may be left at the time of diagnosis of IDDM. Sequence homology studies between β-cell antigen(s) and viral or bacterial proteins may, once such information becomes available, give indications of possible cross-reacting infectious agents.

**Table 4.3** Breakdown of tolerance to self-antigens: autoimmunity

---

(1)  Loss of suppression

(2)  Changes in structure or expression of self-antigens

(3)  Abnormal expression of MHC-class II (HLA-D/Ia) antigens

(4)  Acquisition of abnormal T-cell help

(5)  Polyclonal B-cell activation

(6)  Disturbances in the idiotypic network

---

Chemicals, infectious viruses or bacteria could theoretically modulate an islet cell antigen resulting in altered self. Changes in the concentration of an autoantigen in the circulation or at the cell surface, caused by chemicals or infectious agents and resulting in tissue damage or induction of antigen expression, could lead to imbalance in the homoeostasis of the immune system and evoke an immune response. Quantitative increases in class II expression may play an important role in induction of immunologically mediated disease[75]. Furthermore, certain Ia antigens may have a better ability to associate with a given antigen[76] in such a way that they initiate the highest response from T-helper cells. Certain as yet unidentified alleles of the MHC locus in man in linkage disequilibrium with the HLA-DR3/4 tissue types may associate with an invading antigen and/or $\beta$-cell autoantigen-presenting cell in such a way that an immune response to an otherwise tolerated $\beta$-cell antigen is induced. That the class II antigens in fact play a very important role in the generation of autoimmunity is indicated by the observations that a mutation in mouse class II antigen determinant can change a susceptible mouse strain into an experimental autoimmune Myasthenia Gravis resistant strain[77]. Furthermore, monoclonal antibodies to class II antigens were shown to prevent experimentally induced autoimmunity in animals[78,79], an approach which recently was used to prevent diabetes in db/db mice[80].

Theories have been put forward to suggest that endocrine autoimmunity may be initiated by an aberrant expression of MHC class II antigens on endocrine cells, which then act as antigen-presenting cells for their own surface antigens[81]. However, the prospective studies of pancreas of the BB-rat indicate that Ia antigen expression on $\beta$-cells is a late event in the destruction process[65]. Whether Ia expression in islets is an initiating factor for an autoimmune reaction against $\beta$-cells or whether such expression is instrumental for maintaining a chronic antigen expression and inflammation in the islets is a matter for debate.

## POSSIBLE MECHANISMS OF AUTOIMMUNE ß-CELL DESTRUCTION

Although the exact mechanisms involved in the pathogenesis of IDDM are not clear, it is possible to speculate as to the sequence of events that may lead to the onset of the disease. One can envisage that a key event leading to an immune reaction against the $\beta$-cell may be the acquisition of T-helper cells to viral or bacterial antigens (presented during an infection) that cross-react with a $\beta$-cell surface component (e.g. the $M_r$ 64000 antigen). However, other environmental factors may act to initiate the autoimmune $\beta$-cell destruction.

Events leading to the clinical onset of IDDM can be considered to progress in four phases. The first phase consists of a bodywide immune response to a virus or bacteria having antigenic epitopes that cross-react with a $\beta$-cell surface antigen. A sensitization of T-helper cells possessing receptors to the foreign agent results in the activation of B-lymphocytes and the secretion of antibodies that recognize the $\beta$-cell autoantigen. Thus, already at this stage, low levels of ICSA may be circulating. The viral infection also causes increased levels of $\gamma$-interferon and an increased expression of Ia antigens both on cells of the immune system and on vascular epithelium.

In the second phase the immune response is aimed at the $\beta$-cells in the pancreatic islets. Primary damage to the $\beta$-cells takes place either by interaction of antibody (ICSA) with complement or killer cells or by the action of cytotoxic T-cells. At present there is no experimental evidence to implicate a role for cytotoxic T-cells in the pathogenesis of IDDM, whereas the cytotoxic effect of ICSA and complement is well documented[34-36]. Recent data indicate that the lymphokine interleukin 1, a T-cell growth factor that is released by macrophages, has a cytotoxic effect on islet cells at low concentrations[82]. This effect may enhance the damage of $\beta$-cells. $\beta$-cell specific cell surface antigens in association with Ia antigens are presented locally on vascular endothelium and/or incoming macrophages and cross-reacting T-helper cells home to the pancreas resulting in an enhanced immune response to the autoantigen. There is an increase in ICSA in the circulation and an infiltration of lymphocytes forming an insulitis can be detected. $\beta$-cells may express Ia antigens. The persistent reactivation of a $\beta$-cell specific immune response occurs and the $\beta$-cell killing reaches levels where the release of cytoplasmic components is extensive.

In the third phase there is a secondary immune response to the islet cell cytoplasmic components that are released and ICCA appear in the circulation. A polyclonal T- and B-lymphocyte response may follow the presentation of cytoplasmic antigens on vascular endothelium and/or macrophages or be a non-specific result of the viral or bacterial infection. Continuous non-specific secondary inflammation takes place.

The final phase can develop after several renewals of the environmental assault that occur during the first phase or after a slow acting, but persistent destruction of $\beta$-cells following the first assault. $\beta$-cell death reaches a limit at which the remaining $\beta$-cell mass can no longer meet the insulin requirements of the body and the clinical symptoms of diabetes appear.

It can be speculated that the magnitude and control of the immune response is regulated by genetically determined factors such that only in susceptible individuals does the autoimmune reaction progress to an extent where IDDM appears. In resistant individuals the reaction may never proceed past the first phase.

## PREVENTION OF IDDM

### Identification of genetically susceptible individuals

Molecular cloning of the genes from the class II region in man may eventually yield the structure of determinants which confer IDDM susceptibility. The use of genetic markers for such susceptibility factors will enable the identification of individuals at risk. A simple assay to measure circulating levels of autoantibodies to a $\beta$-cell autoantigen can then be used to detect a primary aberrant immune reaction to $\beta$-cells at an early stage where $\beta$-cell loss is minimal and specific intervention may still be feasible.

### Immune intervention to prevent destruction of ß-cells

In the BB-rat several ways of manipulating the immune system can decrease or prevent the incidence of IDDM[64]. In deciding strategies for immune therapies in man one must bear in mind that an aberrant immune reaction to $\beta$-cells may be a transient phenomenon which can be regulated by the individual himself before a major loss of $\beta$-cells resulting in IDDM has occurred. Furthermore, since insulin is established as a therapy for IDDM, any attempts at preventing the disease must provide a quality of life and life expectancy that exceeds that for this treatment; preventative methods that involve detrimental side-effects are not acceptable. Therefore specific methods are required that eliminate the aberrant immune response to $\beta$-cells without generally depressing the immune system, with unforeseen side-effects.

In other autoimmune diseases where the autoantigen is known and obtainable in large quantities, ways of specifically generating tolerance to an autoantigen and preventing detrimental autoimmune response have already been successfully employed in animal models[83-88]. Once $\beta$-cell autoantigen(s) involved in the pathogenesis of IDDM have been identified and purified in sufficient quantities, similar trials can begin to develop a specific therapy for the prevention of the disease in susceptible individuals.

## References

1. Gepts, W. and LeCompte, P. M. (1981). The pancreatic islets in diabetes. *Am. J. Med.*, **70**, 105–15

2. Gepts, W. (1965). Pathologic anatomy of the pancreas in juvenile diabetes mellitus. *Diabetes*, **14**, 619–33

3. Gepts, W. and De Mey, J. (1978). Islet cell survival determined by morphology. *Diabetes*, **27** (Suppl. 1), 251–61

4. Foulis, A. K. and Stewart, J. A. (1984). The pancreas in recent-onset Type I (insulin dependent) diabetes mellitus: insulin content of islets, insulitis and associated changes in the exocrine acinar tissue. *Diabetologia*, **26**, 456–61

5. Nerup, J., Andersen, O. O., Bendixen, G., Egeberg, J. and Poulsen, J. E. (1973). Anti-pancreatic cellular hypersensitivity in diabetes mellitus. Antigenic activity of fetal calf pancreas and correlation with clinical type of diabetes. *Acta Allergologica*, **28**, 223–30

6. Herold, K. C., Huen, A. H.-J., Rubenstein, A. H. and Lernmark, Å. (1984). Humoral abnormalities in type I (insulin-dependent) diabetes mellitus. In Andreani, D., Di Mario, U., Federlin, K. F. and Heding, L. G. (eds.) *Immunology in Diabetes*. pp. 105–20. (London: Kimpton Medical Publications)

7. Nerup, J. and Lernmark, Å. (1981). Autoimmunity in diabetes mellitus. *Am. J. Med.*, **70**, 135–41

8. Gorsuch, A. N., Spencer, K. M., Lister, J., McNally, J. M., Dean, B. M., Bottazzo, G. F. and Cudworth, A. G. (1981). The natural history of Type I (insulin-dependent) diabetes mellitus: evidence for a long prediabetic period. *Lancet*, **2**, 1363–5

9. Gorsuch, A. N., Spencer, K. M., Lister, J., Wolf, E., Bottazzo, G. F. and Cudworth, A. G. (1982). Can future Type I diabetes be predicted? *Diabetes*, **31**, 862–6

10. Irvine, W. J., Gray, R. S. and Steel, J. M. (1980). Islet cell antibody as a marker for early stage Type I diabetes mellitus. In Irvine, W. J. (ed.) *Immunology of Diabetes*. pp. 117–54. (Edinburgh: Teviot Scientific Publications)

11. Srikanta, S., Ganda, O. P., Eisenbarth, G. S. and Saeldner, J. S. (1983). Islet cell antibodies and beta cell function in monozygotic triplets and twins initially discordant for Type I diabetes mellitus. *N. Engl. J. Med.*, **308**, 322–5

12. Platz, P., Jakobsen, B. K., Morling, M., Ryder, L. P., Svejgaard, A., Thomsen, M., Christy, M., Kromann, H., Benn, J., Nerup, J., Green, A. and Hauge, M. (1981). HLA-D and DR-antigens in genetic analysis of insulin-dependent diabetes mellitus. *Diabetologia*, **21**, 108–15

13. Cudworth, A. G. and Wolf, E. (1982). The genetic susceptibility to Type I (insulin-dependent) diabetes mellitus. *Clin. Endocrinol. Metab.*, **11**, 389–408

14. Marner, B., Knutson, C., Lernmark, Å., Nerup, J. and the Hagedorn Study Group (1984). Immunological investigations: islet cell antibodies. In Larner, J. L. and Pohl, S. L. (eds.) *Methods in Diabetes Research.* Vol. 1, pp. 181–94. (New York: John Wiley & Sons)

15. Dobersen, M. J. (1984). A $^{51}$Cr release microcytotoxicity assay for islet cell surface antibodies. In Larner, J. L. and Pohl, S. L. (eds.) *Methods in Diabetes Research.* Vol. 1, pp. 123–7. (New York: John Wiley & Sons)

16. Baekkeskov, S. (1984). Radiolabelling and immunoprecipitation of islet cell antigens. In Larner, J. L. and Pohl, S. L. (eds.) *Methods in Diabetes Research*, Vol. 1, pp. 129–40. (New York: John Wiley & Sons)

17. Bottazzo, G. F., Florin-Christensen, A. and Doniach, D. (1974). Islet cell antibodies in

diabetes mellitus with autoimmune polyendocrine deficiencies. *Lancet*, **2**, 1279–82

18. MacCuish, A. C., Irvine, W. J., Baines, E. W. and Duncan, L. J. (1974). Antibodies to pancreatic islet cells in insulin-dependent diabetics with coexistent autoimmune disease. *Lancet*, **2**, 1529–31

19. Del Prete, G. F., Betterle, C. and Padovan, D. (1977). Incidence of islet-cell autoantibodies in different types of diabetes mellitus. *Diabetes*, **26**, 909–15

20. Lendrum, R., Walker, G., Cudworth, A. G., Theophanides, C., Pyke, D. A., Bloom, A. J. and Gamble, D. R. (1976). Islet cell antibodies in diabetes mellitus. *Lancet*, **2**, 1273–6

21. Notsu, K., Oka, N., Note, S., Nabeya, N., Kuno, S. and Sakurami, T. (1985). Islet cell antibodies in the Japanese population and subjects with Type 1 (insulin-dependent) diabetes. *Diabetologia*, **28**, 660–2

22. Irvine, W. J., McCallum, C. J., Gray, R. S., Campbell, G. J., Duncan, L. J. P., Farquhar, J. W., Vaughan, H. and Morris, P. J. (1977). Pancreatic islet cell antibodies in diabetes mellitus correlated with the duration and type of diabetes, coexistent autoimmune disease and HLA-type. *Diabetes*, **26**, 138–47

23. Bottazzo, G. F., Mann, J. I., Thorogood, M., Baum, J. D. and Doniach, D. (1978). Autoimmunity in juvenile diabetes and their families. *Br. Med. J.*, **1**, 165–8

24. Srikanta, S., Ganda, O. P., Jackson, R. A., Gleason, R. E., Kaldany, A., Garovoy, M. R., Milford, E. L., Carpenter, C. B., Soeldner, J. S. and Eisenbarth, G. S. (1983). Type I diabetes mellitus in monozygotic twins: chronic progressive beta cell dysfunction. *Ann. Int. Med.*, **99**, 320–7

25. Marner, B., Agner, T., Binder, C., Lernmark, Å., Nerup, J., Mandrup-Poulsen, T. and Walldorff, S. (1985). Increased reduction in fasting C-peptide is associated with islet cell antibodies in Type 1 (insulin-dependent) diabetic patients. *Diabetologia*, **28**, 875–80

26. Bottazzo, G. F. and Gleichmann, H. (1986). Immunology and diabetes workshops. Report of the first international Workshop on standardisation of cytoplasmic islet cell antibodies. *Diabetologia*, **29**, (In press)

27. Lernmark, Å., Freedman, Z. R., Hofmann, C., Rubenstein, A. H., Steiner, D. F., Jackson, R. L., Winter, R. J. and Traisman, H. S. (1978). Islet cell surface antibodies in juvenile diabetes mellitus. *N. Engl. J. Med.*, **299**, 375–80

28. MacLaren, N. K., Huang, S-W. and Fogh, J. (1975). Antibody to cultured human insulinoma cells in insulin-dependent diabetes. *Lancet*, **1**, 997–1000

29. Lernmark, Å., Hagglof, B., Freedman, Z. R., Irvine, W. J., Ludvigsson, J. and Holmgren, G. (1981). A prospective analysis of antibodies reactive with pancreatic islet cells in insulin-dependent diabetic children. *Diabetologia*, **20**, 471–4

30. Van de Winkel, M., Smets, G., Gepts, W. and Pipeleers, D. G. (1982). Islet cell surface antibodies from insulin-dependent diabetics bind specifically to pancreatic $\beta$-cells. *J. Clin. Invest.*, **70**, 41–79

31. Pujol-Borrell, R., Khoury, E. L. and Bottazzo, G. F. (1982). Islet cell surface antibodies in Type I (insulin-dependent) diabetes mellitus: use of human fetal pancreas cultures as substrate. *Diabetologia*, **22**, 89–95

32. Lernmark, Å. and Baekkeskov, S. (1981). Islet cell antibodies – theoretical and practical implications. *Diabetologia*, **21**, 431–5

33. Huen, A. H-J., Haneda, M., Freedman, Z., Lernmark, Å. and Rubenstein, A. H. (1983). Quantitative determination of islet cell surface antibodies using $^{125}$I-protein A. *Diabetes*, **32**, 460–5

34. Dobersen, M. J., Scharff, J. E., Ginsberg-Fellner, F. and Notkins, A. L. (1980). Cytotoxic autoantibodies to beta-cells in the serum of patients with insulin-dependent diabetes mellitus. *N. Engl. J. Med.*, **303**, 1493–8

35. Toguchi, Y., Ginsberg-Fellner, F. and Rubinstein, P. (1985). Cytotoxic islet cell surface antibodies (ICSA) in patients with Type I diabetes and their first-degree relatives. *Diabetes*, **34**, 855–60

36. Rittenhouse, H. G., Oxender, D. L., Pek, S. and Ar, D. (1980). Complement-mediated cytotoxic effects on pancreatic islets with sera from diabetic patients. *Diabetes*, **29**, 317–22

37. Dobersen, M. J. and Scharff, J. E. (1982). Preferential lysis of pancreatic $\beta$-cells by islet cell surface antibodies. *Diabetes*, **31**, 439–62

38. Kanatsuna, T., Baekkeskov, S., Lernmark, Å. and Ludvigsson, J. (1983). Immunoglobulin from insulin-dependent diabetic children inhibits glucose-induced insulin release. *Diabetes*,

**32**, 520-4

39. Svenningsen, A., Dyrberg, T., Gerling, I., Lernmark, Å., Mackay, P. and Rabinovitch, A. (1983). Inhibition of insulin release after passive transfer of immunoglobulin from insulin-dependent diabetic children to mice. *J. Clin. Endocrinol. Metab.*, **57**, 1301-4

40. Vialettes, B., Rousset, B. and Vague, Ph. (1983). Tubulin antibodies in recent onset Type I diabetes. *Diabetologia*, **25**, 202

41. Maron, R., Elias, D., Bartelt, M. de J., Bruining, G. J., van Rood, J. J., Shechter, Y. and Cohen, I. R. (1983). Autoantibodies to the insulin receptor in juvenile onset insulin-dependent diabetes. *Nature (London)*, **303**, 817-8

42. Huang, S. W. and MacLaren, N. K. (1978). Antibodies to nucleic acids in juvenile-onset diabetes. *Diabetes*, **27**, 1105-11

43. Huang, S. W., Hallquist-Haedt, L., Rich, S. and Barbosa, J. (1981). Prevalence of antibodies to nucleic acids in insulin-dependent diabetes and their relatives. *Diabetes*, **30**, 873-4

44. MacCuish, A. C. and Irvine, W. J. (1975). Autoimmunological aspects of diabetes mellitus. *Clin. Endocrinol. Metab.*, **4**, 435-71

45. Papadopoulos, G. K., Petersen, J., Andersen, V., Lernmark, Å., Marner, B., Nerup, J. and Binder, C. (1983). Spontaneous *in vitro* immunoglobulin secretion at the diagnosis of insulin-dependent diabetes. *Acta Endocrinologica*, **105**, 521-7

46. Baekkeskov, S., Nielsen, J. H., Marner, B., Bilde, T., Ludvigsson, J. and Lernmark, Å. (1982). Autoantibodies in newly diagnosed diabetic children immunoprecipitate human pancreatic islet cell proteins. *Nature (London)*, **298**, 167-9

47. Baekkeskov, S., Hansen, J., Bruining, G. J., Molenaar, J. L. and Lernmark, Å. (1985). Antibodies to a $M_r$ 64000 human islet cell antigen precede onset of IDDM in man. *Diabetes Res. Clin. Pract.*, Suppl. 1, 531

48. Baekkeskov, S., Kristensen, J. K., Srikanta, S., Bruining, G. J., Mandrup-Poulsen, T., de Beaufort, C., Soeldner, J. S., Eisenbarth, G., Lindgren, F. and Lernmark, Å. Antibodies to a $M_r$ 64000 human islet cell antigen precede the clinical onset of insulin dependent diabetes. (submitted for publication)

49. Baekkeskov, S. (1986). Immunoreactivity to a $M_r$ 64000 human islet cell antigen in sera from insulin dependent diabetes mellitus patients and individuals with abnormal glucose tolerance. *Molecular Biol. Med.* (In press)

50. Palmer, J. P., Clemons, P., Lyen, K., Tatpati, O., Raghu, P. K. and Paquette, T. L. (1983). Insulin antibodies in insulin-dependent diabetics before insulin treatment. *Science*, **222**, 1337-9

51. Arslanian, S. A., Becker, D. J., Rabin, B., Atchison, R., Eberhardt, M., Cavender, D., Dorman, J. and Drash, A. L. (1985). Correlates of insulin antibodies in newly diagnosed children with insulin-dependent diabetes before insulin therapy. *Diabetes*, **34**, 926-30

52. Trowsdale, J., Young, J. A. T., Kelly, A. P., Austin, P. J., Carson, S., Meunier, H., So, A., Erlich, H. A., Spielman, R. S., Bodmer, J. and Bodmer, W. F. (1985). Structure, sequence and polymorphism in the HLA-D region. In Moller, G. (ed.) *Immunological Reviews.* Vol. 85, pp. 5-43. (Copenhagen: Munksgaard)

53. Owerbach, D., Lernmark, Å., Platz, P., Ryder, L. P., Rask, L., Peterson, P. A. and Ludvigsson, J. (1983). HLA-D region β-chain DNA endonuclease fragments differ between HLA-DR identical healthy and insulin-dependent diabetic individuals. *Nature (London)*, **303**, 815-7

54. Owerbach, D. Hägglöf, B., Lernmark, Å. and Holmgren, G. (1984). Susceptibility to insulin-dependent diabetes defined by restriction enzyme polymorphism of HLA-D region genomic DNA. *Diabetes*, **33**, 958-65

55. Michelsen, B. (1985). Difference in restriction fragment length polymorphism between HLA-DR identical control and insulin-dependent diabetics is related to a HLA-DQ beta-chain gene. *Diabetes Res. Clin. Prac.*, Suppl. 1, 378

56. Barnett, A. H., Eff, C., Leslie, R. D. G. and Pyke, D. A. (1981). Diabetes in identical twins. *Diabetologia*, **20**, 87-93

57. Johnston, C., Pyke, D. A., Cudworth, A. G. and Wolf, E. (1983). HLA-DR typing in identical twins with insulin-dependent diabetes: difference between concordant and discordant pairs. *Br. Med. J.*, **286**, 253-5

58. Rubinstein, P., Walker, M. E., Fedun, N., Witt, M. E., Cooper, L. E. and Ginsberg-Fellner,

F. (1982). The HLA-system in congenital rubella patients with and without diabetes. *Diabetes*, **31**, 1088–91

59. Yoon, J. W., Austin, M., Onodera, T. and Notkins, A. L. (1979). Virus-induced diabetes mellitus: isolation of a virus from the pancreas of a child with diabetic ketoacidosis. *N. Engl. J. Med.*, **300**, 1173–9

60. Toniolo, A. and Onodera, T. (1984). Viruses and diabetes. In Andreani, D., Di Mario, U., Federlin, K. F. and Heding, L. G. (eds.) *Immunology in Diabetes*. pp. 71–93. (London: Kimpton Medical Publications)

61. Onodera, T., Toniolo, A., Ray, W. R., Jenson, A. B., Knazek, A. and Notkins, A. L. (1983). Virus induced diabetes mellitus. XX. Polyendocrinopathy and autoimmunity. *J. Exp. Med.*, **153**, 1457–73

62. Toniolo, A., Onodera, T., Yoon, J. W. and Notkins, A. L. (1980). Induction of diabetes by cumulative environmental insults from viruses and chemicals. *Nature (London)*, **288**, 383–5

63. Bottazzo, G. F., Dean, B. M., McNally, J. M., MacKay, E. H., Swift, P. G. F. and Gamble, D. R. (1985). *In situ* characterization of autoimmune phenomena and expression of HLA molecules in the pancreas in diabetic insulitis. *N. Eng. J. Med.*, **313**, 353–60

64. Marliss, E. B., Nakhooda, A. F., Poussier, P. and Sima, A. A. F. (1982). The diabetic syndrome of the 'BB' Wistar rat: possible relevance to Type I (insulin-dependent) diabetes in man. *Diabetologia*, **22**, 225–32

65. Dean, B. M., Walker, R., Bone, A. J., Baird, J. D. and Cooke, A. (1985). Pre-diabetes in the spontaneously diabetic BB/E rat: lymphocyte subpopulations in the pancreatic infiltrate and expression of rat MHC class II molecules in endocrine cells. *Diabetologia*, **28**, 464–6

66. Melchers, F. and Andersson, J. (1984). B-cell activation: three steps and their variations. *Cell*, **37**, 715–20

67. Unanue, E. R., Beller, D. I., Lu, C. Y. and Allen, P. M. (1984). Antigen presentation: comments on its regulation and mechanism. *J. Immunol.*, **132**, 1–5

68. Gammon, G., Dunn, K., Shastri, N., Oki, A., Wilbur, S. and Sercarz, E. E. (1986). Neonatal T-cell tolerance to minimal immunogenic peptides is caused by clonal inactivation. *Nature (London)*, **319**, 413–5

69. Prabhakar, B. S., Saegusa, J., Onodera, T. and Notkins, A. L. (1984). Lymphocytes capable of making monoclonal autoantibodies that react with multiple organs are a common feature of the normal B-cell repertoire. *J. Immunol.*, **133**, 2815–7

70. Esquivel, P. S., Rose, N. R. and Kong, Y. M. (1977). Induction of autoimmunity in good and poor responder mice with mouse thyroglobulin and lipopolysaccharide. *J. Exp. Med.*, **145**, 1250

71. Jerne, N. K. (1974). Towards a network theory of the immune system. *Ann. Immunol.*, *(Paris)*, **125**, 378–89

72. Shechter, Y., Maron, R., Elias, D. and Cohen, I. R. (1982). Autoantibodies to insulin receptor spontaneously develop as antiidiotypes in mice immunized with insulin. *Science*, **216**, 542–5

73. Lernmark, Å. (1984). Cell-mediated immunity in insulin-dependent (Type I) diabetes: Update 84. In Andreani, D., di Mario, U., Federlin, K. F. and Heding, L. G. (eds.) *Immunology in Diabetes*. pp. 121–31 (London Kimpton Medical)

74. Weiss, M., Ingbar, S. H., Winblad, S. and Kasper, D. L. (1983). Demonstration of a saturable binding site for thyrotropin in *Yersinia enterocolitica*. *Science*, **219**, 1331–3

75. Janeway, C. A., Bottomly, K., Babich, J., Conrad, P., Conzen, S., Jones, B., Kaye, J., Katz, M., McVay, L., Murphy, D. B. and Tite, J. (1984). Quantitative variation in Ia antigen expression plays a central role in immune regulation. *Immunology Today*, **5**, 99–105

76. Babbitt, B. P., Allen, P. M., Matsueda, G., Haber, E. and Unanue, E. R. (1985). Binding of immunogenic peptides to Ia histocompatibility molecules. *Nature (London)*, **317**, 359–61

77. Christadoss, P., Lindstrom, J. M., Melvold, R. W. and Talal, N. (1985). Mutation at I-A beta chain prevents experimental autoimmune Myasthenia Gravis. *Immunogenetics*, **21**, 33–8

78. Steinman, L., Rosenbaum, J. T., Sriram, S. and McDevitt, H. O. (1981). *In vivo* effects of antibodies to immune response gene products: prevention of experimental allergic encephalitis. *Proc. Natl. Acad. Sci. USA.*, **78**, 7111–4

79. Waldor, M. K., Sriram, S., McDevitt, H. O. and Steinman, L. (1983). *In vivo* therapy with

monoclonal anti-Ia antibody suppresses immune responses to acetylcholine receptor. *Proc. Natl. Acad. Sci. USA.*, **80**, 2713–7

80. Singh, B. and Cliffe, W. J. (1986). Treatment of diabetic (db/db) mice with anti-class II MHC monoclonal antibodies. *Ann. N. Y. Acad. Sci.* (In press)

81. Bottazzo, G. F., Pujol-Borrell, R., Hanafusa, T. and Feldmann, M. (1983). Role of aberrant HLA-DR expression and antigen presentation in induction of endocrine autoimmunity. *Lancet*, **1**, 1115–9

82. Mandrup-Poulsen, T., Bendtzen, K., Nerup, J., Dinarello, C. A., Svenson, M. and Nielsen, J. H. (1986). Affinity-purified human interleukin I is cytotoxic to isolated islets of Langerhans. *Diabetologia*, **29**, 63–7

83. Braley-Mullen, H., Tompson, J. G., Sharp, G. C. and Kyriakos, M. (1980). Suppression of experimental autoimmune thyroiditis in guinea pigs by pretreatment with thyroglobulin-coupled spleen cells. *Cell Immunol.*, **51**, 408–13

84. Schoen, R. T., Greene, M. I. and Trentham, D. E. (1982). Antigen-specific suppression of Type II collagen-induced arthritis by collagen-coupled spleen cells. *J. Immunol.*, **128**, 717–9

85. Hohlfeld, R., Toyka, K. V., Heininger, K., Grosse-Wilde, H. and Kalies, I. (1984). Autoimmune human T lymphocytes specific for acetylcholine receptor. *Nature (London)*, **310**, 244–6

86. Rennie, P., McGregor, A. M., Wright, J., Weetman, A. P. and Hall, R. (1983). An immunotoxin of a ricin chain conjugated to thyroglobulin selectively suppresses the antithyroglobulin autoantibody response. *Lancet*, **1**, 1338–40

87. Holoshitz, J., Frankel, A., Ben-Nun, A. and Cohen, I. R. (1983). Autoimmune encephalomyelitis (EAE) mediated and prevented by T lymphocyte lines directed against diverse antigenic determinants of myelin basic protein. Vaccination is determinant specific. *J. Immunol.*, **131**, 2810

88. Sriram, S., Schwartz, G. and Steinman, L. (1983). Administration of myelin basic protein-coupled spleen cells prevents experimental allergic encephalitis. *Cell Immunol.*, **75**, 378–82

# 5
# Insulin Antibodies

**A. KURTZ**

There are several reasons for the continuing interest in the immunological response to insulin. The insulin molecule has been extensively studied and its tertiary structure is fully documented; insulin is the most frequently injected highly purified polypeptide used in medicine, and it is readily available, as are species variants, chemically modified insulins and molecular fragments. Most research over the years has been concerned with the immunological response to injected insulin: usually the production of insulin-binding immunoglobulin G (IgG). The unravelling of the autoimmune nature of the pathology of Type I diabetes has created interest in the occurrence of spontaneous antibodies to insulin.

Insulin preparations have changed considerably over the years. Before the early 1970s insulin was usually prepared by recrystallization; gel chromatography separated these insulins into 'a', 'b' and 'c' components[1]. The 'a' component was high molecular weight material which, when isolated and tested in animals, produced antibodies which cross-reacted with insulin. The 'b' component was proinsulin and non-dissociable insulin dimer. The content of proinsulin was often 10000 parts/$10^6$ or more; both proinsulin and dimer were immunogenic and produced antibodies reacting with insulin. The 'c' component contained the insulin together with arginine insulin and insulins chemically modified during manufacture (desamido insulin and the ethyl ester). Recrystallized insulin preparations also contained glucagon (discovered as an impurity in insulin), pancreatic polypeptide, somatostatin and vasoactive intestinal polypeptide; all of which were immunogenic[2,3]. Purification procedures now include gel chromatography and ion exchange chromatography which allow production of insulin from animal pancreas of near 100% purity; small amounts of desamido insulin and dimers form on storage and may be detected in most insulin preparations[4]. Other pancreatic hormones are undetectable. Similar purification methods are used for insulins produced by recombinant DNA technology and such preparations are free of bacterial or yeast proteins.

Over the last decade there have been dramatic changes in insulin use in the United Kingdom; these changes are illustrated in Figures 5.1–3. The most striking changes have been the increase of the purity of insulins used, the reduction of usage of beef insulin with a change to pork and human insulins, and the increasing use of isophane insulin.

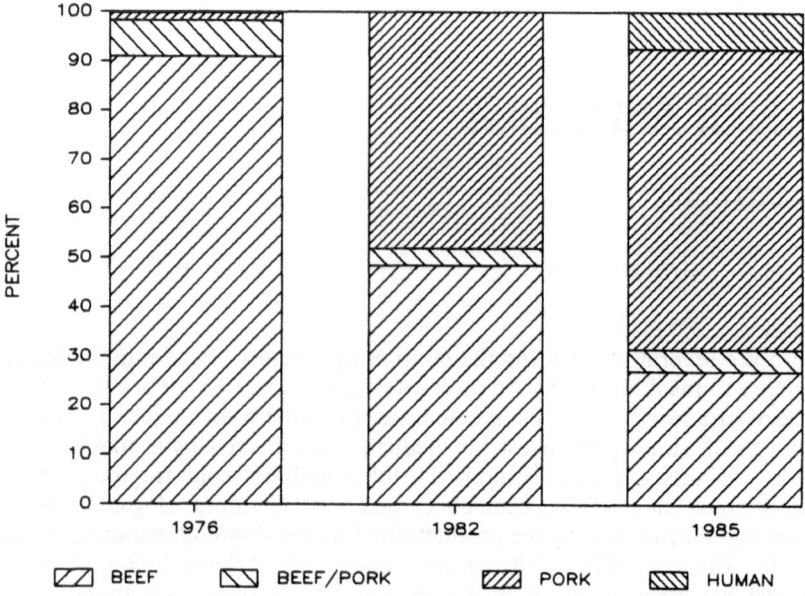

**Figure 5.1** Changes in insulin source

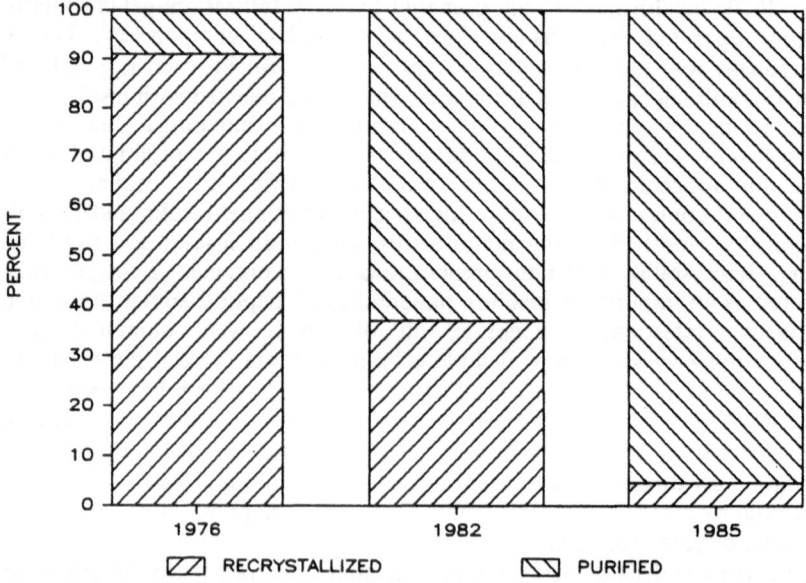

**Figure 5.2** Changes in insulin purity

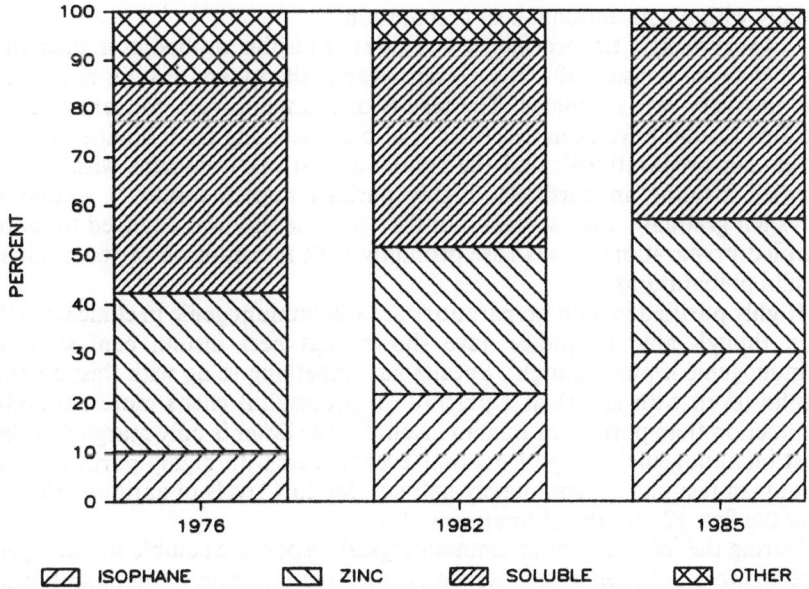

**Figure 5.3** Changes in type of insulin used

In the early years of insulin use observations were made of local and generalized allergic reactions and of resistance to insulin[5]. Insulin resistance caused by insulin neutralizing antibodies was first reported in 1938 in a patient undergoing insulin-shock treatment for a psychiatric disorder[6]. Antibody-mediated insulin resistance in an insulin-treated diabetic was first documented in 1942; a patient developed antibodies which, when tested in mice, neutralized beef/pork insulin but did not neutralize human insulin[7]. The general occurrence of insulin antibodies in insulin-treated patients (both diabetics and schizophrenics) was described in 1956[8]. Antibody-mediated insulin resistance was never common. A series of 29 patients was reported in 1967[9]; the presence of antibodies was confirmed by passive cutaneous anaphylaxis. Insulin requirements were high; all subjects needed more than 200 units/day, and 15 needed more than 500 units/day. Sixteen were treated with prednisone and all experienced dramatic and sustained reduction in insulin requirements. Currently insulin resistance related to insulin antibodies should be considered if the daily insulin dose exceeds 2 units/kg; confirmation of the diagnosis rests now on finding a high level of insulin binding by serum using radiolabelled insulin and one of several different separation techniques[10]. Good concordance for assays of this general type has been reported[11]. Insulin-antibody assays can easily show whether one type of insulin is less avidly bound than another[12-14]; sensitivity may well be shown to a poorly bound insulin. Fish insulin, sulphated insulin, desalanated pork and beef insulins, highly purified pork insulin and recently 'human' insulin have all been considered in this context. Most patients who have developed insulin resistance have been Type II diabetics treated intermittently with insulin, usually with a conventional beef preparation[15]

Not surprisingly the prevalence and titres of insulin antibodies in diabetics have changed considerably over recent years. Allergy and insulin resistance are now very rare problems. The results of changing from conventional to purified insulin have been described[15]; also of changing from bovine to pork or human preparations[3]; and the results of starting treatment with highly purified insulins, in particular highly purified human insulin[16]. Antibody titres fell gradually over several months when therapy was changed to more purified preparations; titres rose promptly with reinstitution of the original insulin preparations.

Highly purified insulin preparations are still immunogenic in clinical use[15], even though animal studies have shown that beef insulin can be non-immunogenic if pure enough[4]. Species has something to do with this; bovine insulin (even with less than 1 part/$10^6$ of proinsulin) elicits more antibody production than porcine or human insulin[17]. The latter is only marginally the least immunogenic[16]. In patients only ever treated with highly purified pork or human insulins approximately half develop low levels of antibody slowly over the first 12 months of treatment.

During the initiation of an immunological response a soluble immunogen is recognized as 'foreign' and 'served up' to T-lymphocytes by an immunogen presenting cell. The site recognized is the carrier determinant, an area on the molecule which renders it immunogenic and which may well be different to the epitope or haptenic determinant to which the antibody binds[18]. With the availability of high purity insulins, studies of the carrier determinants involved in eliciting immunological responses became feasible; impure preparations clearly contained multiple immunogens. Using insulins of different species and various fragments of insulins, studies in mice showed that recognition of carrier determinants was under the control of the immune response gene Ir (located within the H-2 region of the major histocompatability region on chromosome 17). Pork, beef, sheep and horse insulins gave quite different immunological responses in various inbred strains of mice[18].

Genetic factors also influence the antibody response to insulin in diabetics. Histocompatibility antigens and IgG heavy chain allotypes (Gm) are both associated with the magnitude of the response[15,19]. The B8 and DR3 haplotypes tend to be associated with low antibody titres; the DR4 haplotype with average titres; and the B15 and DR7 haplotypes with high titres. Gm xag is associated with high titres too. In general, antibody titres vary widely amongst diabetics reflecting the heterogeneity of their genetic make-up, ages and treatment regimens.

In beef and sheep insulins the amino acids in the A-chain at positions 8–10, and in the B-chain at position 30, are different from human insulin. Pork and human insulins have the same A-chain sequence. The A-chain loop is clearly a potential carrier determinant. In general, two or more carrier determinants are needed to trigger an immune response[18]. Animal studies would suggest that bovine insulin is likely to be a good immunogen in man, that porcine is likely to be a poor immunogen and that human insulin should be non-immunogenic; pork and human insulin differ only at B30 (alanine in pork and threonine in human insulin). However, the actual immunogen in insulin formulations is most probably modified insulin[4]; high molecular weight polymers which can form under conditions of storage or manufacture may be present in small amounts that are undetectable by chromatography or nephelometry. Denatured insulin can retain its ability to induce an immunological response but is no longer bound by immunoglobulin. Monomeric insulin of whatever species may be only a very weak immunogen requiring physicochemical alteration to produce carrier determinants; however, antibody binds to monomeric insulin. Insulin may also act as a hapten; in the immunological response to isophane insulin antibodies are formed, if they are formed at all, to both protamine and insulin[20]. A study of lymphocyte proliferation in diabetics showed that the initiating immunogen was much more specific than was the final insulin-antibody reaction[21]. T-cell responses are specific for primary amino acid sequences on the immunogen; the restricted nature of the T-cell recognition process needs emphasis.

The original contention of Berson and Yalow[22] was that insulin antibody and insulin interacted to produce a soluble non-precipitating complex which did not activate complement, and in which the reaction of each insulin molecule with antibody was independent of the reaction of other insulin and antibody molecules. The Law of Mass Action and the theoretical analysis proposed by Scatchard[23] were therefore appropriate and have been applied in many studies. It is worth noting that the technique of radioimmunoassay developed from these observations on insulin antibodies. Bound insulin is usually biologically available following dissociation from antibody. In the syndrome of antibody-mediated insulin resistance something different seems to happen. Circulating levels of insulin antibody are very high and it is impossible to achieve an effective concentration of free insulin; this is a paradox as it should be possible if enough insulin is given. Our studies suggest that large insulin-antibody complexes are formed by antibodies which recognize several distinct epitopes on the insulin molecule. Such complexes contain two or more antibody molecules and by virtue of their size are removed from the circulation by the reticuloendothelial system. The insulin is destroyed instead of dissociating back into the free insulin pool (Figure 5.4). Up to a certain point, increasing the insulin concentration results in increasingly stable complexes without an increase in the free insulin concentration. This phenomenon has been described in the radioimmunoassay literature as 'hooking' or co-operativity[24,25] and can be created in vitro with combinations of monoclonal antibodies which recognize independent epitopes. Figure 5.5 shows this phenomenon in serum from a patient with insulin resistance with a 'normal' response after the patient received a short course of prednisone. In a clinical study in the same patient infusions of insulin with measurement of the free and bound insulin concentrations in serum showed a similar phenomenon (Figure 5.6); the response after prednisone treatment was also 'normal'. In the guinea pig large insulin-antibody complexes have been demonstrated by ultracentrifugation[26]; the guinea pig is unusual in that it has quite a different insulin structure compared to other mammals and it therefore recognizes, immunologically, more epitopes on beef or pork insulin than does the average diabetic patient. For

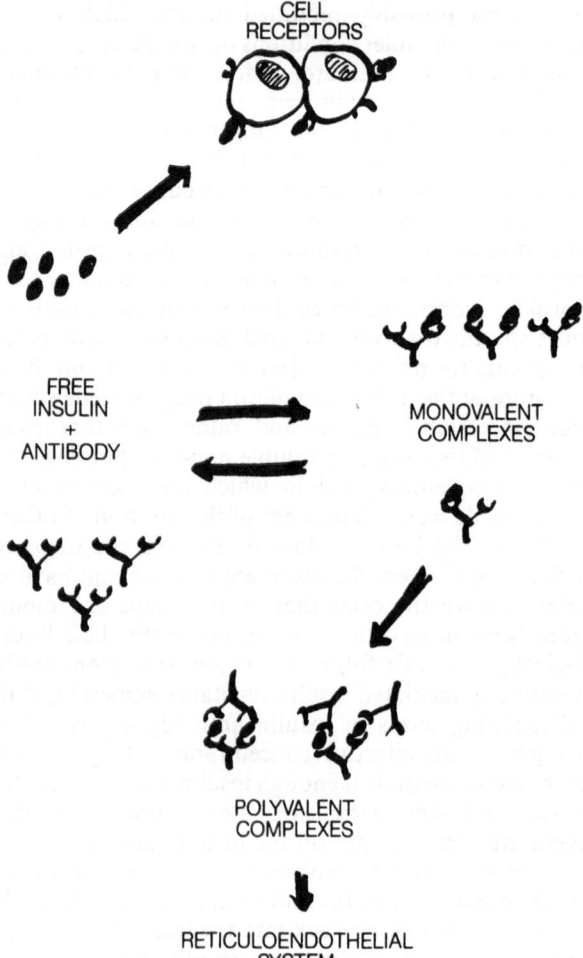

**Figure 5.4** Diagrammatic representation of the interaction of insulin and insulin antibody

the guinea pig the first 16 amino acids of the B-chain of bovine insulin contain all the immunogenic information in the whole molecule as judged by stimulation of T-cell proliferation and expression of T-cell helper activity. It is not surprising that guinea pigs have usually produced the best insulin antisera for radioimmunoassays.

Cross-reaction has been found invariably when antibodies resulting from insulin treatment have been tested with different insulin species[12,13]: by this I mean that binding, by an antiserum, of any species of labelled insulin can be entirely prevented by unlabelled insulin of any species. For a given antiserum the affinity constants can be quite different for different insulin species;

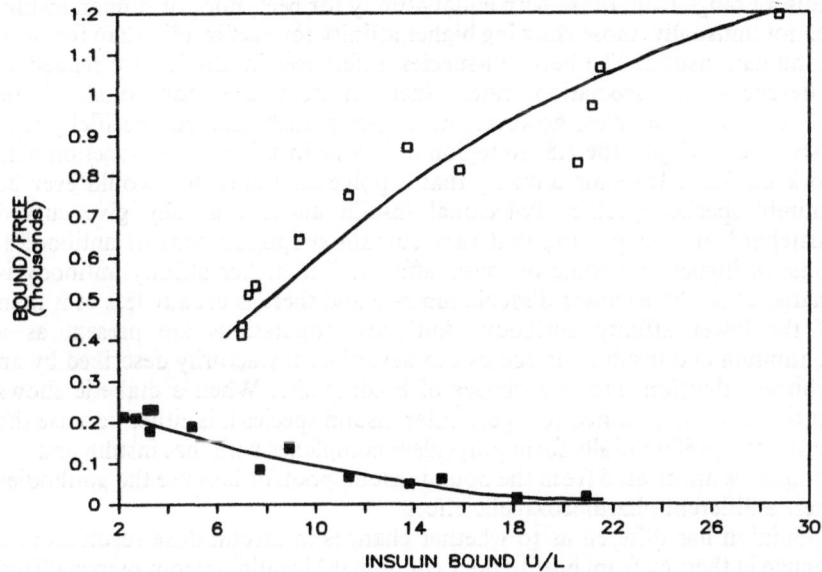

**Figure 5.5** Scatchard plot for serum from a patient with insulin resistance before prednisone treatment (□) after treatment (■). Serum dilution 4 μl/ml, assayed after acid dialysis to remove endogenous insulin. The initial rise in bound/free indicates 'cooperativity' or complex formation

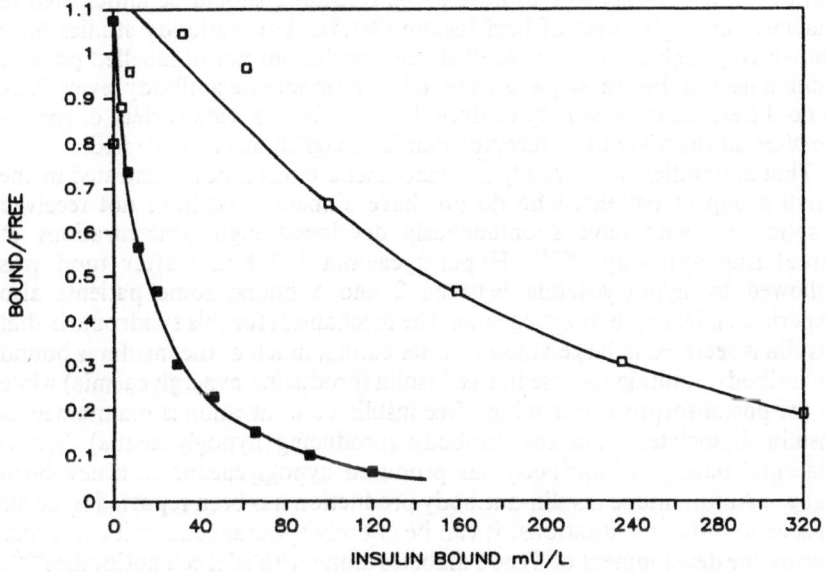

**Figure 5.6** *In vivo* 'Scatchard plot' before prednisone treatment (□) and after treatment (■). The bound and free insulin concentrations in serum were measured during an infusion of insulin. Note the increase in bound/free with increasing bound insulin which indicates 'cooperativity' or complex formation

antisera range from those with equal affinity for beef, pork or human insulin to, not unusually, those showing higher affinity for beef insulin than for pork or human insulin. The between-species differences in affinity are related to differences in association rate. Such antisera are polyclonal. Some monoclonal antibodies, however, have shown such marked specificity that they react with just the A8–10 region of bovine insulin with no reaction with pork insulin[27]. It seems unlikely that a polyclonal antibody would ever be entirely species specific. Polyclonal insulin antisera usually give curved Scatchard plots indicating that they contain subpopulations of antibodies, some of higher and some of lower affinity. The higher affinity antibody is characterized by a slower dissociation rate and there is usually less of it than of the lower affinity antibody. Antibody populations are present as a continuum and insulin antibodies can never be satisfactorily described by an arbitrary division into two classes of binding site. When a diabetic shows partial resistance limited to a particular insulin species it is either because the antibodies preferentially form polyvalent complexes with that insulin and the complexes are cleared from the bound insulin pool, or because the antibodies exert a different pharmacokinetic effect.

Opinion has differed as to whether changes in insulin dose result from a change in therapy from beef to pork (or human) insulin or from recrystallized to purified insulin[5,15]; low levels of insulin antibodies, forming monovalent complexes, probably have no effect on insulin clearance or dose. A few patients have shown partial resistance to beef insulin and, when given pork insulin, have experienced hypoglycaemia and have needed a reduced dose of pork insulin[14,28]. This type of differential resistance should be anticipated in diabetics on high doses of beef insulin ($>1.5\,U/kg$); antibody studies have shown very high binding of labelled beef insulin but not of labelled pork or human insulin. For those patients with low or moderate antibody levels there is no difference in sensitivity or dose. Insulins from a wide variety of species do after all show identical receptor binding (hagfish insulin excepted).

That antibodies can have a 'pharmacokinetic' effect is best illustrated by the small group of patients who do not have diabetes, and have not received insulin, but who have spontaneously developed high concentrations of circulating antibody[17,28–31]. Hyperglycaemia 1–2 hours after food was followed by hypoglycaemia between 2 and 5 hours; some patients also experienced fasting hypoglycaemia. The mechanism for this syndrome is that insulin is secreted in large amounts after eating; much of the insulin is bound to antibody, limiting the rise in free insulin (producing hyperglycaemia) while in the postabsorptive state a high free insulin concentration is maintained as insulin dissociates from the antibody (producing hypoglycaemia). Transplacental passage of antibody has produced hypoglycaemia in a new-born baby[32]. Autoimmune insulin-antibody production has been reported to occur in several different situations. It can be entirely spontaneous or it can occur during the development of Type I diabetes along with islet cell antibodies[33,34]. Insulin antibodies have been reported to develop in mice when viral infection leads to diabetes[35]. Immunosuppression blocks both the production of the antibody and the development of diabetes. Drugs have been associated with the production of autoimmune insulin antibodies; they include methimazole[30], penicillamine[36] and procainamide plus hydralazine[37]. Methimazole and penicillamine both have thiol groups which can interact with thiol groups in proteins; penicillamine, procainamide and hydralazine are all associated with a wide range of autoimmune disorders.

Clinical 'pharmacokinetic' effects have also been reported, if somewhat rarely, in insulin-treated patients. Delayed severe hypoglycaemia occurred in a patient with a very high antibody level; insulin antibody complexes stored large amounts of insulin which was released over many days[38]. In a study in which antibodies were indirectly assessed by determination of the circulating half-life of radioactively labelled insulin, treatment regimens did correlate with the half-life[39]: subjects with long 'half-lives', i.e. slow clearance of insulin from the large pool of bound insulin in the circulation, often managed on one injection of soluble insulin daily. Those with short 'half-lives' required more frequent injections or longer acting insulin (or both). Currently, insulin antibodies seldom cause clinical problems; in the past problems and effects were more frequently seen when antibody titres were in general much higher. Large amounts of insulin may frequently be 'stored' in the circulation by antibodies; bound insulin concentrations ranged up to 20 U/l in a group of 'ordinary' diabetics[40]. This store of insulin can exceed that at subcutaneous depots. Insulin antibody can act as a buffer[41]; this can be beneficial if other sources of insulin fail, or a nuisance if intended pulses of insulin are absorbed. The former effect was shown in a study in which insulin was given intravenously (i.e. subcutaneous depots were depleted) and the infusion then stopped[40]. Free insulin concentrations remained steady and deterioration of diabetic control was prevented for up to 12 hours in subjects with moderately high antibody titres. 'Blunting' of free insulin peaks has seldom been specifically demonstrated. Insulin is absorbed all too slowly from subcutaneous injection sites and the effect of antibody binding on the size and timing of the free insulin peak following insulin injection is clinically inapparent. In other words, absorption is the rate-limiting step and it predominates over the buffering effect, which might be apparent clinically if insulin pulses were given intravenously[28]. By trial and error most patients achieve a measure of diabetic control in such a way that many variables are consciously or unconsciously taken into account. An effect of antibody is just one factor; diet, exercise, insulin dose, type of insulin, site of injection, variability of absorption, precision of dosage, etc. are others. The use of highly purified insulins over recent years has certainly markedly reduced insulin antibody levels in most diabetics and has reduced the incidence of the 'genuine' immunological problems: insulin resistance, cutaneous reactions (either of the urticarial IgE mediated type or the delayed IgG mediated type), lipoatrophy and anaphylaxis. Insulin antibodies have been put forward as possible candidates in the causation of microvascular and macrovascular complications of diabetes. The fact that diabetics untreated with insulin are prone to these complications suggests that a contribution of antibody, or of antibody-bound insulin, to the development of complications is unlikely to be major. Several studies have exonerated insulin antibodies from an association with microvascular complications[5].

In several areas methodology requires comment. One of the undoubted but unmentioned effects of insulin antibody is interference with measurements of insulin by radioimmunoassay which has led to the relatively primitive understanding we have of insulin pharmacokinetics. Assays for free insulin are used but are of uncertain validity as there is no theoretically and technically sound method which can produce accurate results that would allow the preparation of standards and the validation of 'routine' methods. Several different methods have been proposed for free insulin assay[42-45]. The simplest is:

(1)  rapid separation of plasma after venesection;
(2)  rapid separation of free insulin from the antibody-bound insulin by precipitating the immunoglobulin with polyethylene glycol;
(3)  storage of the sample at $-20°C$;
(4)  radioimmunoassay.

Problems are introduced if serum is fractionated after storage (frozen), when erroneous and variable elevation of free insulin occurs; or if ethanol is used to separate bound from free insulin, when the free insulin results are very much higher than with other methods. Another method is to use steady-state gel filtration to remove the high molecular weight fraction (i.e. the antibody-bound insulin) from the low molecular weight fraction (i.e. insulin)[46]. The results obtained by the best methods are physiologically sensible in that most free insulin values are in the range 5–25 mU/l for random samples from insulin-dependent diabetics; free insulin concentrations are independent of the antibody titre or the total insulin concentration.

Measurement of total (mainly bound) insulin is technically satisfactory[44], but the results, for a group of patients, simply reflect the wide range of antibody levels in different diabetics. A difference between determinations of free and total insulin concentrations indicates the presence of insulin antibodies. Direct methods for the determination of insulin antibody fall into two main groups, solid phase methods and the traditional liquid phase 'radioimmunoassay' in which [125]iodine-labelled insulin is incubated with serum, and the bound and free moieties subsequently separated by one method or another[3,8,10]. Different methods can give comparable results[11] and all are sensitive enough to detect antibody if the total insulin exceeds the free insulin, i.e. quite sensitive enough for any clinical purpose. Of this group of methods the most specific includes a second antibody separation step. The material actually measured is IgG immunoglobulin, because it is specifically precipated by an anti-human IgG antiserum, and as it binds insulin it can only be anti-insulin antibody (IgG). Less specific separation methods (e.g. electrophoresis, charcoal or polyethylene glycol) actually give similar results which provides a large measure of validation for the methods in general. Argument has raged over whether insulin should be stripped from serum before antibody determination[10]. This is usually done with acidification to break the insulin-antibody bond followed by charcoal treatment to remove the insulin by adsorption; dialysis at low pH is an alternative. The effect of this procedure is to increase the apparent antibody level in sera with high, and otherwise easily measurable levels. With lower antibody levels there is not much difference and it should not be forgotten that the procedure may destroy some antibody. Consideration of the Law of Mass Action, ($K_d$ = [I*AB]/[I] [AB], where I = free insulin, AB = free antibody, and I*AB = insulin-antibody complex), leads to the conclusion that the majority of insulin-binding sites in the circulation are unoccupied. High affinity binding sites are relatively more occupied than low affinity sites. At a free insulin concentration of $10 \, mU/1$ ($6.7 \times 10^{-11} \, mol/1$) 50% binding site occupancy would indicate an average dissociation constant of $1.5 \times 10^{10} \, 1/mol$ and in practice the affinity is lower than this. Reported dissociation constants range from $10^{10} \, 1/mol$ for higher affinity sites to $10^7 \, 1/mol$ for the lower affinity component. In a system in which antibodies with differing affinities coexist equilibrium may only be reached slowly. Berson and Yalow described the gradual transfer of the insulin from low affinity to high affinity antibody[22]. This occurs because both high and low affinity antibody react with insulin at the same rate but the dissociation rates are markedly different.

With very low antibody levels or with absent antibody misclassification of samples is not unknown[10,11]. Non-immune sera do give non-specific responses in all assays. Clearly in the best assays the non-specific response is small in comparison to the specific response obtained with immune sera (i.e. there is a high signal-to-noise ratio). Defining the non-immune response is not simple as it is distributed logarithmically; errors are introduced if the 'cut-off' point is incorrectly chosen. In a diabetic population antibody titres (expressed as percent ligand bound) are not distributed normally; the distribution is skewed and may be approximately normalized by logarithmic transformation. An advantage of liquid phase methodology is that analysis of data using Scatchard plots or variants thereof, are possible and theoretically sound. Disadvantages are that the assays are relatively slow, that radioactive material is used and that the detection limit for antibody is limited both by the average affinity constant of the antibody and by the relatively low specific activity of radioactively labelled ligands (by comparison with enzyme, chemiluminescent or fluorescent labels). Alternative methods are now entering the arena. Solid phase methods are appropriate for specific detection of antibody but there are pitfalls. Enzyme-linked immunosorbent assays (ELISA) have been used[47].

(1)   A plastic well is coated with a monolayer of insulin;
(2)   Diluted serum is then put in the well and the insulin antibody binds to the insulin monolayer;
(3)   All other serum constituents are then washed away;
(4)   Finally the antibody is detected using an enzyme-labelled anti-human IgG.

Although this sounds very 'specific' it is very difficult to ensure that IgG is not non-specifically bound to the plastic surface or that IgG directed to IgG (e.g. rheumatoid factor) is not interfering. In other words the principal danger is of false-positive detection of insulin antibody. In insulin allergy specific IgE can be detected using the Radioallergosorbent Test RAST[48]. Insulin immobilized on a solid phase binds antibody (IgG, IgM, etc.) and bound IgE is specifically detected with radiolabelled anti-IgE. As with the ELISA technique cross-reaction can only be assessed indirectly[49]. To do this, serum samples are incubated with different species of insulin before the test is carried out, and cross-reaction assessed by determining the extent to which blocking of the test response occurs. The advantages of solid phase methods are assay speed, avoidance of radioactivity and theoretically unlimited sensitivity. Similar methodology can also be used to detect IgM or IgE antibodies. Solid phase methods are not suitable for Scatchard type analysis, for cross-reaction studies, except in an indirect fashion, or for measurement of affinity constants. Dissociation rates can be determined. These constraints can make validation rather difficult. Whatever method of antibody determination is used the units used for reporting results remain a problem; no true unit exists. Percent bound, bound/free, optical density, counts per minute and 'mU'/l are not interconvertible.

Attention has been focused on the occurrence of spontaneous insulin antibodies at or before the presentation of clinical diabetes. The natural history of Type I diabetes makes it clear that important autoimmune phenomena happen well in advance of clinical disease; insulin antibodies do occur in this context. Insulin antibodies may be another marker of incipient Type I diabetes in addition to islet cell antibodies. Hormonal immunogens might be proinsulin, C-peptide or insulin; the human sequences for C-peptide and proinsulin are very different from those in the pork and beef polypeptides so that the finding of antibodies to the human sequences would be clear evidence of autoimmunity. The differences in insulin sequence are small and cross-reaction with the animal insulins is to be expected even with an autoimmune immunogenic response. An autoantibody might show higher affinity for human than for pork insulin; for that to happen the major haptenic determinant recognized by the antibody would be the B30 threonine. The most common epitopes[50] are A4, A18–A19, B3 and B30. There will inevitably be doubts expressed that exogenous insulin was involved as has been the case with patients with the spontaneous insulin antibody syndrome[17]; however, autoimmune antibodies are here to stay.

## References

1. Schlichtkrull, J., Brange, J., Christiansen, Aa. H., Hallund, O., Heding, L. G. and Jorgensen, K. H. (1972). Clinical aspects of insulin – antigenicity. *Diabetes*, Suppl. 2, 649–56
2. Bloom, S. R., West, A. M., Polak, J. M., Barnes, A. J. and Adrian, T. E. (1978). Hormonal contaminants of insulin. In Bloom, S. R. and Grossman, M. I. (eds.) *Gut Hormones*. pp. 318–22. (Edinburgh: Churchill Livingstone)
3. Kurtz, A. B., Matthews, J. A., Mustaffa, B. E., Daggett, P. R. and Nabarro, J. D. N. (1980). Decrease of antibodies to insulin, proinsulin and contaminating hormones after changing treatment from conventional beef to purified pork insulin. *Diabetologia*, **18**, 147–50
4. Hansen, B., Hoiriis Nielsen, J. and Welinder, B. (1981). Immunogenicity of insulin in relation to its physicochemical properties. In Keck, K. and Erb, P. (eds.) *Basic and Clinical Aspects of Immunity to Insulin*. pp. 335–52. (Berlin: de Gruyter)
5. Kurtz, A. B. and Nabarro, J. D. N. (1980). Circulating insulin-binding antibodies. *Diabetologia*, **19**, 329–34
6. Banting, F. G., Franks, W. R. and Gairns, S. (1938). Anti-insulin activity of serum of insulin-treated patient. *Am. J. Psych.*, **95**, 562–5
7. Lowell, F. C. (1944). Immunologic studies in insulin resistance. II. The presence of a

neutralizing factor in blood exhibiting some characteristics of an antibody. *J. Clin. Invest.*, **23**, 233–40

8. Berson, S. A., Yalow, R. S., Bauman, A., Rothschild, M. A. and Newerly, K. (1956). Insulin [131]I metabolism in human subjects. Demonstration of insulin binding globulin in circulation of insulin treated subjects. *J. Clin. Invest.*, **35**, 170–90

9. Oakley, W. G., Jones, V. E. and Cunliffe, A. C. (1967). Insulin resistance. *Br. Med. J.*, **2**, 134–8

10. Reeves, W. G. (1983). Insulin antibody determination: theoretical and practical considerations. *Diabetologia*, **24**, 399–403

11. Kurtz, A. B., Reeves, W. G., Smith, W. C. and Spradlin, C. T. (1984). Inter-laboratory insulin antibody workshop: a report of a collaborative study in Europe and the United States. *Diabetologia*, **27**, 300A

12. Berson, S. A. and Yalow, R. S. (1959). Species-specificity of human anti-beef, pork insulin serum. *J. Clin. Invest.*, **38**, 2017–25

13. Kurtz, A. B., Matthews, J. A. and Nabarro, J. D. N. (1978). Insulin-binding antibody: reaction differences with bovine and porcine insulins. *Diabetologia*, **15**, 19–22

14. Devlin, J. G. and Brien, T. G. (1965). Relationship between differential antibody binding capacity and clinical requirements of beef and pork insulin. *Metabolism*, **14**, 1034–6

15. Reeves, W. G. (1985). Immunological aspects of therapy. In Alberti, K. G. M. M. and Krall, L. P. (eds.) *The Diabetes Annual*. Vol. 1, pp. 67–81. (Amsterdam: Elsevier)

16. Fineberg, S. E., Galloway, J. A., Fineberg, N. S., Rathbun, M. J. and Hufferd, S. (1983). Immunogenicity of recombinant DNA human insulin. *Diabetologia*, **25**, 465

17. Goldman, J., Baldwin, D., Rubenstein, A. H., Klink, D. D., Blackard, W. G., Fisher, L. K., Roe, T. F. and Schnure, J. J. (1979). Characterization of circulating insulin and proinsulin-binding antibodies in autoimmune hypoglycaemia. *J. Clin. Invest.*, **63**, 1050–9

18. Keck, K. (1981). Insulin as a tool for the study of immunological problems. In Keck, K. and Erb, P. (eds.) *Basic and Clinical Aspects of Immunity to Insulin*. pp. 3–16. (Berlin: de Gruyter)

19. Nakao, Y., Matsumoto, H., Miyazaki, T., Mizuno, N., Arima, N., Wakisaka, A., Okimoto, K., Akazawa, Y., Tsuji, K. and Fujita, T. (1981). IgG heavychain (Gm) allotypes and immune response to insulin-requiring diabetes mellitus. *N. Engl. J. Med.*, **304**, 407–9

20. Kurtz, A. B., Gray, R. S., Markanday, S. and Nabarro, J. D. N. (1983). Circulating IgG antibody to protamine in patients treated with protamine-insulins. *Diabetologia*, **25**, 322–4

21. Kurtz, A. B., Di Silvio, L. and Lydyard, P. (1985). Lymphocyte proliferation as a test of the immune response to insulin in diabetics. *Diabetes Res.*, **2**, 175–8

22. Berson, S. A. and Yalow, R. S. (1959). Quantitative aspects of the reaction between insulin and insulin-binding antibody. *J. Clin. Invest.*, **38**, 1996–2016

23. Scatchard, G. (1949). The attraction of proteins for small molecules and ions. *Ann. N. Y. Acad. Sci.*, **51**, 660–73

24. Matsukura, S., West, C. D., Ichikawa, Y., Jubiz, W., Harada, G. and Tyler, F. H. (1971). A new phenomenon of usefulness in the radioimmunoassay of plasma adrenocorticotropic hormone. *J. Lab. Clin. Med.*, **77**, 490–500

25. Weintraub, B. D., Rosen, S., McCammon, J. A. and Perlman, R. L. (1973). Apparent cooperativity in radioimmunoassay of human chorionic gonadotrophin. *Endocrinology*, **92**, 1250–5

26. Folling, I. (1976). Insulin anti-insulin complexes. *Acta Endocrinol. (Kbh).*, (Suppl 205), 199–209

27. Schroer, J. (1981). Mouse hybridoma antibody recognition of the insulin molecule. In Keck, K. and Erb, P. (eds.) *Basic and Clinical Aspects of Immunity to Insulin*. pp. 183–200. (Berlin: de Gruyter)

28. Kurtz, A. B., Harrington, M. G., Matthews, J. A. and Nabarro, J. D. N. (1979). Factitious diabetes and antibody mediated resistance to beef insulin. *Diabetologia*, **16**, 65–7

29. Folling, I. and Norman, N. (1972). Hyperglycaemia, hypoglycaemia attacks and production of anti-insulin antibodies without previous known immunization. *Diabetes*, **21**, 814–26

30. Hirata, Y. (1977). Spontaneous insulin antibodies and hypoglycaemia. In Bajaj, J. S. (ed.) *Diabetes*. pp. 278–84. (Amsterdam: Excerpta Medica)

31. Kruse, V. (1981). Effect of insulin-binding antibodies on free insulin in plasma and tissue after subcutaneous injection. A model study. In Keck, K. and Erb, P. (eds.) *Basic and

*Clinical Aspects of Immunity to Insulin.* pp. 319–34. (Berlin: de Gruyter)

32. Nakagawa, S., Suda, N., Kudo, M. and Kawasaki, M. (1973). A new type of hypoglycaemia in a newborn infant. *Diabetologia,* 9, 367–75

33. Palmer, J. P., Asplin, C. M., Clemons, P., Lyen, K., Tatpati, O., Raghu, P. K. and Paquette, T. L. (1983). Insulin antibodies in insulin-dependent diabetics before insulin treatment. *Science,* 222, 1337–9

34. Soeldner, J. S., Tuttleman, M., Srikanta, S., Ganda, O. P. and Eisenbarth, G. S. (1985). Insulin-dependent diabetes mellitus and autoimmunity: islet-cell autoantibodies, insulin autoantibodies, and beta-cell failure. *N. Engl. J. Med.,* 313, 893

35. Onodera, T., Ray, U. R., Melez, K. A., Suzuki, H., Tonolio, A. and Notkins, A. L. (1982). Virus-induced diabetes mellitus: autoimmunity and polyendocrine disease prevented by immunosuppression. *Nature (London),* 297, 66–8

36. Benson, E. A., Healy, L. A. and Barron, E. J. (1985). Insulin antibodies in patients receiving penicillamine. *Am. J. Med.,* 78, 857–60

37. Blackshear, P. J., Rofner, H. E., Kriauciunas, K. A. M. and Kahn, C. R. (1983). Reactive hypoglycaemia and insulin autoantibodies in drug induced lupus erythematosus. *Ann. Intern. Med.,* 99, 182–4

38. Harwood, R. (1960). Insulin-binding antibodies and 'spontaneous' hypoglycemia. *N. Engl. J. Med.,* 262, 978–9

39. Bolinger, R. E., Morris, J. H., McKnight, F. G. and Diederich, D. A. (1964). Disappearance of [131]I-labelled insulin from plasma as a guide to management of diabetes. *N. Engl. J. Med.,* 270, 767–70

40. Vaughan, N. J. A., Matthews, J. A., Kurtz, A. B. and Nabarro, J. D. N. (1983). The bioavailability of circulating antibody-bound insulin following insulin withdrawal in type 1 (insulin-dependent) diabetes. *Diabetologia,* 24, 355–8

41. Dixon, K., Exon, P. D. and Malins, J. M. (1975). Insulin antibodies and the control of diabetes. *Q. J. Med.,* 44, 543–53

42. Heding, L. G. (1969). Determination of free and antibody-bound insulin in insulin treated diabetic patients. *Horm. Metab. Res.,* 1, 145–6

43. Nakagawa, S., Nakayama, H., Sasaki, T., Yoshino, K., Yu, Y. Y., Shinozaki, K., Aoki, S. and Mashio, K. (1973). A simple method for the determination of serum free insulin levels in insulin-treated patients. *Diabetes,* 22, 590–600

44. Kuzuya, H., Blix, P. M., Horwitz, D. L., Steiner, D. F. and Rubenstein, A. H. (1977). Determination of free and total insulin and C-peptide in insulin-treated diabetics. *Diabetes,* 26, 22–9

45. Gerbitz, K. D. and Sumner, J. (1981). Distribution of insulin in blood of type 1 diabetics. *Diabetologia,* 21, 274

46. Asplin, C. M., Goldie, D. J. and Hartog, M. (1977). The measurement of serum free insulin by steady-state gel filtration. *Clin. Chim. Acta,* 75, 393–9

47. Nell, L. J., Virta, V. J. and Thomas, J. T. (1985). Application of a rapid enzyme-linked immunosorbent microassay (ELIZA) to study human anti-insulin antibody. *Diabetes,* 34, 60–6

48. Wide, L. (1973). Clinical significance of measurement of reaginic (IgE) antibody by RAST. *Clin. Allergy,* 3, 583–95

49. Carini, C., Brostoff, J. and Kurtz, A. B. (1982). An anaphylactic reaction to highly purified pork insulin. Confirmation by RAST and RAST inhibition. *Diabetologia,* 22, 324–6

50. Karsson, F., Harrison, L. C., Khan, C. R., Itin, A. and Roth, J. (1982). Subpopulations of antibodies directed against evolutionarily conserved regions of the insulin molecule in insulin-treated patients. *Diabetologia,* 23, 488–93

# 6
# Immunogenetics of Diabetes

## A. H. BARNETT

## INTRODUCTION

Much of the confusion that has arisen from studies of the genetics of diabetes mellitus arises from the fact that, until recently, diabetes was regarded as a single disease. It is now clear that there are at least two major types of diabetes which are aetiologically distinct, although they have similar long-term complications. The recent WHO classification of diabetes includes these two categories:

(1)  Type I, insulin dependent or ketosis prone;
(2)  Type II, non-insulin dependent or non-ketosis prone.

The evidence that these two conditions are separate entities is summarized in Table 6.1. It is precisely these differences which give clues to their pathogenesis.

The studies of identical twins, where at least one twin is diabetic, provided some early indication of basic differences between the two types of disease. Perhaps the most celebrated study is that from the King's College Hospital diabetic unit. Over the past two decades, this unit has been collecting diabetic twins in order to elucidate the relative roles of genetic and environmental factors in the aetiology of diabetes[1]. Two hundred pairs are reported of which 147 are Type I and 53 type II diabetics. About half of the Type I pairs are discordant for the disease, i.e. one has diabetes and the other has not. It is likely that the great majority of these pairs will remain discordant since most have been discordant for over 10 years and some for over 20 or even 30 years, without any deterioration in glucose tolerance in the non-diabetic co-twins. Most of the concordant pairs, however, become concordant within 5 years and almost certainly within 10 years of diagnosis of the index twin. These data suggest that genetic factors alone cannot be the cause of Type I diabetes (since the twins are genetically identical). This discordance rate for Type I diabetes is probably an underestimate since there is a bias towards referral of concordant pairs, i.e. they are at least twice as likely to be noticed and referred when compared with discordant pairs. Estimates from this study and other twin studies suggest that the true

**Table 6.1** Differences between Type I and Type II diabetes

|  | *Type I* | *Type II* |
|---|---|---|
| Histology | Inflammatory cell infiltration and destruction of pancreatic β-cell | Normal or almost normal |
| Progression | Complete β-cell failure, absolute requirement for insulin | Often little progression, usually non-insulin requiring |
| Islet cell antibodies | Present in majority at diagnosis (>70% of subjects) | Very low incidence (<10% of subjects) |
| HLA-associations | Characteristic, particularly HLA DR3 and DR4 | Not present |
| T-cell abnormalities | Present at diagnosis | No association |
| Association with other autoimmune diseases | Present | No association |
| Concordance rates in identical twins | 30–50% | 90% |

There is good evidence that genetic factors are involved in both types of diabetes, but they are clearly of a different nature. Immunogenetic factors are important in Type I diabetes; the nature of the genetic factor for Type II diabetes is unknown.

discordance rate for Type I diabetes is something of the order of 65–70%.

The findings for Type II diabetes are rather different. About 90% of pairs are concordant for this disease and for those who are still discordant, the index twin has only been diagnosed relatively recently. It might be argued that this high concordance rate is due to a bias in ascertainment since concordant twins are twice as likely to be recognized as discordant ones. This is probably not the case since many twin pairs were actually referred as being discordant and it was only after glucose tolerance testing of the 'non-diabetic' co-twin that the pairs were discovered to be concordant. Environmental factors are unlikely to explain the high concordance rate since most of the twins are elderly and have been living apart for many years. In addition, the concordance rates for non-identical twins are much lower, although they presumably had similar degrees of environmental exposure in early life. Interestingly, when the non-diabetic co-twins from the discordant pairs of identical twins were further studied, they were found to have abnormalities of intermediary metabolites and reduced insulin secretion, although their blood glucose levels did not yet fulfil the criteria for the diagnosis of diabetes. Presumably, these subjects will go on to develop diabetes in time. It seems clear, therefore, that Type II diabetes has a very strong inherited component and, indeed, genetic factors probably predominate in its aetiology.

Although Type I diabetes cannot be caused entirely by genetic factors, more recent studies suggest that there is an important immunogenetic component. There is, however, no evidence that immunological factors play a part in the pathogenesis of Type II diabetes except in certain very rare clinical syndromes characterized by severe insulin resistance due to anti-insulin receptor antibodies (e.g. associated with acanthosis nigricans). The twin studies suggest a strong genetic component of the aetiology of Type II diabetes, but cannot determine what that component is. Since there is no evidence for an immunological basis for Type II diabetes, it will not be considered further in this chapter.

## IMMUNOGENETICS OF TYPE I DIABETES

The major susceptibility to Type I diabetes is conferred by a gene or genes at a locus or loci closely linked to the HLA region. The HLA system is located on the short arm of chromosome 6 and is concerned with immune response (Figure 6.1). It can be subdivided into three regions – HLA-A, B and C loci coding for class I antigens; D region coding for three sets of class II molecules: DP, DQ, DR in man (Ia in mouse); genes coding for complement proteins (Bf, C2 and C4), class III molecules. Apart from the complement components, the products of these genes are expressed in the cell membranes of lymphocytes and other cells. HLA-A, B and C molecules are found on all nucleated cells and platelets, whereas HLA-D/DR molecules have a more limited distribution and are found only on endothelial cells, Langerhans cells, some epithelial cells and activated T-lymphocytes. They do not appear to be expressed on normal pancreatic $\beta$-cells. DR molecules are important in initiating immune response by presenting foreign antigens to T-cells.

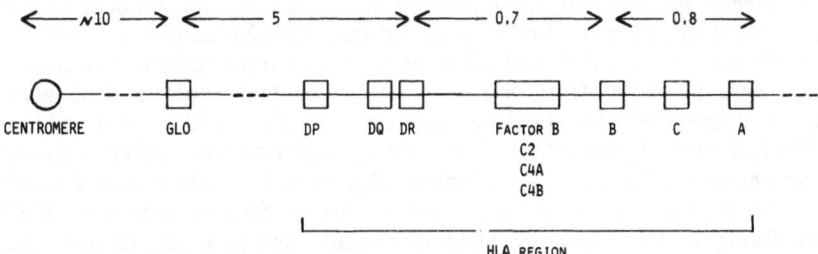

**Figure 6.1** The major histocompatibility complex and the locus for red cell glyoxalase 1 (GLO) on the short arm of chromosome 6. The distances between the loci are in centimorgans. Class I loci include the HLA A, B and C loci. Class II loci include the DP, DQ and DR loci. Class III loci include the complement loci – factor B, C2, C4A and C4B

A currently favoured hypothesis is that Type I diabetes is caused by some environmental factor (perhaps a virus or viruses) initiating an immune-mediated destructive process of the pancreatic $\beta$-cell in a genetically predisposed individual. This form of the disease has been labelled Type Ia to distinguish it from the less common (<20%) Type Ib which may be a more primary autoimmune form of the disease. Type Ib diabetes often has a later onset and is associated with persistence of islet cell antibodies and other organ-specific autoimmune diseases. The immunogenetic characteristics of these two forms, however, show considerable overlap. It is, perhaps, important to stress at this stage that Type I diabetes *per se* is not inherited – rather it is the susceptibility to develop the disease which is inherited. What actually converts genetic susceptibility to development of disease remains speculative and will form part of the discussion in this chapter. The current state of knowledge concerning the immunogenetics of Type I diabetes will now be considered in more detail covering genetic susceptibility including HLA and non-HLA associations, the role of viruses and other environmental factors, humoral and cellular immune factors and autoimmunity.

## THE GENETIC SUSCEPTIBILITY TO TYPE I DIABETES

### Class I and II associations

Associations of Type I diabetes with certain HLA-B locus antigens were first reported in the mid-1970s[2,3]. Positive associations with HLA B15, B8 and, to a lesser extent, B18 and B40 were described, and some studies showed a negative association with B7. More recently, stronger associations have been reported with HLA-DR3 and DR4 and these appear to provide a more primary association with the disease. Population studies, most notably the 'Barts-Windsor prospective family study', have confirmed these associations[4]. This study was started in 1978 to compare the immunogenetic characteristics of the siblings of Type I diabetics in relation to their susceptibility to develop the disease. One hundred and sixty families were ascertained through Type I diabetics attending clinics in East Berkshire and surrounding districts. They were selected on the basis of the presence of at least one non-diabetic sibling below the age of 20 years. For various reasons, only 123 families were studied and of these HLA-A, B, C and DR genotypes were obtained on 116 families. Data were available from healthy random control subjects. The great majority (almost 98%) of the diabetics possessed either DR3 or DR4 and half (51%) had both. This confirmed the findings reported from other countries using phenotype frequencies, including subjects with widely different ethnic origins (e.g. Basques, African and American Blacks. Similar findings for DR4 were found in the Japanese; DR3 is virtually absent from the Japanese population, but an increase in DRW8 has been reported.) Wolf and co-workers have reported a relative risk for development of Type I diabetes of 5.0 and 6.8 for DR3 and DR4 respectively, with an approximate additive relative risk of 14.3 for the presence of both DR3 and DR4 (others report this figure even higher in the region of 20–40 times)[4].

Although DR3 and/or DR4 occur in very high frequency in this disease population, the frequency of these antigens in the non-diabetic population is over 50%. Why then does Type I diabetes, with a prevalence of about 0.3%, mainly affect the DR3 and DR4 positive population? It is possible that these molecules themselves are directly involved in the pathogenesis of Type I diabetes. DR molecules, however, are probably not expressed on healthy islet cells, but might be expressed after damage. An alternative, and now more likely, explanation is that some subset of DR3 or DR4 or a closely linked, but distinct locus, bears the diabetogenic gene(s). This concept is supported by the recent techniques of restriction fragment length polymorphism (RFLP) analysis utilizing specific D-region DNA probes. Furthermore, epidemiological studies have suggested that not all DR3 or DR4 bearing chromosomes are increased in frequency in Type I diabetes – only certain haplotypes bearing these antigens are associated[5].

The strong association with both DR3 and DR4 (at least in Caucasoids) suggests that there may be two separate susceptibility genes, each in linkage disequilibrium* with DR3 and DR4 operating at the same or different loci. Interestingly, homozygosity for DR3 or DR4 does not confer a double dose of susceptibility to diabetes. This observation together with the high frequency of DR3, DR4 heterozygotes argues against a single gene in linkage disequilibrium with both DR3 and DR4. The interactive effect of both DR3 and DR4 is supported by studies of identical twins – a preliminary communication suggests that there are about twice as many concordant pairs (both twins diabetic) who are DR3/DR4 heterozygous compared with discordant pairs (only one twin diabetic after 5 years diagnosis)[6].

The most consistent negative association with Type I diabetes has been reported with DR2 – it is difficult to establish whether this implies a specific protective effect, but a gene or genes in linkage disequilibrium with DR2 might confer protection against islet cell damage.

For reasons outlined, it seems unlikely that DR3 or DR4 are more than disease susceptibility markers and they do not constitute the 'diabetogenic' gene(s). The techniques of molecular biology have recently been utilized to determine whether stronger associations than those with DR3 or DR4 antigens exist.

## cDNA probing studies

Class II molecules are coded for in the HLA-D region and contain two subunits – $\alpha$- and $\beta$-chains of about 34000 and 28000 molecular weight respectively. These proteins are expressed on the surface of immune competent cells and are concerned with regulation of immune response. Present data suggest that the DP and DQ loci both encode two $\alpha$- and two $\beta$-chains each. The DR locus probably encodes one $\alpha$- and possibly a variable number of $\beta$-chains. Lernmark and co-workers have used a cloned probe for one of the HLA-DQ $\beta$-chain genes in restriction fragment length polymorphism (RFLP) analysis. The technique was applied to homozygous tissue typing cells, HLA-DR identical control and diabetic individuals and to a linkage analysis in HLA-DR typed control and diabetic families. Polymorphism detected by this probe was associated with HLA-DR, but HLA-DR identical control and Type I diabetics differed in the presence of

---

*Linkage disequilibrium – the co-occurrence of alleles at separate but closely linked loci at a frequency different from that expected on the basis of individual allelic frequencies.

certain restriction fragments. Thus a HLA DR4-linked restriction fragment (Bam HI 3.7 kb) was more commonly associated with DR3 and/or DR4 positive non-diabetics than with HLA-DR identical Type I patients[7]. The difference between patients and controls was due to the absence of a Bam HI restriction site within a DQ $\beta$-chain intervening sequence[8]. Another group, using the restriction enzyme Taq 1, has reported a particular RFLP pattern in 11 of 12 DR3/DR4 Type I patients and in none of 12 DR-matched controls[9]. This was estimated to indicate a relative risk of over 400 compared with (at most) 40 using DR3/DR4 serological markers!

If these preliminary reports are confirmed, then it appears that cDNA probes may better define the risk of developing the disease. Initial observations suggest that Type I diabetes is either more closely associated with the HLA-DQ $\beta$-chain gene or again that this particular genomic sequence is in close linkage with a diabetes susceptibility gene(s).

### Class III associations (complement factors)

Complement is a complex system of different proteins concerned with humoral immunity, the components of which act in sequence usually after stimulation by antigen/antibody complexes. They are concerned with viral neutralization, clearance of immune complexes and play a role in inflammation. Genes coding for the complement proteins are situated between the HLA B and D loci (see Figure 6.1).

Type I diabetes is associated with a rare allele of the Bf (properdin factor) system – BfF1 – this is in strong linkage disequilibrium with DR3 and forms part of an extended haplotype (see later) which is associated with Type I diabetes. Associations with certain alleles of the second component of complement are described and will not be discussed further.

Associations of Type I diabetes with certain phenotypes of the fourth component of complement (C4) are now well described[10]. The C4 protein is coded for by two separate loci, C4A and C4B, and both loci are extremely polymorphic. There are at least 13 different alleles for the A protein and 22 for the B protein including a null ('silent' or non-expressed) allele at each locus (termed A or B Quantity zero – AQ0 or BQ0 respectively). We have found that Type I diabetics have an increased frequency of homozygous A null alleles (13%) and of the rare C4B3 allotype (17%) when compared with non-diabetics (frequency for both <1%)[11] and this is similar to data published elsewhere. It is important to point out, however, that C4A null is in linkage disequilibrium with DR3 and C4B3 with DR4 – indeed, both phenotypes occur within the commonly reported extended haplotype sequences associated with Type I diabetes. It is, however, interesting to speculate (with regard to the known functional roles of complement) as to whether absolute or relative C4 deficiency might contribute *per se* to the pathogenesis of Type I diabetes.

### Extended haplotypes

The association of Type I diabetes with DR3 and DR4 can be interpreted, as already discussed, as a reflection of linkage disequilibrium with immune response genes directly involved in its pathogenesis. An alternative hypothesis is that the association is due to differences in immune responsiveness in relation to different HLA haplotypes. Indeed, the complement associations described could be interpreted to support either hypothesis. A common feature of the HLA genes in Type I diabetes is the finding of relatively invariable patterns over a considerable portion of the chromosome in many patients. These have been termed 'extended haplotypes'.

Family studies have been instrumental in defining certain extended haplotypes commonly associated with Type I diabetes. HLA-genotyping of families provides accurate information on the four different parental haplotypes and their inheritance by the offspring. The probability of any randomly chosen pair of siblings being HLA-identical (i.e. inheriting the same haplotypes), haploidentical (inheriting one haplotype in common) or non-identical (neither haplotype in common) is 25%, 50% and 25% respectively. The observed distribution of haplotypes in families with two or more Type I diabetic siblings is markedly disturbed from that expected. Review of the literature from a number of European countries and the US suggests that 57% of pairs of affected siblings are HLA-identical, 38% are haploidentical and only 5% are non-identical[12].

The most recent study has described three 'extended haplotypes' that confer significant increased susceptibility to Type I diabetes[13] (Table 6.2).

**Table 6.2** Extended HLA-haplotypes increased in frequency in Type I diabetes

| B | Bf | C2 | C4A | C4B | DR |
|---|-----|-----|-------|------|-----|
| B8 | BfS | C2C | C4AQ0 | C4B1 | DR3 |
| B15 | BfS | C2C | C4A3 | C4B3 | DR4 |
| B18 | BfF1 | C2C | C4A3 | C4BQ0 | DR3 |

These extended haplotypes are reported to confer a relative risk of 2.4, 10.2 and 10.6 respectively in the North American Caucasoid population under study. For relative situation of these loci on chromosome 6 see Figure 6.1.

This finding of associations of 'extended haplotypes' with Type I diabetes and, indeed, a recent report of relative risk less than unity for DR3 in the absence of certain components of the extended haplotype[5], could be explained on the basis of several different components of the haplotype contributing to the pathogenesis of the disease. An alternative explanation, however, is that there is a single-susceptibility gene in linkage disequilibrium with multiple-gene complexes. Clearly, studies of extended haplotypes provide an alternative approach to gene probing in studying the mode of inheritance and genetics of Type I diabetes.

## Non-HLA susceptibility

The major susceptibility to Type I diabetes is found within the HLA region. There has also been a report of an association with red cell glyoxalase 1

(GLO) phenotype coded for on chromosome 6 near the centromere, but this has never been confirmed. A significant association with the fast acetylator phenotype has been described, but the locus controlling acetylator status is not known.

The genes coding for the immunoglobulin heavy chain (Gm) are situated on chromosome 14. Interactions between Gm, HLA-DR and Type I diabetes have been described. This suggests that genetic predisposition to Type I diabetes may be partially determined by alleles at the Gm locus or a locus in linkage disequilibrium with Gm interacting with alleles at the HLA-DR locus (or a locus in linkage disequilibrium with HLA-DR). These findings, however, have not been confirmed by other workers[14].

Insulin gene polymorphism has also been associated with Type I diabetes. In particular, 70% of juvenile cases have been associated with class I alleles[15].

## VIRUSES AND TYPE I DIABETES

It is clear from the studies of identical twins that the true concordance rate for Type I diabetes is well under 50%. This indicates that non-genetic (environmental) factors must also be involved in its pathogenesis. Both toxins and hormonal imbalance have been implicated in the development of diabetes. Investigators have reported an association between the ingestion of trace amounts of N-nitroso-compounds in food and diabetes in childhood when ingested close to the time of conception[16]. The most consistent hypothesis, however, first proposed a century ago, suggests that viruses are the environmental factors most commonly involved. More recently, animal models of virus-induced Type I diabetes have been described. Evidence for involvement of an infective agent in humans comes from the age and seasonal distributions, family clustering and temporal relationships between viral illness and diagnosis of diabetes. The age distribution at diagnosis is quite characteristic – epidemiological studies have demonstrated that incidence increases steadily from age 9 months with a peak at 10–12 years, and a smaller peak at 5 years (coincident with changing or starting school for many children).

Most striking, however, is the difference in seasonal distribution for diagnosis of Type I diabetes. In a recent review, it was reported that autumn and winter peaks in diabetes incidence have been observed in six different countries in both northern and southern hemispheres[17]. It is, however, of interest that the annual variation of Type I diabetes is fairly small and changes are not correlated with the prevalence of any particular infectious agent within the population. These observations are against any single virus being responsible for any appreciable number of the cases of diabetes. There have, however, been a few well-documented reports of a temporal relationship between a number of infectious diseases and the onset of clinical symptoms of diabetes. Indeed, most of the common childhood illnesses have been so associated.

There have also been reports of 'outbreaks' of Type I diabetes. Clustering of cases temporally and geographically has been reported from a number of countries, most notably in Sweden. Gamble has commented upon the many different viral illnesses occurring within 1 month prior to the onset of symptoms in a large retrospective study – about 25% of Type I diabetics reported such an illness prior to clinical symptoms of disease[17]. This suggests that many viruses might act as a trigger in the pathogenesis of diabetes or, alternatively, that they have no role at all.

Family studies have both supported and refuted the concept of a virus (or viruses) having pathogenic importance in Type I diabetes. Studies of identical twins have failed to show a significant difference in viral antibody titres within or between concordant and discordant pairs. Other, more traditional family studies have been suggestive and, indeed, familial clusters of cases have been well described. Rarely, however, have specific viruses been implicated.

A prospective study[18] (based on the Barts-Windsor prospective family study) has suggested Type I diabetes has a much longer latency period before development of overt diabetes than previously thought. This has been taken to suggest that the role of viruses is either non-specific or the final insult in the process of $\beta$-cell destruction.

The viruses which have most consistently been reported in association with Type I diabetes are mumps, rubella and Coxsackie B. The evidence for mumps involvement is circumstantial and mumps alone could only account for a tiny proportion of cases. Symptomatic diabetes associated with serological evidence of recent Coxsackie B infection (especially B4) is well documented[19], although other studies have shown no relationship.

It is hardly surprising that the data available is confusing and often inconclusive. The Type I diabetic population is undoubtedly heterogeneous – in different subsets of patients the disease may result from different pathogenetic mechanisms. Different susceptibility factors (including HLA phenotype) are likely to operate and, indeed, the association of HLA with immune response is likely to mean that hyper-responsiveness to some antigens could be associated with certain HLA types. Spurious associations with raised antiviral antibody titre might then arise. Prospective family data including HLA identical non-diabetic siblings might overcome this problem. Other problems, however, include the imprecise nature of the latency period between initiation of $\beta$-cell injury and clinical expression of disease. It is, therefore, obvious that, although environmental factors are involved in the pathogenesis of Type I diabetes, the frequency and mechanisms by which viral illness might lead to its development are unresolved. The concept of an underlying viral aetiology is, however, exciting and worth pursuing since this approach may offer the possibility of active immunization and, perhaps, prevention.

## AUTOIMMUNITY IN TYPE I DIABETES

Inflammatory cell infiltration of the islet of Langerhans was reported at the turn of the century from postmortem specimens of patients dying from untreated ketotic diabetes. It was not until 1965, however, that Gepts reported major abnormalities in the $\beta$-cells. $\beta$-Cell destruction is highly specific and the other pancreatic endocrine cells are unaffected. It appears that $\beta$-cells are lost in association with a specific autoimmune reaction, possibly provoked by an external agent, e.g. virus, controlled by certain HLA-D region genes, and directed specifically against molecules expressed solely on the $\beta$-cell. The roles of both humoral and cellular immunity in relation to the pathogenesis of Type I diabetes have been studied extensively in recent years.

## Islet cell antibodies

Islet cell antibodies (ICA) were first described by Bottazzo et al.[20] and MacCuish et al., in 1974, having been detected by indirect immunofluorescence on frozen sections of fresh human pancreas. They occur in over 70% of newly diagnosed Type I diabetics and are primarily of the IgG class. Immunofluorescence studies demonstrate reactions with the cytoplasmic components of all islet cell types, and ICAs have not been shown to cause complement-mediated $\beta$-cell lysis in vitro. It is unlikely that they have any pathogenetic role in Type I diabetes.

More recently, complement fixing islet cell antibodies (CF-ICA) have been described[21]. They are present in most diabetics who are ICA positive, but often in lower titre and they are IgG. They selectively stain $\beta$-cells and may be cytotoxic.

Antibodies of the IgG class directed against the surface of islet cells – islet cell surface antibodies (ICSA) – have also been demonstrated by an indirect immunofluorescence technique on dispersed islets from mice and rats[22]. At diagnosis, about 70% of Type I diabetics have ICSA, the prevalence diminishing with increasing duration of disease. They can mediate complement-dependent $\beta$-cell cytotoxicity, and impair $\beta$-cell function in vitro. Immunoglobulin from ICSA-containing sera from Type I diabetics can inhibit proinsulin synthesis as well as glucose-induced release from rat islet cells. Confirmation of these studies using human $\beta$-cells is awaited.

## Predictive significance of ICA

Various studies have demonstrated that ICA is highly predictive of Type I diabetes in individuals who are at increased risk of developing the disease (e.g. first degree relatives of Type I diabetics). In the Barts-Windsor prospective study of 582 first-degree relatives of Type I diabetics, six became diabetic over 3 years and all were ICA positive[18]. In another study, of 16 ICA-positive non-diabetics over 5 years, three developed diabetes and CF-ICA in particular was a good predictive factor[23]. Others[24] have reported that the probability of developing diabetes in a healthy sibling or parent who is CF-ICA positive is 73%. ICA-positivity appears to be also predictive of those patients on oral hypoglycaemics who will eventually require insulin therapy.

First-degree relatives of Type I diabetics may have ICA for many months and occasionally years before the development of overt diabetes. Even at this stage, however, there may be an absence of the first phase insulin response and selective loss of insulin release to intravenous glucose. Thus the immune attack on the $\beta$-cell may occur long before clinical manifestations of disease.

It is, however, equally clear that the presence of ICA and even other manifestations of the immune response do not inevitably predict the development of Type I diabetes. Recently, Bottazzo and co-workers have described the presence of CF-ICA in 20 of 685 unaffected first-degree relatives of children with Type I diabetes[25]. During a 5 year follow-up, seven of the 20 subjects became diabetic, one continued to show CF-ICA without metabolic abnormality, *but* 12 subjects lost them without the disease developing. Pyke and co-workers have also studied ICA and activation of T-lymphocytes in two groups of Type I diabetics and their non-diabetic identical co-twins. They examined 12 pairs in which the diabetic twin was diagnosed within 5 years (in only about four of these pairs is the non-diabetic co-twin likely to become diabetic) and ten pairs with long discordance for the disease (in none of these is the non-diabetic co-twin likely to become diabetic). In the short duration group all 12 diabetics and ten of their non-diabetic co-twins had ICA or activated T-lymphocytes or both. In the long duration group, however, who were selected because all of the non-diabetic co-twins had previously shown ICA, only two of these non-diabetic twins still had ICA or activated T-lymphocytes. This suggests that the same immunological changes can occur in the genetically identical non-diabetic co-twins of diabetics, but may remit without leading to the disease. So what limits the immune-mediated damage in those twins in whom the damage has remitted? Clearly, it can hardly depend on genetic predisposition alone since this study was performed on genetically identical twins!

## ß-Cell autoantigen(s)

The strong association of the islet cell surface antibody (ICSA) with newly diagnosed Type I diabetes and its possible pathogenetic role begs the question 'which antigen(s) are these antibodies recognizing?' Lernmark and co-workers have recently identified a protein with a molecular weight of 64 000 (64K), by techniques of sodium dodecyl sulphate gel electrophoresis and autoradiography, which is immunoprecipitated by sera from eight out of ten newly diagnosed diabetic children[26]. Thus, antibodies from Type I diabetics detect at least one human islet cell protein. Cross-reactivity with Type I diabetes sera and rat pancreatic islets has also been demonstrated. This autoantigen is thought to be a pancreatic $\beta$-cell specific membrane component since the presence of antibodies against the 64K protein coincide with ICSA, which is also $\beta$-cell specific, in the sera of Type I diabetic patients. Interestingly, preliminary observations suggest that autoantibodies against this component may be present long before the diagnosis of diabetes and even before the appearance of ICA. Attempts are now being made to isolate, characterize and sequence this antigen.

## Associations of ICA with other organ specific endocrine disorders

Titres of ICA usually decline fairly rapidly after diagnosis of diabetes, perhaps mirroring the rate of $\beta$-cell destruction (although this is still controversial). ICA is present in about 70% of newly diagnosed Type I diabetics, but declines to 40% after a year and 15% after 5 years. Those showing persistence of ICA are more likely to be HLA-B8-DR3 positive. As discussed previously, it has been proposed that Type I diabetes can be subdivided into Types Ia and Ib. Type Ia accounts for 85–90% of cases and tends to occur at a young age, often showing seasonal variation, in subjects who are more commonly HLA-B15-DR4 and with non-persistence of ICA. Type Ib, however, is more common in females and is associated with B8-DR3 and persistence of ICA. It is often associated with other organ specific autoimmune disorders, especially thyroid disease[20], and even if the diseases are not clinically manifest, characteristic organ specific antibodies are often found. Indeed, it is reported that 15% of patients with idiopathic Addison's disease and 7–10% of patients with autoimmune thyroid disease have Type I diabetes. Since there is a high prevalence of thyroid autoimmunity in the general population, specific relationships are hard to define. Whether these diseases have a common pathogenetic mechanism or whether they have different aetiologies with a common genetic background is still undetermined.

## CELL-MEDIATED IMMUNITY IN TYPE I DIABETES

The pancreatic islets of newly diagnosed Type I diabetics show typical inflammatory changes or 'insulitis'. The fact that lymphocytes seem to be attracted by an antigen present in $\beta$-cells, but not in the other endocrine cells, supports the concept that 'insulitis' may be involved in the progressive destruction of insulin secreting cells. It is likely that cell-mediated immune mechanisms are as important for the initiation of 'insulitis' as humoral responses.

Human T-lymphocytes can be divided into two functional categories – effector T-cells which mediate the functions of cell-mediated immunity (cytotoxic lymphocytes) and immunoregulator T-cells (helper and suppressor cells) which influence the differentiation of B-lymphocytes to synthesize immunoglobulin and regulate effector T-cell activity. Approximately 5% of peripheral blood lymphocytes do not meet the criteria for either T or B lymphocytes – these have been given various labels including K-cells, defined as killer cells responsible for antibody-dependent cell-mediated cytotoxicity. K-cells kill non-specifically, but the destruction can be made specific by the reactivity of the antibodies involved. They are involved in the elimination of virus-infected cells and allograft rejection.

Nerup and colleagues first reported positive leukocyte migration inhibition tests in patients with recent onset Type I diabetes using an antigen extracted from human or animal pancreas. Many studies have since been reported examining lymphocyte subsets in these patients. There have been consistent reports of increases in K-cell numbers, decreased specific and non-specific suppressor cell function and the presence of activated T-cells[27]. These abnormalities tend to disappear within a few months of diagnosis. Receptors for the Fc part of IgG are expressed on already activated T-cells, and this subset appears to be the one increased in some genetically and immunologically susceptible, non-diabetic, first-degree relatives of Type I diabetics. Since a proportion of these subjects will go on to develop the disease, it is suggested that lymphocytes with Fc-IgG receptors might have pathogenetic importance.

Recently, Bottazzo and colleagues have reported studies on fresh-frozen pancreas obtained from a newly diagnosed diabetic child who died within 24 hours of diagnosis[28]. The expected 'insulitis' was found, and the majority of islets were devoid of insulin-secreting cells, whereas glucagon- and somatostatin-secreting cells were well preserved. The majority of infiltrating mononuclear cells were found to be T-lymphocytes. A number of lymphocyte populations were represented, mostly cytotoxic/suppressor lymphocytes and killer lymphocytes. Most of the autoreactive T-lymphocytes expressed HLA-DR antigens, indicating that they were 'activated' T-cells and suggesting a specific immune response directed against islet antigens. A striking feature was that IgG was present inside the cytoplasm of islet cells, suggesting penetration of antibodies following injury to the cell membranes. (Similar events have been described in autoimmune thyroiditis and nephritis.)

Based on studies of autoimmune thyroid disease and some preliminary studies in Type I diabetes, Bottazzo and colleagues have suggested that β-cells might express DR inappropriately in diabetic insulitis (this has been shown for thyrocytes in Graves' disease and Hashimoto's thyroiditis)[28]. Immune responses are thought to be initiated by HLA-DR positive cells presenting antigens to T-lymphocytes. They have suggested a new hypothesis explaining induction of autoimmunity in endocrine organs. It is postulated that interferon, which is the best inducer of DR-antigen expression, could be stimulated by viruses (or other environmental agents), which are present in relevant endocrine glands of genetically predisposed individuals without causing signs of infection. This might then trigger a series of events with aberrant DR expression, presentation of surface autoantigens and induction of autoreactive T-cells. These would then activate effector B- and T-lymphocytes. Subsequent development of overt autoimmune disease might then depend on a number of other factors such as abnormalities of the suppressor T-cell pathway (well documented in autoimmunity). These workers consider that this hypothesis might explain vague associations with viral infections and long latency periods before disease induction. It would also provide an explanation for DR-associations with various autoimmune diseases, including Type I diabetes.

## IMMUNOTHERAPY OF TYPE I DIABETES

Diabetes can be prevented or reversed by immunotherapy in the BB rat. A 1-month course of antilymphocyte serum or whole body X-irradiation will prevent the development of diabetes and reverse it in one-third of animals after development of the disease. Other approaches, including administration of cyclosporin A and neonatal thymectomy, have similar effects. There are, however, major immunological differences in this model in comparison with Type I diabetes, and results in humans have been much less exciting or convincing. There appear to be two major factors confounding current approaches:

(1)     At diagnosis, about 90% of pancreatic $\beta$-cells are already destroyed and abnormalities of the remaining cells are present. By this stage, the process is likely to be irreversible, although a small proportion of patients will continue to have residual insulin secretion for many years.

(2)     Lack of specificity of the immunosuppressive agents used.

Of the trials that have been carried out, none has been particularly convincing. In a study from New Zealand, 1 year's treatment with prednisone $(0.25\,\mathrm{mg\,kg^{-1}\,day^{-1}})$ in 17 children with recent onset diabetes was associated with increased urinary C-peptide excretion when compared with a control group. Overall, control did not improve and insulin requirements did not change appreciably.

Various studies using plasmapheresis have produced variable results, some suggesting improvement with occasional temporary remission of insulin requirement. Several patients have been treated with a combination of antilymphocyte globulin, plasmapheresis (both over the first month), azathioprine and prednisone, the latter two drugs initially given in high dosage with a prolonged period on smaller dose[29]. One patient had a prolonged remission off insulin, but eventually this had to be re-started.

Immunotherapy with levamisole and interferon have produced very disappointing results. Other trials using antithymocyte globulin and prednisone have caused short-term improvements in glucose tolerance and reversal of the need for insulin therapy, but many side-effects have been recorded. Pilot studies using cyclosporin A are underway, but initial reports give no evidence for any long-term dramatic improvement.

Studies already discussed have indicated that only about 50% of CF-ICA positive first-degree relatives of Type I diabetics will go on to develop the disease. It is clear, therefore, that prediction of who will develop Type I diabetes cannot be done with any great degree of accuracy. In addition, the precision of the immune response to recognize and destroy foreign antigens has not been met by availability of current agents to affect the immune response. In view of the potentially serious side-effects associated with currently available drugs, and their overall lack of specificity, serious questions need to be asked concerning the efficacy of such drug administration in future studies.

## IMMUNOGENETICS OF DIABETIC MICROVASCULAR DISEASE

Duration of diabetes and quality of metabolic control are probably the major determinants of susceptibility to microangiopathy. Approximately 20% of Type I diabetics, however, do not develop clinically evident complications even after 30 years of disease[30]. Indeed, the rate of development and severity of complications between individuals is very variable despite often apparently similar control. The Danes have described a syndrome of 'malignant' microangiopathy, which occurs in about one-third of their Type I diabetics. It is characterized by early onset and extreme severity of complications with poor prognosis, whereas the remaining two-thirds of patients have a more benign course. The concept of other, particularly genetic, susceptibility factors has, therefore, arisen.

Support for a possible immunogenetic association with microangiopathy comes from studies demonstrating raised values of circulating immune complexes and insulin-binding capacity in retinopathy and linear deposition of IgG on the glomerular basement membrane in nephropathy. Whether circulating immune complexes have a pathogenic role in microangiopathy is still controversial. In view of these findings, and the known associations of Type I diabetes with certain HLA loci, there have been many studies of the relationship between HLA and microangiopathy. There have been a number of reports of significant associations between HLA B8, B15 and DR4 and retinopathy and/or nephropathy, but this has not been confirmed by others[30]. Recently, an association between the B3 allotype of the fourth component of complement and microangiopathy has been reported[11]. C4B3 is in linkage disequilibrium with DR4 and which association is primary, if either, is still under study. A similar association with a phenotype of the immunoglobulin heavy chain markers on chromosome 14 (Gm zafnbg) has also been reported[31]. Both complement and the immunoglobulins are concerned with humoral immunity and statistical analysis of the data suggests that the association with both factors is additive, but independent. Whilst it is possible that these phenotypes have a direct effect on the development of microangiopathy, it is, perhaps, more likely that immunogenetic susceptibility to microangiopathy is located in other immune function genes in linkage disequilibrium with either the Gm or C4B loci respectively. It is possible that the action of such genes will at least partly explain the variable rate of development of complications in patients with apparently similar control.

## THE FUTURE

Many of the earlier studies have reported 'associations' with Type I diabetes, but recent work has moved towards 'mechanisms' of disease development. A greater understanding of the immunological aspects in the early stages of Type I diabetes is a key also to understanding the pathogenesis of the disease. DNA probing of the HLA-D region in particular, and perhaps other parts of the HLA-system, will further emphasize the extreme polymorphism of these regions. Studies within and between populations of Type I diabetics will undoubtedly provide further evidence for genetic heterogeneity and, hopefully, will aid in understanding the disease process. Clarification as to whether susceptibility to the disease is controlled by a single gene or genes or whether a combination of different haplotypes is required for such susceptibility is needed.

Further studies of the autoantigen thought to be a pancreatic β-cell specific membrane component are awaited. Attempts are being made to isolate, characterize and sequence this antigen and other antigens are being looked for.

Many attempts, mostly unsuccessful, to influence the course of Type I diabetes by immunotherapy have been made. Better markers for development of Type I diabetes and more specific immunosuppressive agents are required. Molecular cloning of the genes for antigens, antibodies and lymphocyte receptors, as well as HLA antigens, is an important tool for analysis of those components involved in the development of an immune response to an antigen. It has been suggested that production of more specific immuno-suppressive agents might also be possible utilizing these techniques[32]. Indeed, it is likely that recent developments in molecular biology will not only provide a greater understanding of the pathogenesis of Type I, but might also provide a means of prevention and treatment.

## SUMMARY

Diabetes mellitus can be subdivided into two major types which are aetiologically distinct. Studies of identical twins suggest that Type II or non-insulin-dependent diabetes has a strong inherited component, but cannot determine what the component is. There is no evidence for immunological disturbance in this disease. Type I or insulin-dependent diabetes, however, appears to be caused by an environmental agent (or agents), combined with an autoimmune reaction resulting in pancreatic $\beta$-cell destruction in a genetically predisposed individual. The precise events involved, however, are still obscure. In the majority of cases, two genes, or clusters of genes, in linkage disequilibrium with HLA DR3 or DR4, control susceptibility to the disease. Different types of antibodies against islet cells have been observed in susceptible individuals, but complement fixing islet cell antibodies, CF-ICA, seem (at present) to be the most predictive for Type I diabetes. CF-ICA selectively stain $\beta$-cells and are cytotoxic. Islet cell surface antibodies, ICSA, have also recently been described and these can mediate complement-dependent $\beta$-cell cytotoxicity, and impair $\beta$-cell function *in vitro*. The antigen provoking production of ICA has not been characterized. Most recently, by using sera from recently diagnosed Type I diabetics, a large band of 64 000 molecular weight has been obtained by immunoprecipitating proteins from human islet cells.

Although ICA are markers for sensitization towards islet cells, this does not necessarily mean the development of the disease. Cell-mediated immune events appear to be most important at this stage and cellular abnormalities can be demonstrated in both newly diagnosed Type I diabetics, but also in genetically susceptible, otherwise normal, first-degree relatives of Type I diabetics. There are now consistent reports in new Type I diabetics of increases in K-cell numbers, decreased specific and non-specific sup-pressor cell function and the presence of activated T-cells. Receptors for the Fc part of IgG are expressed on already activated T-cells, and this subset appears to be the one increased in some genetically and immunologically susceptible, non-diabetic, first-degree relatives of Type I diabetics. Since some of these subjects will go on to develop the disease, lymphocytes with Fc-IgG receptors might have pathogenetic importance. Recent reports suggest that $\beta$-cell destruction is very specific, with sparing of glucagon- and somatostatin-secreting cells. Most of the autoreactive T-lymphocytes found as part of the insulitis express HLA-DR molecules, indicating that they are activated T-cells and suggesting a specific immune response directed against islet antigens. Recent hypotheses as to the mechanism of autoimmune destruction have included the suggestion that $\beta$-cells might express DR inappropriately in diabetic insulitis. Environmental agents might then trigger a series of events with aberrant DR expression, presentation of surface autoantigens and induction of autoreactive T-helper cells. These would then activate effector B- and T-lymphocytes. Subsequent development of autoimmune disease might then depend on a number of other factors such as abnormalities of the suppressor T-cell pathway. This hypothesis might explain vague associations with viral infections and the long latency period before disease induction.

The very strong evidence for an immunogenetic basis of Type I diabetes offers a possible means of prevention or treatment by immunosuppression. Results have so far been disappointing, probably because treatment is instituted too late and because of the lack of specificity of immunosuppressive agents used. Better markers for development of Type I diabetes and more specific immunosuppressive agents are required. The techniques of molecular biology might be utilized to produce more specific agents, in addition to providing a greater understanding of the aetiology of Type I diabetes.

## ACKNOWLEDGEMENTS

I am most grateful to Dr J. A. Fletcher and Dr A. R. Bradwell for advice on the preparation of this manuscript. I am also grateful to Dr D. A. Pyke for allowing me to quote unpublished data from his unit and to Dr G. F. Bottazzo for useful discussion.

### References

1.  Barnett, A. H., Eff, C., Leslie, R. D. G. and Pyke, D. A. (1981). Diabetes in identical twins: a study of 200 pairs. *Diabetologia*, **20**, 87–93
2.  Nerup, J., Platz, P., Anderson, O. O., Christy, M., Lyngsoe, J., Poulsen, J. E., Ryder, L. P., Staub-Neilsen, L., Thomsen, M. and Svejgaard, A. (1974). HLA antigens and diabetes mellitus. *Lancet*, **2**, 864–6
3.  Cudworth, A. G. and Woodrow, J. C. (1975). HLA system and diabetes mellitus. *Diabetes*, **24**, 345–9
4.  Wolf, E., Spencer, K. M. and Cudworth, A. G. (1983). The genetic susceptibility to type I (insulin dependent) diabetes: analysis of the HLA-DR association. *Diabetologia*, **24**, 224–30
5.  Raum, D., Awdeh, Z. and Yunis, E. (1984). Extended major histocompatibility complex haplotypes in Type I diabetes mellitus. *J. Clin. Invest.*, **74**, 449–54
6.  Johnston, C., Pyke, D. A., Cudworth, A. G. and Wolf, E. (1982). Does the development of Type I (insulin dependent) diabetes depend upon one or two alleles? Studies of HLA-DR3 and DR4 in identical twins. *Diabetologia*, **22**, 388
7.  Owerbach, D., Lernmark, A., Platz, P., Ryder, L. P., Rask, L., Paterson, P. A. and Ludvigsson, J. (1983). HLA-D region beta chain DNA endonuclease fragments differ between HLA-DR identical, healthy and insulin dependent diabetic individuals. *Nature*, (*London*), **303**, 815–7
8.  Michelsen, B., Kastern, W., Lernmark, A. and Owerbach, D. (1985). Identification of an HLA-DQ beta-chain related genomic sequence associated with insulin dependent diabetes. *Biomed. Biochim. Acta*, **44**, 33–6

9. Dausset, J. and Cohen, D. (1984). In Albert, E. D. *et al.*, (eds.) *Histocompatibility Testing.* pp. 22-8. (Berlin, Heidelberg: Springer Verlag)

10. McCluskey, J., McCann, V. J., Kay, P. H., Zilko, P. J., Christiansen, F. T., O'Neill, G. J. and Dawkins, R. L. (1983). HLA and complement allotypes in type I (insulin dependent) diabetes. *Diabetologia*, **24**, 162-5

11. Mijovic, C., Fletcher, J. A., Bradwell, A. R., Harvey, T. and Barnett, A. H. (1985). Relation of gene expression (allotypes) of the fourth component of complement to insulin dependent diabetes and its microangiopathic complications. *Br. Med. J.*, **291**, 9-10

12. Gorsuch, A. N., Spencer, K. M., Wolf, E. and Cudworth, A. G. (1982). HLA and family studies. In Kobberling, J. and Tattersall, R. B. (eds.) *The Genetics of Diabetes Mellitus*, 2nd Edn., pp. 42-53. (London: Academic Press)

13. Rich, S., O'Neill, G., Dalmasso, A. P., Nerl, C. and Barbosa, J. (1985). Complement and HLA. Further definition of high-risk haplotypes in insulin-dependent diabetes. *Diabetes*, **34**, 504-9

14. Bertrams, J. and Baur, M. P. (1985). No interaction between HLA and immunoglobulin IgG heavy chain allotypes in early onset Type I diabetes. *J. Immunogenet.*, **12**, 81-6

15. Hitman, G. A., Tarn, A. C., Williams, L. G., Bottazzo, G. F., Gale, E. A. M. and Galton, D. J. (1986). Genetic analysis of type I diabetes mellitus. In Laron, Z. and Karp, M. (eds.) *Future Trends in Juvenile Diabetes. Paed. Adolesc. Endocr.* Vol. 15. (Basle: S. Karger) (In press)

16. Helgason, T. and Jonasson, M. R. (1981). Evidence for a food additive as a cause of ketosis-prone diabetes. *Lancet*, **2**, 716-20

17. Gamble, D. R. (1980). The epidemiology of insulin dependent diabetes with reference to the relationship of virus infection to its aetiology. *Epidemiol. Rev.*, **2**, 49-70

18. Gorsuch, A. N., Lister, J., Dean, B. M., Spencer, K. M., McNally, J. M. and Bottazzo, G. F. (1981). Evidence for a long prediabetic period in type I (insulin-dependent) diabetes mellitus. *Lancet*, **1**, 1363-5

19. King, M. L., Shaikh, A., Bidwell, D., Voller, A. and Banatvala, J. E. (1983). Coxsackie-B-virus-specific IgM responses in children with insulin-dependent (juvenile-onset; Type I) diabetes mellitus. *Lancet*, **1**, 1397-9

20. Bottazzo, G. F., Florin-Christensen, A. and Doniach, D. (1974). Islet cell antibodies in diabetes mellitus with autoimmune polyendocrine deficiencies. *Lancet*, **2**. 1279-82

21. Bottazzo, G. F., Gorsuch, A. N., Dean, B., Cudworth, A. G. and Doniach, D. (1980) Complement-fixing islet-cell antibodies in Type I diabetes: possible monitors of active beta-cell damage. *Lancet*, **1**, 668-72

22. Lernmark, A., Freedman, Z. R., Hoffman, C., Rubenstein, A. H., Steiner, D. F., Jackson, R. L., Winter, R. J. and Traisman, H. A. (1978). Islet cell surface antibodies in juvenile diabetes mellitus. *N. Engl. J. Med.*, **299**, 375-80

23. Betterle, C., Zanette, F., Tiengo, A. and Trevison, A. (1982). Five year follow-up of non-diabetes with islet cell antibodies. *Lancet*, **1**, 284-5

24. Gorsuch, A. N., Spencer, K. M., Lister, J., Wolf, E., Bottazzo, G. F. and Cudworth, A. G. (1982). Can future Type I diabetes be predicted? A study in families of affected children. *Diabetes*, **31**, 862-6

25. Spencer, K. M., Tarn, A., Dean, B. M., Lister, J. and Bottazzo, G. F. (1984). Fluctuating islet-cell autoimmunity in unaffected relatives of patients with insulin-dependent diabetes. *Lancet*, **1**, 764-6

26. Baekkeskov, S., Nielsen, J. H., Marner, B., Bilde, T., Ludvigsson, J. and Lernmark, A. (1982). Autoantibodies in newly diagnosed diabetic children immunoprecipitate specific human pancreatic islet cell proteins. *Nature (London)*, **298**, 167-9

27. Sensi, M., Pozzilli, P., Gorsuch, A. N., Bottazzo, G. F. and Cudworth, A. G. (1981). Increased killer cell activity in insulin dependent (Type I) diabetes. *Diabetologia*, **20**, 106-9

28. Bottazzo, G. F. (1984). B-cell damage in diabetic insulitis: are we approaching a solution? *Diabetologia*, **26**, 241-9

29. Leslie, R. D. G. and Pyke, D. A. (1980). Immunosuppression of acute insulin-dependent diabetes. In Irvine, W. J. (ed.) *Immunology of Diabetes.* pp. 345-7. (Edinburgh: Teviot Scientific Publications)

30. Barbosa, J. and Saner, B. (1984). Do genetic factors play a role in pathogenesis of microangiopathy? *Diabetologia*, **27**, 487-92

31. Mijovic, C., Fletcher, J., Bradwell, A. R. and Barnett, A. H. (1986). Immunoglobulin heavy chain phenotypes in diabetic microangiopathy - evidence for an immunogenetic predisposition. *Clin. Sci.*, **70**, 56
32. Lernmark, A. (1985). Molecular biology of Type I (insulin-dependent) diabetes mellitus. *Diabetologia*, **28**, 195-203

# 7
# Immunogenetics of Graves' Disease

**H. TAMAI, L. F. KUMAGAI AND S. NAGATAKI**

## INTRODUCTION

The actual aetiology of Graves' disease, like that of Hashimoto's chronic thyroiditis, remains unknown. The condition of hyperthyroidism was initially recognized by Parry in 1786 and recorded cases were published in 1825[1]. Subsequently, Graves, from whom the eponym has been derived, described three cases in greater detail in 1835[2]. Basedow also described the condition in great detail in 1840[3]. It is recognized that females are affected by Graves' disease much more commonly than males, as is true for virtually all thyroidal disorders, the reported ratios varying from 4:1 to 10:1. The familial occurrence of hyperthyroidism has been recognized by several investigators for many years. Bartels found evidence of a familial disposition in 60% of cases with Graves' disease[4]. Pedigrees have been published that have shown a high incidence of Graves' disease in families; however, a definitive pattern of inheritance has not been established. Although hereditary factors appear to be involved in the pathogenesis of Graves' disease, it is apparent that a combination of several genetic and environmental determinants are involved rather than a single gene as being a predominant factor. The twin and clinical family studies initially demonstrated the important role of hereditary factors in Graves' disease. The investigation of autoantibodies and immunogenetic markers have further supported the hereditary importance. Furthermore, the greater rate of concordance of hyperthyroidism among monozygotic twins is also indicative of hereditary determinants in this condition. Retrospective studies of unselected twins demonstrated that about 50% of monozygotic pairs are concordant for hyperthyroidism in contrast to less than 5% of dizygotic pairs[5].

Graves' disease is one of the autoimmune disorders associated with immunogenetic influences. Therefore, it was felt that further clarification of the immunogenetics involved in Graves' disease would be gained by studying the relationship between Graves' disease and specific HLA and Gm determinants in a large number of families.

## FAMILY STUDIES AS A BASIS FOR IMMUNOGENETIC INVESTIGATIONS IN GRAVES' DISEASE

Consanguineous occurrence of Graves' disease has led to the suggestion that hereditary constitutional factors may be important in its pathogenesis. In our studies[6,7], a total of 206 clinically and biochemically euthyroid subjects representing families who had two or more thyrotoxic patients within the second degree was studied. 69 subjects were followed for 6 months to 5 years, and determinations of serum concentrations of $T_4$, $T_3$, TSH, TRH tests and $T_3$ suppression tests were performed once every 6 or 12 months. Results of thyroidal abnormalities found at the initial visit in the 206 euthyroid subjects with family histories of Graves' disease are shown in Table 7.1. Among 206 individuals who had TRH tests at the initial visit, 29 (14%) exhibited a less than normal response, 150 (73%) had normal responses, and 27 (13%) demonstrated increased responses. $T_3$ suppression tests were performed in 117 of 206 subjects; eight (7%) were $T_3$ non-suppressible and all others were $T_3$ suppressible. Three subjects became clinically and biochemically thyrotoxic and two subjects became hypothyroid during the follow-up period. Our data suggested that hyperthyroidism or hypothyroidism occurs frequently among euthyroid relatives who have a family history of Graves' disease, and that thyrotoxicosis occurs frequently in TRH hyporesponders. Chopra et al.[8] studied thyroid function, antithyroidal antibodies and human major histocompatibility locus antigens in first-degree relatives (parents, siblings, and children) of patients with Graves' disease and Hashimoto's thyroiditis. The most common abnormalities in Graves' relatives were the observations of positive antithyroidal antibodies (25 of 75, 34%) and supranormal TSH responses to TRH (12 of 44, 27%). Less common abnormalities were goitre (10 of 92, 11%), ophthalmopathy (1 of 92, 1.1%), $T_3$ non-suppressibility (2 of 48, 4.2%), elevated baseline serum TSHs (4 of 80, 5%), subnormal responses to TRH (2 of 44, 4.5%), and detectable LATS-protector (3 of 47, 6.4%). Ingbar et al.[9] also studied peripheral thyroxine turnover in 12 clinically euthyroid relatives of five thyrotoxic patients. Circulating thyroxine half-lives were significantly diminished. Although thyroidal radioactive iodine uptakes averaged 61% in this group, basal metabolic rates and protein bound iodine values were normal. Thus two distinct abnormalities in the metabolism of iodine were found in certain eumetabolic relatives of patients with Graves' disease: (1) an augmented rate of peripheral degradation of thyroxine, and (2) an increased thyroidal avidity for iodine. As shown in our study[10], the clinical picture and serum antithyroidal antibodies in 16 pairs of siblings with Graves' disease were compared with age- and sex-matched groups of 32 patients with Graves' disease who did not have a family history of any thyroidal disease (control patients). There were significant differences in the frequency and mean titres of antibodies to thyroglobulin between paired-sibling patients and controls. Lymphoid follicles and epithelial degeneration were observed more often in the thyroids of paired sibling patients than in those of the controls. Moreover, there was a strong tendency of increased lymphocyte and plasma cell infiltration in the thyroids of the paired sibling patients with Graves' disease. Several studies have also demonstrated that both Graves' disease and

**Table 7.1** Thyroid abnormalities in 206 euthyroid relatives with a family history of Graves' disease[7]

| Thyroid abnormalities | No. of subjects |
|---|---|
| Abnormal response to TRH | 56/206 (27.1) |
| No response or hyporesponse | 29/206 (14.1) |
| Hyper-response | 27/206 (13.1) |
| T₃ non-suppressibility | 8/117 (6.8) |
| Positive antithyroid antibody | |
| TGHA* | 43/206 (20.7) |
| MCHA† | 114/206 (55.2) |

The percentages of the total number of subjects are in parentheses.
* Antithyroglobulin haemagglutination antibodies (positive titre, $\geq 2\times 10^2$).
† Antithyroid microsomal haemagglutination antibodies (positive titre, $\geq 2\times 10^2$).

Hashimoto's thyroiditis are commonly found in near relatives of patients with Hashimoto's thyroiditis. Actually, our results from earlier studies in euthyroid Graves' disease suggested that thyroid function tests in subjects with euthyroid Graves' disease are quite variable and that euthyroid Graves' disease, Graves' disease, and Hashimoto's thyroiditis are closely related to each other and cannot be clearly separated before the clinical onset of each disease[11]. Banovac et al.[12] reported that none of 76 euthyroid relatives of patients with Graves' disease had either detectable LATS or thyroid-stimulating antibodies (TSAb) in their sera, but seven of 41 sera were slightly positive for TSH-binding inhibiting antibodies (TBIAb). The first hint that autoimmune antibodies might be involved with the pathogenesis of Graves' disease came with the discovery that LATS was associated with the Ig fraction of serum proteins[13,14]. In 50 relatives of ten families, thyroidal diseases were found in 20%, positive LATS-IgG responses in 30%, and thyroid antibodies in 23%[15]. These authors suggested the existence of a thyroid metabolic abnormality in the families of patients with thyrotoxicosis and argued against LATS as being the cause of the hyperthyroidism of Graves' disease. Bartels reported extensive studies in many Copenhagen families[4] with a history of hyperthyroidism. He investigated 204 propositi with Graves' disease and 21 with toxic nodular goitre. The incidence of Graves' disease among female relatives was greater than one would expect in a control population. The increased incidence of both hyperthyroid disorders was thought to be due to hereditary factors in the above studies because not only mothers and daughters, but also aunts were affected, so that more than environmental factors alone were thought to be involved[16]. The sera of parents and siblings of 74 patients with diffuse toxic goitre were examined for antithyroidal antibodies[17]. The incidence of antithyroglobulin and antimicrosomal antibodies in 57 mothers and 101 daughters was significantly higher than in the controls. These data also suggested that there is a hereditary influence on the production of antithyroidal antibodies. Organ-specific autoimmune diseases are found with increased frequency not only in patients with Graves' disease, but also among their relatives. Subclinical serological evidence of autoimmunity is found in relatives even more commonly than clinical disease[18]. Graves' disease and thyroid antibodies have been observed more often than expected among patients with Down's syndrome and their maternal relatives[19,20]. The biological implications of these associations are unclear, but it is possible that common pathogenetic mechanisms are involved in the development of chromosomal aberrations and thyroidal autoimmunity[21]. As previously mentioned, many family studies, especially euthyroid relatives of patients with Graves' disease, have been reported. Thyroidal abnormalities have been demonstrated among euthyroid relatives with a significantly higher incidence than in normal unrelated subjects. There are very few long-term follow-up studies showing the relationship between thyroidal abnormalities found in euthyroid relatives and the development of Graves' disease. These studies are being accumulated and will be reported at a future date.

## TSH RECEPTOR ANTIBODIES AND HLA DISEASE ASSOCIATIONS

### TSH receptor antibodies

The concept of a genetic origin or predisposition to Graves' disease and also to Hashimoto's thyroiditis, has been strongly suggested[4,22], and studied mainly by determining defects in immune surveillance[13,23]. Present concepts suggest that TSH receptor antibodies may be the result of antigen-specific suppressor cell defects, thus allowing the unabated production of TSH receptor antibodies[24,25]. Numerous investigators have reported high and varying incidences of positive results of increased TSH receptor antibodies in untreated or active Graves' disease[26-30]. The interlaboratory variations in results may be due to a number of factors, e.g. variations in TSH receptor antibody assay methodology, membrane preparative techniques, the source and species of thyroid glands, and purity of radioiodinated TSH. Despite many variable factors, the aforementioned studies have reported TSH receptor antibodies in about 70–80% of untreated Graves' patients. Various technical factors and differences in the degree of sensitivity of various assays may account for the lack of detection in the remaining subjects. The undetectability of TSH receptor antibodies could also be indicative of important pathophysiological variations in Graves' disease[31]. Mukhtar et al.[32] investigated the effect of various therapeutic modalities on TBIAb levels. The frequency of TBIAb in patients treated by carbimazole (4–18 months) was 53%; by radioiodine (6 months–4 years post-therapy) was 50% and by subtotal thyroidectomy (4–12 months postoperatively) was 17%. Antithyroidal drugs per se may reduce TSH receptor antibody levels directly[31]. McGregor et al.[33] demonstrated that irradiation of peripheral blood lymphocytes inhibited their ability to generate IgG and thyroglobulin antibodies in culture. On the other hand, if intrathyroidal lymphocytes are the major source of TSH receptor antibodies, then levels of the latter probably should decrease more rapidly after surgery than has been observed[31].

## TSH receptor antibodies as determined by thyroid stimulating assay

Zakarija *et al.*[34] correlated thyroid-stimulating antibodies (TSAb) with the clinical course in 187 patients with Graves' disease. In 64 patients with newly diagnosed hyperthyroidism, 59 were positive; 36 of 38 patients tested early in therapy were also positive. The incidence of positive results of thyroid-stimulating immunoglobulins in Graves' disease has been reported[35-39] to vary between 61 and 91%. Rapaport *et al.*[40] demonstrated that 57 of 61 patients with untreated hyperthyroid Graves' disease were TSAb positive (93%) using a sensitive, specific and practical bioassay. TSAb was undetectable in all normal subjects and in patients with Hashimoto's thyroiditis, non-toxic goitre, and toxic nodular goitre. Atkinson and Kendall-Taylor[41] reported a thyroid stimulation assay in which $T_3$ incremental increases were measured after the *in vitro* incubation of porcine thyroid tissues with serum. Forty-four of 49 serum samples in Graves' patients were positive. Smythe *et al.*[42] concluded that idiopathic non-toxic goitre, toxic nodular goitre with functioning nodules (Plummer's disease), and Graves' disease shared, in part, a common pathogenesis according to determinations of TSAb using a highly sensitive cytochemical section bioassay. The most persuasive study supporting the usefulness of TSH receptor antibody measurements is that of Zakarija *et al.*[34]. Twenty-eight patients received antithyroidal drug therapy and thyroid-stimulating antibodies were measured at the cessation of therapy. Thirteen patients were negative and 12 of 15 relapsed patients were positive. Davis *et al.*[43] demonstrated that after discontinuing antithyroidal drugs after 6 months of treatment, 16 patients relapsed within 6 months of stopping therapy, and all patients with high levels of thyroid-stimulating antibodies (TSAb) at the time of drug withdrawal relapsed within 2 months, whereas all patients with low or undetectable TSAb activity at the time of drug discontinuation remained in remission. The data indicated, therefore, that an accurate and useful predictor of the early clinical course of Graves' disease, after withdrawal of antithyroidal drugs, could be made in patients with high or low levels of TSAb. The clinical usefulness in long-term predictability, however, has not proven to be nearly as good.

## TSH receptor blocking antibodies

Interest in the understanding of TSH receptor blocking antibodies was initiated by the report of Matsuura *et al.*[44] in 1980 of a hypothyroid mother who was maintained euthyroid with exogenous thyroid hormone throughout pregnancy and gave birth to two hypothyroid sons. The authors astutely reasoned that the mother and offspring could have anti-TSH receptor antibodies that were blocking TSH action and thereby resulting in hypothyroidism. They confirmed their hypothesis by measuring the ability of antibodies contained in the $\gamma$-globulin fractions from the three subjects to inhibit [$^{125}$I]TSH binding to human thyroid membranes. Several other investigators have extended these findings and have demonstrated the presence of TSH receptor blocking antibodies in the sera of 15–25% of adult primary hypothyroid patients[28,45-48]. Therefore, the concept that clinical hypothyroidism can result from the occurrence of TSH receptor blocking antibodies appears to be established.

Burman and Baker[31] described in their recent review that if the foregoing is correct, our concept, that all primary hypothyroidism results from thyroid damage rendering the gland incapable of generating sufficient $T_4$ and $T_3$ to maintain euthyroidism and resulting in increased serum TSH levels, must be altered. They also suggested that the clinical utility of TSH receptor antibodies would be useful in the following: (1) to help diagnose Graves' disease when the aetiological diagnosis of hyperthyroidism may be in doubt; (The diagnosis of Graves' disease has implications with regards to remission, response to antithyroidal drugs and to radioiodine, and with regards to family counselling); (2) to help diagnose Graves' disease in patients with ophthalmopathy or proptosis, especially in patients with unilateral proptosis; (3) to help predict the possibility that an infant will be born with hypothyroidism or hyperthyroidism, albeit either neonatal condition is very infrequent.

## HLA

HLA is a region on chromosome 6 which includes several genetic loci. The effects of most of these genes are expressed on cell surfaces. HLA is structurally and functionally homologous to the major histocompatability region in mice (where it is called H-2). Many biologically important functions including qualitative and quantitative control of immune responses to certain antigens, killing of virus-infected cells, and synthesis of several complement components have been associated with the major histocompatability complex of several species[49,50]. Irvine et al.[51] have observed a difference in the frequency of HLA-B8 between patients with recurrent Graves' disease and patients in remission (69% vs. 40%) and an even greater difference when compared with control subjects (28%). A similar conclusion was reached by Beck et al.[52], who noted recurrence rates of 81% and 84% in HLA-B8 and HLA-Dw3 positive patients compared to HLA-B8 and HLA-Dw3 negative patients. The latter patients had recurrence rates of 61% and 59% respectively. On the other hand, McGregor et al.[53] have shown that within a year of stopping a 6-month course of carbimazole treatment, 41 of 65 patients (63%) with Graves' disease had a recurrence. By combined analysis of the HLA-DRw3 status and the level of TSH receptor antibodies at the time of drug withdrawal, relapses or remissions could be predicted in 62 of 65 patients. One hundred and fifty patients with toxic diffuse goitres were HLA typed by Schleusener et al.[54]. One group consisted of 101 patients with concomitant Graves' ophthalmopathy and/or TSH-binding inhibiting antibodies (GBIAb). Forty-nine patients had neither ophthalmopathy nor TBIAb. The former group showed a higher prevalence of HLA-B8 and DR3 antigens compared to a normal control group. The latter group showed a higher frequency of HLApDR5, whereas the HLA-B8 and DR3 antigens were slightly below the normal prevalence. These data indicate an immunogenetic heterogeneity in patients with toxic diffuse goitre. Patients with long-term remission did not show a different prevalence of any of the HLA antigens compared to controls. In contrast, patients with Graves' ophthalmopathy and/or TBIAb activity who relapsed had a significantly higher prevalence of HLA-B8, DR3, whereas patients without TBIAb and eye signs who relapsed had a significantly greater prevalence of HLA-DR5 than the control group. However, Allannic et al.[55] reported different results. They studied 111 unselected patients with hyperthyroidism due to Graves' disease who had been treated with carbimazole for 18 months. Seventy-two patients were followed for 2 years after withdrawal of treatment. Of the 72 patients, 37 relapsed and 35 remained in remission. Forty patients were DR3 positive (20 relapsed) and 32 were DR3 negative (17 relapsed). HLA frequency was not significantly different in relapsed patients or in those who remained in remission. The authors concluded that HLA frequency cannot be used to predict relapse of hyperthyroidism due to Graves' disease. Wenzel and Lente[56] treated Graves' disease patients longitudinally with either PTU, methimazole (MMI), or perchlorate. Five of ten patients receiving PTU and eight of 13 patients receiving MMI attained normal TBIAb levels. TBIAb levels also decreased to normal in 11 of 18 patients receiving perchlorate. In all three groups, however, a decrease in $T_4$ and $T_3$ levels preceded the fall in TBIAb. The authors concluded that the immunomodulating effects of MMI and PTU must be minimal *in vivo* if present at all, assuming that perchlorate was not immunosuppressive. Weetman et al., however, have recently reported in preliminary studies that perchlorate itself decreases immunoglobulin synthesis *in vitro*[57].

## HLA AND IgG HEAVY CHAIN ALLOTYPES (Gm) IN GRAVES' DISEASE

### Population studies of HLA

It is well recognized that inheritance patterns of disease susceptibility can be elucidated if the disease is associated with genetic markers, e.g. red blood cell groups. Such associations are helpful in specific disease diagnosis as well as identifying patients who may be at risk[18]. HLA antigens are genetic markers which are most often associated with autoimmune disorders and are divided into two morphologically and functionally distinct groups: Class I and Class II. Of the Class I human antigens, three different types are noted as A, B and C. The Class II human antigens are composed of three different types, DR, DQ and DP. Each type relates to a different gene in the major histocompatibility complex[31]. The most important function of HLA antigens is the regulation of immune responses to certain antigens. In Graves' disease, significant differences in the frequency of certain HLA antigens compared to that in normal subjects have been reported by many investigators: HL-A8[58], W5[59], HLA-B8[60], HLA-B8, Dw3[61], HLA-B8, Dw3, DRw3[62], HLA-DRw3[54], HLA-DR3, DR5[55], and HLA-DR5[63]. The first evidence of a significant association between HLA8 and Graves' disease in Caucasians was reported by Grumet et al.[58]. Evidence of genetic control of susceptibility to Graves' disease was sought using HLA antigens as genetic markers. Their study was performed in 62 unrelated Caucasian patients with Graves' disease. The frequency of HLA-B8 antigen among the patients was 47% compared to an incidence of 21% in controls. Grumet et al.[59] also described HLA findings in

44 Japanese patients with Graves' disease. The frequency of the W5 antigen among the Japanese patients (57%) was significantly greater than among controls (20%). They concluded that the occurrence of different HLA antigens in association with the same disease in different ethnic groups indicates that the use of HLA antigens as disease susceptibility markers must be confirmed for each ethnic group under study. Farid et al.[60], in a study of Graves' disease in an isolated and inbred Newfoundland population, reported an increased frequency of patients who apparently had HLA-B8 in both of their haplotypes. They suggested that HLA-B8 homozygosity confers an increased risk for Graves' disease compared to HLA-B8 heterozygocity. We found[63] in a study of 30 unrelated probands in Japanese families that the antigen frequency of HLA-DR5 was significantly increased, 30%, compared with 5% in a control group ($p < 3.0 \times 10^{-3}$). The association between Graves' disease and HLA-DR5 indicated that an HLA-linked disease susceptibility gene was in strong linkage disequilibrium with HLA-DR5 (Table 7.2). The HLA-DRw3, class II antigen, has an increased incidence of 60% in Caucasian Graves' disease patients compared to 11% of the control population. One might postulate that due to their pivotal role in antigen presentation, a particular class II antigen might facilitate the development or propagation of an autoimmune response to thyroid antigens. Several studies have shown that Graves' disease patients who have DRw3 antigenic determinants develop the disease earlier and have more recalcitrant disease which is less likely to respond to medical antithyroid therapy[31,52,55,58,64-66].

**Table 7.2** Association between Graves' disease and HLA[63]

| HLA-antigens | Graves' disease (n = 30) | Control group (n = 80) | $\chi^2$ | Pc | RR |
|---|---|---|---|---|---|
| DR5 | 9(30.0%) | 4( 5.0%) | 13.08 | $<3.0 \times 10^{-3}$ | 8.14 |
| DRw8 | 11(36.7%) | 13(16.3%) | 5.82 | NS | 3.07 |

DR5 and DRw8 were determined using 11 and 5 sera, respectively, from the 8th International Histocompatibility Workshop[18]. *Pc*: *P* multiplied by the number of HLA-DR antigens studied. *RR*, relative risk.

## Population studies of Gm

Two groups of immune response genes have been identified and studied extensively in humans and in animals. One group is linked to the major histocompatibility complex (MHC) and the other is grouped to genes which control immunoglobulin (Ig) allotypic determinants of·the heavy (H) chain group[67-69]. Furthermore, genes controlling the idiotypes of specific antibodies have been shown to be linked with the IgG H-chain gene complex[70,71]. Nakao et al.[72] found in 1980 that the Gm (1, 2, 21) haplotype was increased in patients with Graves' disease or Hashimoto's thyroiditis. Farid et al.[73] also reported that the Gm haplotype, Gmf,b or Gmf,n,b was found in all 40 patients with Graves' disease studied contrasted with 35 of 40 controls and 20 of 31 patients with Hashimoto's thyroiditis. The difference in incidence in the Gm haplotype between the two groups with autoimmune thyroid disease was significant. These results suggested that thyroid-stimulating antibodies may be allotypically restricted and that Gm typing is likely to be a useful genetic marker for Graves' disease, in addition to HLA and phenylthiocarbamide (PTC) testing. The frequencies of the antigens, HLA-B8 and DR3, are increased in Caucasians with Graves' disease[62]; however, the existence of HLA-B8, DRw3-negative patients with Graves' disease and the lack of any association with HLA-B8 or DRw3 in Japanese patients point out the difficulty in interpretation of association of HLA antigens and Graves' disease[72,74]. Therefore, the existence of a polygenic background in Graves' disease represents a reasonable hypothesis in explaining disease susceptibility. The Gm genes may be in chromosome 14 and they cannot be very close to the HLA region[75]. Nakao et al.[72] therefore postulated that their data suggested the existence of disease-susceptible genes linked to Gm genes, and different from the HLA-linked susceptibility genes.

## Family studies of HLA and Gm haplotypes

Family studies represent an excellent approach to investigating associations between HLA antigens and diseases; however, they are generally more difficult to perform because they require kinships in which two or more siblings or other relatives (but not a parent and single child, who always share one haplotype) are affected with the same disease. Family studies have an important asset in their ability to provide information about the inheritance of disease susceptibility. Since complete HLA haplotypes are almost always inherited as a unit, family studies can be used to demonstrate HLA-linked disease-predisposing genes even if they are not associated with any detectable antigen in the population[18]. Therefore, to identify the genes governing susceptibility to Graves' disease, we studied a large number of Japanese families as described below[76]. We found evidence for the existence of two genes controlling the susceptibility to Graves' disease, one closely linked to HLA, the other linked to the gene coding for the Gm allotype[63]. Our studies[76] were performed in 243 members of 37 families in which two or more first-degree relatives had hyperthyroid Graves' disease, hereafter referred to as Graves' disease. In 27 families, 173 members were studied; 70 (40%) of them had Graves' disease and none had Hashimoto's disease. In the other ten families with 70 members, 26 (37%) had Graves' disease and 14 (20%) had Hashimoto's thyroiditis among first-degree relatives. After the complete analysis of HLA and Gm haplotypes for all members studied in each family, the particular HLA and Gm haplotypes that were found to be concordant in two members with Graves' disease in each family were defined as being the disease-associated haplotypes. The data in the remaining members of the families were then examined to determine those in whom one or both of the disease-associated haplotypes was present or those in whom both were lacking. The findings were correlated with the presence or absence of thyroid disease. Representative examples of this type of analysis are shown in Figures 7.1 and 7.2. Figure 7.1 shows the association between Graves' disease and

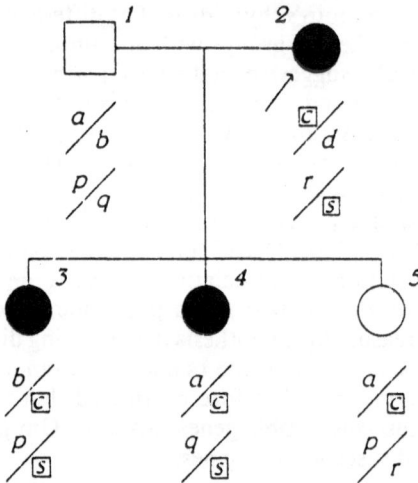

**Figure 7.1** A family with Graves' disease. ●, Graves' disease; a) HLA-A9, B22, Cw1-; b) HLA-A9, B51, Cw3; c) HLA-A26, B40, Cw3; d) HLA-A-, B-, C-; p, Gm (1, 21, 17, 26); q, Gm (1, 11, 13, 15, 16, 17); r, Gm (1, 11, 13, 10, 15, 16, 17); s, Gm (1, 2, 21, 17, 26). From ref. 76

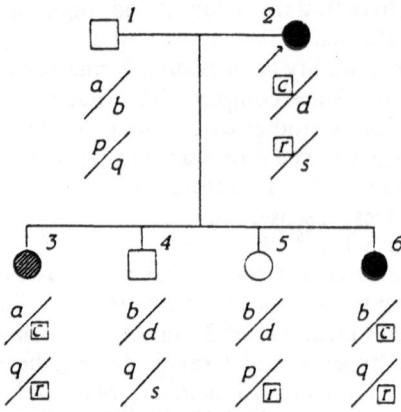

**Figure 7.2** A family with Graves' and Hashimoto's diseases. ●, Graves' disease; ◧, Hashimoto's disease; a) HLA-A2, B40, Cw3; b) HLA-A9, Bw51, Cw-; c) HLA-A26, B40, Cw-; d) HLA-A-, B7, Cw-; p, Gm (1, 3, 5, 13, 23); q, Gm (1, 13, 15, 16, 17); r, Gm (1, 2, 21, 17, 26); s, Gm (1, 17, 21). From ref. 76

HLA and Gm haplotypes in a representative family. Haplotypes of HLA (a,b,c, and d) and haplotypes of Gm (p,q,r, and s) were determined by analysing HLA-A, -B, and -C antigens and Gm haplotypes in all members of the family. The disease-associated haplotypes of HLA and Gm were identified by determining concordant haplotypes in two members with Graves' disease. In the family depicted, the disease-associated haplotypes of HLA-(c) and

Gm(s) were identified in patients 2 and 3. Another sibling (no. 4) had the disease-associated haplotypes of both HLA and Gm and also had Graves' disease. The other sibling (no. 5) had only the disease-associated HLA haplotype and did not have Graves' disease. We found that all affected siblings except one female shared the disease-associated haplotypes with both HLA and Gm. However, siblings who shared the disease-associated haplotypes did not necessarily have overt clinical disease. Table 7.3 shows the occurrence of thyroid disease in all members of 37 families in which two or more first-degree relatives had Graves' disease. Among 96 patients with Graves' disease, 74 patients (two members in each family) served as the basis for identifying the disease-associated haplotypes. Among the remaining 22 patients with Graves' disease, 21 had the disease-associated haplotypes of both HLA and Gm and one had only the Gm haplotype. Among 97 subjects who had only one or none of the disease-associated haplotypes of HLA and Gm (16 with HLA, only 39 with Gm only, and 42 with neither HLA nor Gm), only one had Graves' disease. Although not shown, there was no significant difference in the frequency of any HLA antigen or Gm allotype between normal Japanese subjects and the patients with Graves' disease in the above study. We analysed the segregation of Graves' disease and HLA and Gm haplotypes in 15 selected families[63]. Statistical significance of this genetic association between the development of Graves' disease and particular HLA and Gm haplotypes in each family was analysed by the sib-pair method using 62 siblings in the families. Siblings under 10-years-old were excluded from analysis because Graves' disease is rare below this age (Table 7.4). The strong association between the development of Graves' disease and HLA and Gm haplotypes indicated that there might be two genes linked to HLA and Gm respectively, which had a major influence on the development of Graves' disease. As

**Table 7.3** Association among Graves' and Hashimoto's diseases; HLA and Gm haplotypes in 37 families (243 subjects) in which two or more first-degree relatives were affected with Graves' disease. From ref. 76

| | Concordance of disease-associated haplotypes* of | | | | |
|---|---|---|---|---|---|
| | Both HLA and Gm | HLA only | Gm only | Neither HLA nor Gm | Total |
| Graves' disease | 95 (74+21)† | 0 | 1 | 0 | 96 (74+22) |
| Hashimoto's disease | 14 | 0 | 0 | 0 | 14 |
| Others | 37 | 16 | 38 | 42 | 133 |
| Total | 146 | 16 | 39 | 42 | 243 |

*After complete analysis of HLA and Gm haplotypes in all members studied in each family, the particular HLA and Gm haplotypes that were found to be concordant in two members with Graves' disease in each family were defined as being the disease-associated haplotypes.
†Seventy-four members with Graves' disease (two in each family) served as the basis for determining the disease-associated haplotypes.

**Table 7.4** Association between Graves' disease and HLA and Gm haplotypes in 15 families. From ref. 63

| | | Disease-associated haplotypes of HLA and Gm allotype | | |
| | | Positive* | Negative† | p |
| --- | --- | --- | --- | --- |
| Total sib | Affected | 17 | 1 | |
| (n = 62) | Unaffected | 15 | 14 | $<2.0 \times 10^{-3}$ |
| | | | | |
| Female sib | Affected | 14 | 1 | |
| (n = 50) | Unaffected | 8 | 12 | $<2.0 \times 10^{-3}$ |
| | | | | |
| Male sib | Affected | 3 | 0 | |
| (n = 12) | Unaffected | 7 | 2 | NS |

One affected sibling used to determine disease-associated haplotypes in each family was excluded from this analysis. The p value was calculated by Fisher's exact method. NS, not significant.
*Positive for disease-associated HLA and Gm haplotypes.
†Negative for either or both disease-associated HLA haplotype and Gm haplotype.

previously mentioned, in a study of 30 unrelated probands in families, the antigen frequency of 30% of HLA-DR5 was significantly increased, compared to 5% in control groups (Table 7.2). The association between Graves' disease and HLA-DR5 indicated that an HLA-linked disease susceptibility gene was in strong linkage disequilibrium with HLA-DR5. The only other study of large numbers of families was reported by Farid et al.[77]. Fifteen families with sibling or mother–child pairs with Graves' disease were studied and although linkage of Graves' disease to specific HLA-defined haplotypes was apparent, no specific HLA antigen was found to be associated with the disease. It was postulated that although the actual gene associated with Graves' disease was randomly distributed throughout the population, gene expression could be facilitated by DRw3, thus explaining the association with this particular antigen. Adams et al.[78] failed to show involvement of immunoglobulin genes in family studies testing for associated inheritance of Graves' disease and immunoglobulin allotypes. The HLA-D region is assumed to be comparable to the I-region of murine H-2 complex, in which immune response genes (Ir genes), and immune suppression genes (Is genes) are located. Recently, it has become more evident that HLA-linked Ir genes or Is genes exist in man[79,80]. In the murine system, it has been demonstrated that idiotype determinants are linked to heavy-chain constant region allotypic markers[81,82], and the idiotypic determinants of antigen-specific receptors on lymphocyte membranes are likely to have fundamental roles in immune regulation. It was, therefore, assumed that two genes, HLA-linked and Gm-linked, could govern the specific immune response to certain antigens relevant to the development of Graves' disease. The elucidation of antigens and environmental or other factors involved in the pathogenesis of Graves' disease will, in turn, help to clarify the immunogenetic factors controlling the susceptibility to Graves' disease.

## GENETIC CONTROL OF DISEASE SUSCEPTIBILITY

Many authors have noted the occurrence of hyperthyroidism in two or more family members. Bartels[4] found evidence of familial disposition in 60% of cases with toxic diffuse goitre. Because there was increased incidence of hyperthyroidism in the aunts of the affected parents as well as among the daughters and mothers, Bartels concluded that genetic rather than environmental factors were responsible for the increased familial incidence. He considered the data compatible with the hypothesis that one or more recessive genes could cause an underlying instability of the thyroid which could manifest itself in different ways. Similar studies by Martin and Fisher[83] suggested that a recessive gene was responsible in the aetiology of Graves' disease. Family studies in 57 male patients who had undergone subtotal thyroidectomies for either Graves' disease or non-toxic goitre indicated that genetic determinants of a complex nature appeared to contribute to the pathogenesis of both thyroidal disorders[16,84]. Other family studies[16,85] investigated the determination of antithyroidal antibodies in juvenile thyrotoxicosis. Eleven of 12 propositi had elevated antibodies and either antithyroglobulin or antimicrosomal antibodies were found in ten of 11 propositi. The predisposition to form antithyroidal antibodies was postulated to be inherited in dominant fashion in Graves' disease as in Hashimoto's thyroiditis. Howell-Evans *et al.*[17] investigated this problem extensively by determining antithyroidal antibodies in sera of parents and siblings of 74 patients with Graves' disease. The incidence of thyroglobulin and thyroid microsomal antigens in 57 (mothers) and 101 daughters was significantly higher than in the controls, indicating a much greater likelihood of forming antithyroidal antibodies. The authors indicated, however, that the mode of inheritance was not simple and thought that several genes might be involved. The pattern of autoantibody occurrence found in relatives of Graves' disease patients is not consistent with simple autosomal dominant or recessive inheritance[86,87]. Moreover, recessive inheritance is difficult to reconcile with pedigrees showing transmission of Graves' disease through multiple generations[88-91]. Several examples of apparent male to male transmission of Graves' disease rule out X-linked mechanisms in those families[89,92,93]. In our study[94], two genetic models, which could not be distinguished by the affected sib-pair method, were proposed: (1) an HLA-linked recessive gene with a frequency of 0.30 plus a Gm-linked recessive gene with a frequency of 0.10; (2) an HLA-linked dominant gene with a frequency of 0.08 plus a Gm-linked recessive gene with a frequency of 0.10. Within the small recombination fraction between HLA and HLA-linked loci (<5%) perturbation in gene frequency was not significant in our studies. Sasazuki *et al.*[95] reported that the mode of inheritance and gene frequency of HLA-linked disease susceptibility gene were inferred by using the affected sib-pair method developed and utilized by Cudworth and Woodrow[96], Day and Simons[98], Thomson and Bodmer[98], and Svejgaard and Ryder[99]. Sasazuki demonstrated that the dominant model was clearly rejected if their data were analysed with that of Farid and Bear[100]. Of 43 affected sib-pairs, 27 shared two, 14 shared one, and two shared no HLA haplotypes. It was thus possible to identify the HLA-linked recessive gene which had a major effect on the development of Graves' disease[95]. Stenszky et al.[101] showed from clinical and family studies in Hungary, that genetic variation in Graves' disease susceptibility was related to polymorphism at MHC loci. Among 1980 relatives of 534 index patients, 2.9% of the siblings, 2.7% of offspring, and 3.0% of parents had Graves' disease. HLA haplotype combinations in affected sibling pairs were determined from their data and combined with data in the literature, (Farid[102], Chan et al.[103] and Sasazuki et al.[95]). Forty-three, 23, and one affected sibling pairs shared two, one and no HLA haplotypes, respectively. This distribution is inconsistent with simple dominant inheritance of HLA-related susceptibility over a range of gene frequencies (0.2–0.4). The distribution of HLA haplotypes in 33 families related disease susceptibility more strongly to DR than to other loci. The authors suggested that the probability that an individual will be affected with Graves' disease can be predicted, based on sex, HLA genotype, and family history.

## OTHER FACTORS AS A TRIGGER FOR THE ONSET OF GRAVES' DISEASE

Graves' disease is thought to be a multifactorial disease and in addition to hereditary influences, other factors such as 'stress', infections, environmental factors, etc. may play important roles as triggers for the development of Graves' disease. The actual event(s) precipitating Graves' disease remain(s) unknown. The possibility that emotional or chronic stresses may alter the immune system response may be raised because, after obtaining clinical histories, they are associated not infrequently with the onset of the disease. Joasoo et al.[104] found a significantly higher frequency of complement-fixing antibodies to influenza B virus in patients with Graves' disease than in a comparable number of controls.

## CONCLUSION

It appears highly unlikely that Graves' disease is a single entity with a simple pattern of inheritance. Nevertheless, a familial or hereditary predisposition for the development of Graves' disease has been convincingly demonstrated in numerous clinical and family studies. The participation of genetic factors has been clearly shown by the HLA association and twin studies of Graves' disease. There is little doubt that Graves' disease is a multifactorial entity and its aetiology may be heterogeneous. Further investigation of clinical, immunological and immunogenetic factors in members of families with Graves' disease will undoubtedly provide insight into the aetiological heterogeneity of the disorder. From our studies and a review of the literature, it is evident that the development of Graves' disease results from a combination of genetic determinants which involve the immune systems and undetermined factors that 'trigger' the production of thyroid-stimulating immunoglobulins resulting in the onset of hyperthyroid Graves' disease.

# References

1. Parry, C. H. (1825). *Collections from Unpublished Medical Writings of the Late Caleb Hillier Parry.* Vol. 2, p. 111. (London: Underwoods)
2. Graves, R. G. (1835). Newly observed affection of the thyroid gland in females. *Lond. Med. Surg. J.*, 7, 516–20
3. von Basedow, K. A. (1840). Exophthalmos druch Hypertrophie der Zellgewebes in der Augenhöhle. *Wschr. Ges. Heilk.*, 14, 197
4. Bartels, E. D. (1941). *Heredity in Graves' Disease.* (Copenhagen: Munksgaard)
5. Verscheur, O. V. (1958). Die Zwillingsforschung im Dienste der innern Medizin. *Verhand. Deut. Gesell. Inn. Med.*, 64, 262–73
6. Tamai, H., Suematsu, H., Ikemi, Y., Kuma, K., Matsuzuka, F., Kumagai, L. F., Shizume, K. and Nagataki, S. (1978). Responses to TRH and $T_3$ suppression tests in euthyroid subjects with a family history of Graves' disease. *J. Clin. Endocrinol. Metab.*, 47, 475–9
7. Tamai, H., Ohsako, N., Takeno, K., Fukino, O., Takahashi, H., Kuma, K., Kumagai, L. F. and Nagataki, S. (1980). Changes in thyroid function in euthyroid subjects with family history of Graves' disease; a follow-up study of 69 patients. *J. Clin. Endocrinol. Metab.*, 51, 1123–8
8. Chopra, I. J., Solomon, D. H., Chopra, U., Yoshihara, E., Teraski, P. L. and Smith, F. (1977). Abnormalities in thyroid function in relatives of patients with Graves' disease and Hashimoto's thyroiditis: lack of correlation with inheritance of HLA-B8. *J. Clin. Endocrinol. Metab.*, 45, 45–54
9. Ingbar, S. H., Freinkel, N., Dowling, J. T. and Kumagai, L. F. (1965). Abnormalities of iodine metabolism in euthyroid relatives with Graves' disease, *J. Clin. Invest.*, 35, 714
10. Tanaka, T., Katayama, S., Kuma, K., Tamai, T., Matsuzuka, F. and Hidaka, H. (1980). Clinical and pathological significance of sibling Graves' disease. *Acta Endocrinol.*, 94, 498–502
11. Tamai, H., Nakagawa, T., Ohsako, N., Fukino, O., Takahashi, H., Matsuzuka, F., Kuma, K. and Nagataki, S. (1980). Changes in thyroid functions in patients with euthyroid Graves' disease. *J. Clin. Endocrinol. Metab.*, 50, 108–12
12. Banovac, K., Zakarija, M., Mckenzie, J. M., Witte, S. and Sekso, M. (1981). Absence of thyroid stimulating antibody and long acting thyroid stimulator in relatives of Graves' disease patients. *J. Clin. Endocrinol. Metab.*, 53, 651–3
13. Werner, S. C. (1978). Etiology, pathogenesis, immune system, other mechanism, emotional factors. In Werner, S. C. and Ingbar, S. H. (eds.) *The Thyroid: A Fundamental and Clinical Text.* 4th Edn., p. 616. (New York: Harper and Row)
14. Kriss, J. P., Pleshakov, V. and Chien, J. R. (1964). Isolation and identification of the long-acting thyroid stimulator and its relation to hyperthyroidism and circumscribed pretibrial myxedema. *J. Clin. Endocrinol. Metab.*, 24, 1005–11
15. Bonnyns, M., Vanhaelst, J., Golstein, J., Caunchie, C., Ermans, A. M. and Bastenie, P. A. (1973). Long-acting thyroid stimulator and thyroid function in relatives of patients with Graves' disease. *Clin. Endocrinol.*, 2, 277–87
16. Kitchin, F. D. and Weinstein, I. B. (1978). Genetic factors in thyroid disease. In Werner, S. C. and Ingbar, S. H. (eds.) *The Thyroid: A Fundamental and Clinical Text.* 4th Edn., p. 495. (New York: Harper and Row)
17. Howel-Evans, A. W., Woodrow, J. C. and McDougall, C. D. M. (1967). Antibody in families of thyrotoxic patients. *Lancet*, 1, 636–41
18. Friedman, J. M. and Fialkow, P. J. (1978). The genetics of Graves' disease. *Clin. Endocrinol. Metab.*, 7, 47–65
19. Fialkow, P. J., Thuline, H. C., Hecht, F. and Bryant, J. (1971). Familial predisposition to thyroid disease in Down's syndrome: controlled immunoclinical studies. *Am. J. Hum. Gen.*, 23, 67–86
20. Azizi, F., Chandler, H., Bozorgzadeh, H. and Braverman, L. E. (1974). The occurrence of hyperthyroidism in patients with Down's syndrome. *Hosp. Med. J.*, 134, 303–6
21. Fialkow, P. J. (1970). Thyroid autoimmunity and Down's syndrome. *Ann. N. Y. Acad. Sci.*, 171, 500–11
22. Boas, N. F. and Oher, W. B. (1946). Hereditary exophthalmic goitre: report of eleven children in one family. *J. Clin. Endocrinol. Metab.*, 6, 575–82

23. Volpe, R., Farid, N. R., Von Westarp, C. and Row, V. V. (1974). The pathogenesis of Graves' disease and Hashimoto's thyroiditis. *Clin. Endocrinol.*, 3, 239–61
24. Volpe, R. (1981). Auto-immunity in thyroid disease. In Volpe, R. (ed.) *Monographs on Endocrinology, Auto-immunity in the Endocrine System.* p. 108. (New York: Springer-Verlag)
25. Strakosh, R. D., Wenzel, B. E., Row, V. V. and Volpe, R. (1982). Immunology of autoimmune thyroid disease. *N. Engl. J. Med.*, 307, 1499–507
26. McGregor, A. M., Peterson, M. M., Capifferi, R., Evered, D. C., Rees-Smith, B. and Hall, R. (1979). Effects of radioiodine on thyrotropin binding inhibiting immunoglobulin in Graves' disease. *Clin. Endocrinol.*, 11, 437–44
27. Schleusener, H., Kotulla, P., Finke, R., Sorje, H., Meinhold, H., Adlkofer, F. and Wenzel, K. W. (1978). Relationship between thyroid status and Graves' disease - specific immuno- globulin. *J. Clin. Endocrinol. Metab.*, 47, 379–84
28. Endo, K., Kasagi, K., Konishi, J., Ikekubo, K., Okuno, T., Takeda, Y., Mori, T. and Torizuka, K. (1978). Detection and properties of TSH binding inhibitor immunoglobulin in patients with Graves' disease and Hashimoto's thyroiditis. *J. Clin. Endocrinol. Metab.*, 46, 734–9
29. Teng, C. S., Yeung, R. T. T., Khoo, R. K. K. and Alagaratnam, T. T. (1980). A prospective study of the changes in thyrotropin binding inhibitory immunoglobulin in Graves' disease treated by subtotal thyroidectomy or radioactive iodine. *J. Clin. Endocrinol. Metab.*, 50, 1005–10
30. Kishihara, M., Nakao, Y., Baba, Y., Kobayashi, N., Matukura, S., Kuma, K. and Fujita, T. (1981). Interaction between thyrotropin (TSH) binding inhibitor immunoglobulin (TBII) and soluble TSH receptors in fat cell. *J. Clin. Endocrinol. Metab.*, 52, 665–70
31. Burman, K. D. and Baker, J. R. (1985). Immune mechanisms in Graves' disease. *Endocrine Rev.*, 6, 183–232
32. Mukhtar, E. D., Smith, B. R., Pyle, G. A., Hall, R. and Vice, P. (1975). Relation of thyroid-stimulating immunoglobulins to thyroid function and effects of surgery, radioiodine, and antithyroid drug. *Lancet*, 1, 713–5
33. McGregor, A. M., McLachlan, S. M., Rees-Smith, B. and Hall, R. (1979). Effect of irradiation on thyroid-autoantibody production. *Lancet*, 2, 442–4
34. Zakarija, M., McKenzie, J. M. and Banovac, K. (1980). Clinical significance of assay of thyroid stimulating antibody in Graves' disease. *Ann. Int. Med.*, 93, 28–32
35. Beck, K., Feldt-Rasmussen, U., Bliddal, H., Date, J. and Blickert-Toft, M. (1982). The acute changes in thyroid stimulating immunoglobulin, thyroglobulin and thyroglobulin antibodies following subtotal thyroidectomy. *Clin. Endocrinol.*, 16, 235–42
36. Macchia, E., Fenzi, G. F., Monzani, F., Lippi, F., Vitti, P., Grasso, L., Bartalena, L., Baschieri, L. and Pinchera, A. (1981). Comparison between thyroid stimulating and TSH binding inhibiting immunoglobulins of Graves' disease. *Clin. Endocrinol.*, 15, 175–82
37. Kuzuya, N., Chiu, S. C., Ikeda, H., Uchimura, H., Ito, K. and Nagataki, S. (1979). Correlation between thyroid stimulators and 3,5,3'-triiodothyronine suppressibility in patients during treatment for hyperthyroidism with thionamide drug: comparison of assays by thyroid stimulating and thyrotropin displacing activities. *J. Clin. Endocrinol. Metab.*, 48, 706–11
38. Karlsson, F. A. and Dahlberg, P. A. (1981). Thyroid stimulating antibody (TSAb) in patients with Graves' disease undergoing antithyroid drug treatment: indicators of activity of disease. *Clin. Endocrinol.*, 14, 579–85
39. Etienne-Decerf, J. and Winand, R. J. (1981). A sensitive technique for determination of thyroid-stimulating immunoglobulin in unfractionated serum. *Clin. Endocrinol.*, 14, 83–91
40. Rapoport, B., Greenspan, F. S., Filettr, S. and Pepitone, M. (1984). Clinical experience with a human thyroid cell bioassay for thyroid stimulating immunoglobulin. *J. Clin. Endocrinol. Metab.*, 58, 332–8
41. Atkinson, S. and Kendall-Taylor, P. (1981). The stimulation of thyroid hormone secretion *in vitro* by thyroid-stimulating antibodies. *J. Clin. Endocrin. Metab.*, 53, 1263–6
42. Smyth, P. P. A., Neylan, D. and O'Donovan, D. K. (1982). The prevalence of thyroid stimulating antibodies in goitrous disease assessed by cytochemical section bioassay. *J. Clin. Endocrinol. Metab.*, 54, 357–61
43. Davis, T. F., Yeo, P. P. B., Evered, D. C., Clark, F., Smith, B. R. and Hall, R. (1977).

Value of thyroid stimulating antibody determination in predicting short-term thyrotoxic relapse in Graves' disease. *Lancet*, **1**, 1181-2

44. Matsuura, N., Yamada, T., Nohara, Y., Knoishi, J., Kasagi, K., Endo, K., Kojima, H. and Wataya, K. (1980). Familial neonatal transient hypothyroidism due to maternal TSH-binding inhibition immunoglobulin. *N. Engl. J. Med.*, **303**, 738-41

45. Takasu, N., Mori, T., Koizumi, Y., Takeuchi, S. and Yamada, T. (1984). Transient neonatal hypothyroidism due to maternal immunoglobulin that inhibit thyrotropin-binding and post-receptor processes. *J. Clin. Endocrinol. Metab.*, **59**, 142-6

46. Takasu, N., Naka, M., Mori, T. and Yamada, T. (1984). Two types of thyroid function-blocking antibodies in autoimmune atrophic thyroiditis and transient neonatal hypothyroidism due to maternal IgG. *Clin. Endocrinol.*, **21**, 345-55

47. Konishi, J., Iida, Y., Endo, K., Misaki, T., Nohara, Y., Matsuura, N., Mori, T. and Torizuka, K. (1983). Inhibition of thyrotropin-induced adenosin 3'5'-monophosphate increase by immunoglobulins from patients with primary myxedema. *J. Clin. Endocrinol. Metab.*, **57**, 544-9

48. Steel, N. R., Weightman, D. R., Taylor, J. J. and Kendall-Taylor, P. (1984). Blocking activity to action of thyroid stimulating hormone in serum from patients with primary hypothyroidism. *Br. Med. J.*, **288**, 1559-64

49. Frelinger, J. A. and Shreffler, D. C. (1975). The major histocompatibility complex. In Benacerraf, B. (ed.) *Immunogenetics and Immunodeficiency.* p. 81. (Baltimore: University Park Press)

50. Bach, F. H. and Van Rood, J. J. (1976). The major histocompatibility complex – genetics and biology. *N. Engl. J. Med.*, **295**, 806-13

51. Irvine, W. J., Gray, R. J., Moriss, P. J. and Ting, A. (1977). Correlation of HLA and thyroid antibodies with clinical course of thyrotoxicosis treated with antithyroid drugs. *Lancet*, **2**, 898-900

52. Bech, K., Lunholtz, B., Nerup, J., Tomsen, M., Platz, P., Ryder, L. E., Svejgaard, A., Siersbock-Nielsen, K., Hanse, J. M., and Larsen, J. H. (1977). HLA antigens in Graves' disease. *Acta Endocrinol.*, **86**, 510-5

53. McGregor, A. M., Smith, B. R. and Hall, R. (1980). Prediction of relapse in hyperthyroid Graves' disease. *Lancet*, **1**, 1101-3

54. Schleusener, H., Schernthaner, G., Mayr, W. R., Kotulla, P., Bogner, U., Finke, R., Meinhold, H., Koppenhagen, K. and Wenzel, K. W. (1983). HLA-DR3 and HLA-DR5 associated thyrotoxicosis – two different types of toxic diffuse goiter. *J. Clin. Endocrinol. Metab.*, **56**, 781-5

55. Allannic, H., Fauchet, R., Lorcy, Y., Gueguen, M., Guerrier, A. L. and Genetel, B. (1983). A prospective study of the relationship between relapse of hyperthyroid Graves' disease after antithyroid drugs and HLA haplotype. *J. Clin. Endocrinol. Metab.*, **57**, 719-22

56. Wenzel, K. W. and Lente, J. R. (1984). Similar effects of thionamide drugs and perchlorate on thyroid-stimulating immunoglobulin in Graves' disease: evidence against an immunosuppressive action of thionamide drugs. *J. Clin. Endocrinol. Metab.*, **58**, 62-9

57. Weetman, A. P., Gunn, C., Hall, R. and McGregor, A. (1984). Immunosuppression by perchlorate. *Lancet*, **1**, 906

58. Grumet, F. C., Payne, R. O., Konishi, J. and Kriss, J. P. (1974). HL-A antigens as markers for disease susceptibility and autoimmunity in Graves' disease. *J. Clin. Endocrinol. Metab.*, **39**, 1115-9

59. Grumet, F. C., Payne, R. O., Konishi, J., Mori, T. and Kriss, J. P. (1975). HL-A antigens in Japanese patients with Graves' disease. *Tissue Antigen.*, **6**, 347-52

60. Farid, N. R., Barnard, J. M. and Marshall, W. H. (1976). The association of HLA with autoimmune thyroid disease in Newfoundland. The influence of HLA homozygosity in Graves' disease. *Tissue Antigen.*, **8**, 181-9

61. Beck, K., Lumholtz, B., Nerup, J., Thomsen, M., Platz, P., Ryder, L. P., Svejgaard, A., Siersbck-Nielsen, K., Hansen, J. M. and Larsen, J. H. (1977). HLA antigens in Graves' disease. *Acta Endocrinol.*, **86**, 510-6

62. Farid, N. R., Sampson, E. P., Barnard, J. M., Mandeville, R., Lasen, B. and Marshall, W. H. (1979). A study of human leucocyte D locus related antigen in Graves' disease. *J. Clin. Invest.*, **63**, 108-13

63. Uno, H., Sasazuki, T., Tamai, H. and Matsumoto, H. (1981). Two major genes linked to

HLA and Gm control susceptibility to Graves' disease. *Nature (London)*, **292**, 768–70

64. Farid, N. R., Stone, E. and Johnson, G. (1980). Graves' disease and HLA: clinical and epidemiological associations. *Clin. Endocrinol.*, **13**, 535–44
65. Schernthaner, G., Schleusner, H., Kotulla, P., Finke, R., Wenzel, B. and Mayr, W. R. (1981). Prediction of relapse or long term remission in hyperthyroid Graves' disease. *Lancet*, **2**, 323–5
66. Sasazuki, T., Kohno, Y., Iwamoto, L. and Tanimura, M. (1977). HLA-B,D, haplotypes associated with autoimmune disease in Japanese populations. *Tissue Antigens.*, **10**, 218–24
67. Wells, J. V., Fundenberg, H. H. and Mackay, I. R. (1971). Relation of the human antibody response to flagellin to Gm genotypes. *J. Immunol.*, **107**, 1505–11
68. Shreffler, D. C. and Davis, D. C. (1975). The H-2 major histocompatibility complex and immune response region: genetic variations, function, and organization. *Adv. Immunol.*, **20**, 125–9
69. Pandy, J. P., Fudenberg, H. H., Virella, G., Kyong, C. U., Loadholt, C. B. and Galbraith, R. M. (1979). Association between immunoglobulin allotypes and immune response to *Haemophilus influenzae* and *Meningococcus polysaccharides*. *Lancet*, **1**, 190–2
70. Lieberman, K., Potter, M., Humphrey, W., Jr. and Chen, C. C. (1976). Idiotypes of insulin-binding antibodies and myeloma proteins controlled by genes linked to the allotype locus of the mouse. *J. Immunol.*, **117**, 2105–11
71. Pisetski, D. S., Piodran, S. E. and Sachs, D. H. (1978). Genetic control of the immune response to staphylococcal nuclease. *J. Immunol.*, **122**, 842–6
72. Nakao, Y., Matsumoto, H., Miyazaki, T., Nishitani, H., Takasuki, K., Katsukawa, R., Nakayama, S., Izumi, S., Fujita, T. and Tsuji, K. (1980). IgG heavy chain allotypes (Gm) in autoimmune disease. *Clin. Exp. Immunol.*, **42**, 20–6
73. Farid, N. R., Newton, R. M., Noel, E. P. and Marshall, W. H. (1977). Gm phenotype in autoimmune thyroid disease. *J. Immunogenet.*, **4**, 429–32
74. Nakao, Y., Kishihara, M., Baba, Y., Kuma, K., Fukunishi, T. and Imura, H. (1978). HLA antigens in autoimmune thyroid disease. *Arch. Intern. Med.*, **138**, 567–70
75. Smith, M., Krinsky, A., Arredondo-Vega, F., Wang A. L. and Hirschhorn, K. (1981). Confirmation of the assignment of genes for human immunoglobulin heavy chains to chromosome 14 by analyses of Ig synthesis by man-mouse hybridoma. *Eur. J. Immunol.*, **11**, 852–5
76. Tamai, H., Uno, H., Hirota, Y., Matsubayashi, S., Kuma, K., Matsumoto, H., Kumagi, L. F., Sasazuki, T. and Nagataki, S. (1985). Immunogenetics of Hashimoto's and Graves' disease. *J. Clin. Endocrinol. Metab.*, **60**, 62–5
77. Farid, N. R., Barnard, J. M., Marshall, W. H., Woolferey, I. and O'Driscoll, R. F. (1977). Thyroid autoimmune disease in a large Newfoundland family: the influence of HLA. *J. Clin. Endocrinol. Metab.*, **45**, 1165–72
78. Adams, D. D., Adams, Y. J., Knight, J. G., McCall, J., White, P., Parkinson, P., Horrocks, R. and Van Loghen, E. (1983). On nature of the genes influencing the prevalence of Graves' disease. *Life Sci.*, **31**, 3–11
79. Sasazuki, T., Kohno, Y., Iwamoto, I., Tanimura, M. and Naito, S. (1978). Association between an HLA haplotype and low responsiveness to tetanus toxoid in man. *Nature (London)*, **272**, 359–61
80. Sasazuki, T., Kaneko, H., Nishimura, Y., Kaneko, R., Hayama, M. and Ohkuni, H. (1980). An HLA-linked immune suppression gene in man. *J. Exp. Med.*, **152**, 297–313
81. Schwartz, M., Lifshitz, R., Givol, D., Mozes, E. and Haimovich, T. (1978). Cross-reactive idiotypic determinants on murine anti(T.G)-A-L antibodies. *J. Immunol.*, **121**, 421–6
82. Greenberg, L. J., Gray, D. and Yunis, J. E. (1975). Association of HL-A5 and immune responsiveness *in vitro* to streptococcal antigens. *J. Exp. Med.*, **141**, 935–43
83. Martin, L. and Fisher, R. A. (1951). The hereditary and familial aspects of toxic nodular goiter (secondary thyrotoxicosis). *Q. J. Med.*, **20**, 293–8
84. Fraser, G. R. (1963). A genetical study of goiter *Ann. Hum. Genet.*, **26**, 335–40
85. Saxena, K. M. (1965). Inheritance of thyroglobulin antibody in thyrotoxic children. *Lancet*, **1**, 583–6
86. Doniach, D. (1975). Humoral and genetic aspects of thyroid autoimmunity. *Clin. Endocrinol. Metab.*, **4**, 267–85
87. Farid, N. R., Von Westarp, C., Row, V. V. and Volpe, R. (1974). Studies of cell-mediated

immunity (CMI) in relatives of patients with Graves' disease. *J. Clin. Endocrinol. Metab.*, **39**, 778–84

88. Boas, N. F. and Ober, W. B. (1945). Hereditary exophthalmic goiter – report of eleven cases in one family. *J. Clin. Endocrinol. Metab.*, **6**, 575–88

89. Sorensen, E. W. (1958). Thyroid diseases in a family. *Acta Medica Scandinavia*, **162**, 123–7

90. Wilroy, R. S. and Etteldorf, J. N. (1971). Familial hyperthyroidism including two siblings with neonatal Graves' disease. *J. Pediatr.*, **78**, 625–32

91. Hollingsworth, D. R., McKean, M. E. and Roeckel, I. (1974). Goiter, immunological observations, and thyroid function tests in Down's syndrome. *Am. J. Dis. Child.*, **127**, 524–7

92. Mason, A. M. S., Raper, C. G. and Lloyd, P. (1970). Thyrotoxicosis in a father and two sons. *Lancet*, **1**, 81

93. Hollingsworth, D. R., Mabry, C. C. and Eckerd, J. M. (1972). Hereditary aspects of Graves' disease in infancy and childhood. *J. Pediatr.*, **81**, 446–59

94. Sasazuki, T., Uno, H., Yasuda, H., Tamai, H. and Matsumoto, H. (1982). Evidence for HLA-linked and Gm-linked genes in Graves' disease. In Tamir, B. B. (ed.) *Human Genetics*, Part B, p. 65. (New York: Liss)

95. Sasazuki, T., Nishimura, Y., Muto, M. and Ohta, N. (1983). HLA-linked genes controlling immune response and disease susceptibility. *Immunol. Rev.*, **70**, 51–75

96. Cudworth, A. G. and Woodrow, J. C. (1975). Evidence for HLA-linked genes in 'juvenile' diabetes mellitus. *Br. Med. J.*, **3**, 133–5

97. Day, N. E. and Simons, M. J. (1976). Disease susceptibility genes. Their identification by multiple case family studies. *Tissue Antigen*, **8**, 109–19

98. Thomson, G. and Bodmer, W. F. (1977). The genetics of HLA and disease association. In Christianess, T. B. and Feachel, T. M. (eds.) *Measuring Selection in National Populations*. p. 545. (Berlin: Springer-Verlag)

99. Svejgaard, A. and Ryder, L. P. (1981). HLA genotype distribution and genetic models of insulin-dependent diabetes mellitus. *Ann. Hum. Genet.*, **45**, 293–8

100. Farid, N. P. and Bear, J. C. (1983). Autoimmune endocrine disorders and the major histocompatibility complex. In Davis, T. (ed.) *Autoimmune Endocrine Disease*, p. 59. (New York: Wiley and Sons)

101. Stenszky, V., Kozma, L., Balazs, Cs., Rocheitz, Sz., Bear, J. C. and Farid, N. R. (1985). The genetics of Graves' disease: HLA and disease susceptibility. *J. Clin. Endocrinol. Metab.*, **61**, 735–40

102. Farid, N. R. (1981). Graves' disease. In Farid, N. R. (ed.) *HLA in Endocrine and Metabolic Disorders*, p. 85. (New York: Academic Press)

103. Chan, S. H., Yeo, P. P. B., Cheah, J. S. and Lim, P. (1980). HLA haplotype sharing in affected siblings in multiple case Chinese families with thyrotoxicosis. *Tissue Antigen.*, **16**, 258–63

104. Joassoo, A., Robertson, P. and Murray, I. P. C. (1975). Viral antibodies in thyrotoxicosis. *Lancet*, **2**, 125

# 8
# HLA-DR Antigen Expression and Autoimmunity

## A. P. WEETMAN

---

Products of the major histocompatibility complex (MHC) of genes play several key roles in the autoimmune response. Besides being predominantly responsible for the rejection of tissue grafts and graft-versus-host reactions, molecules encoded by MHC genes are directly involved in the recognition of antigen by T-cells. The MHC also determines to a great extent whether or not a particular antigen will evoke an immune response. The chapter begins with a synopsis of MHC antigens and their involvement in the normal immune response, together with a review of the factors involved in antigen presentation. This is followed by a summary of the recent studies which show that a wide variety of cells, including those from endocrine tissues, may express MHC class II antigens, like HLA-DR, under certain conditions. In the last section, the possible consequences of this phenomenon are discussed with regard to endocrine autoimmunity.

## THE MHC AND THE IMMUNE RESPONSE

### Classes of MHC antigens

The MHC is known as HLA (human leukocyte antigen) in man and H-2 (histocompatibility-2) in the mouse[1]. Each complex has a linked set of at least three gene families, which give rise to class I, II and III MHC antigens (Figure 8.1). The genes responsible for class III antigens are implicated in complement synthesis and do not concern us here. Class I antigens are glycoproteins found on the surface of nearly all nucleated cells and platelets; they are encoded by the HLA-A, HLA-B and HLA-C regions in man and by similar genes in the H-2K, H-2D and H-2L regions in the mouse. Class II antigens are different glycoproteins whose cell distribution is restricted normally to macrophages, B-cells, dendritic cells and a small number of T-cells. Genes for these products were originally mapped to the H2-I region in mice, hence the synonymous term Ia (I-region associated) antigens. In man class II antigens are encoded in the HLA-D region. The terms class II and Ia will be used interchangeably in this chapter.

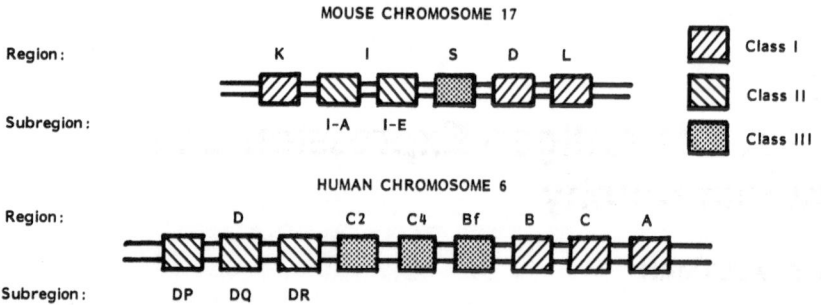

**Figure 8.1** The major histocompatibility complex (MHC) of mouse and man showing the location of regions and subregions. The centromere lies to the left of each of the sequences

## Structure of MHC antigens

### Class I antigens

Each of the three loci for class I antigens encodes a single 45 kd polypeptide which is non-covalently associated with $\beta_2$-microglobulin, a 12 kd protein not encoded by the MHC (Figure 8.2). The class I molecule has five domains of which three, $\alpha_1$, $\alpha_2$ and $\alpha_3$, lie outside the cell membrane with $\beta_2$ microglobulin. The fourth domain lies in the membrane itself and the fifth is intracytoplasmic. The loci that encode class I antigens are highly polymorphic and these allelic forms are expressed by variability in the $\alpha_1$–$\alpha_3$ domains.

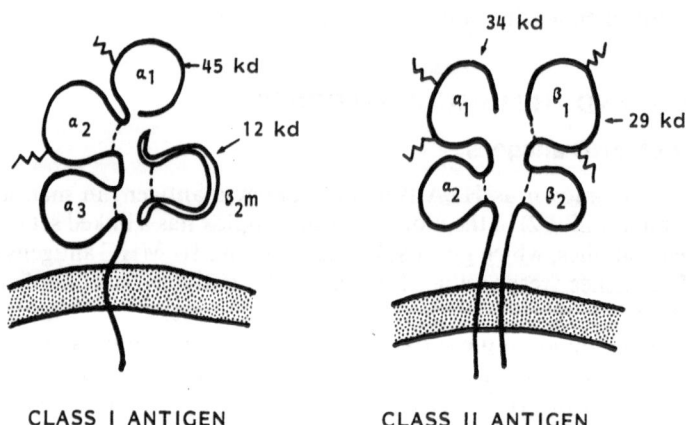

**Figure 8.2** The structure of class I and class II antigens. The major domains of each lie outside the cell; the cell membrane is shown stippled. The dotted lines within a domain represent disulphide bonds; the zig-zag represents the sugar residues of these glycoproteins

## Class II antigens

Class II antigens are encoded by subregions which are termed I-A and I-E in the mouse. Each antigen is composed of two non-covalently bound chains termed $\alpha$(34 kd) and $\beta$(29 kd) giving rise to structures $A_\alpha$ $A_\beta$ or $E_\alpha$ $E_\beta$. Both types of $\beta$-chain are encoded in the I-A region; the $\alpha$-chains arise from appropriately lettered subregions ($A_\alpha$ in I-A, $E_\alpha$ in I-E). Class II molecules resemble the class I 44 kd polypeptide but have only two extracellular domains (Figure 8.2). In man there are three HLA-D subregions, DP (formerly SB), DQ (formerly DC, DS, MB or LB-E) and DR[2]. DQ is homologous to I-A and DR to I-E. In the DR subregion there are genes for a single $\alpha$ and three $\beta$-chains, whereas the DP and DQ subregions each encode two $\alpha$ and two $\beta$-chains. It seems likely that $\alpha$-chains associate primarily with $\beta$-chains of the same family.

## Identification of Class I and II antigens

Although transplantation reactions indicated the presence of MHC antigens in early studies, it is the vigorous antibody formation which accompanies such reactions that has led to the present ability to tissue-type an outbred population like man. Serological determination of class I and some class II MHC antigens is now a standard technique using well characterized sera from pregnant women, immunized against paternal MHC antigens by the fetus, or more recently using monoclonal antibodies. In most tests for aberrant class II antigen expression detailed below, monoclonal antibodies against non-polymorphic parts of the antigen are used, usually in combination with immunofluorescence techniques to assess antibody binding.

Historically however, class II antigens were recognized by their ability to stimulate a mixed lymphocyte reaction (MLR) in which T-cells proliferate in response to non-compatible class II antigens on second-party B-cells and monocytes. Modifications of the MLR are still used, for instance, to detect DP antigens. Clearly, in the MLR the antigen is recognized by a T-cell, whereas serological testing relies on B-cell recognition of the antigen. It is now known that many apparently discrete antigens defined serologically are in fact heterologous when T-cells are used to identify them. Such discrimination is possible because of differences between the determinants recognized by B-and T-cell antigen receptors.

## Function

Perhaps evolving from a primitive mechanism for recognizing members of the same species, MHC antigens have become key restriction elements in the recognition of antigens by T-cells. This means, in short, that T-cells respond to an antigen X in association with one particular allelic product of the MHC and not another[1,3]. Restriction is achieved by a T-cell surface receptor specific for both MHC antigen and X; current evidence favours the existence of a single T-cell receptor for both molecules[4].

A second important concept is that, broadly speaking, class I MHC antigens are restriction elements for cytotoxic T-cells and class II MHC antigens are restriction elements for helper T-cells. In man, this dichotomy correlates even better with whether the T-cell bears cell surface antigens which react with OKT8 or OKT4 monoclonal antibodies. An elegant model has been proposed in which these monoclonal antibodies are considered to identify T-cell surface glycoproteins capable of binding to non-polymorphic regions of class I (for OKT8) and class II (for OKT4) antigens[5]. The antigen-specific T-cell receptor may then bind to the relevant antigen and polymorphic determinants on the MHC antigen (Figure 8.3). Thus in an immune response, the class of the MHC antigen is important in determining which subset of T-cells is stimulated, and the polymorphic region of each class of MHC antigen is important as a restriction element.

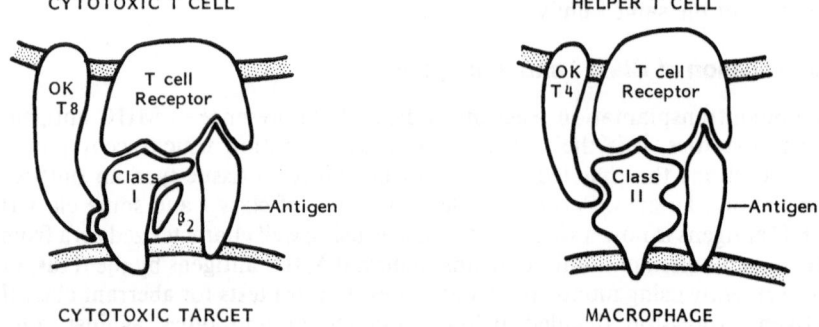

**Figure 8.3** Interaction of class I molecule (left) or class II molecule (right) with both the T-cell receptor for antigen and the OKT8 or OKT4 molecule. This interpretation is based on the currently favoured single receptor model for T-cell recognition of antigen and MHC molecule

Against this background, it seems that the main physiological role for class I antigens is to restrict the killing of antigen-bearing target cells by OKT8-positive cytotoxic T-cells. For instance, virally-infected cells will only be lysed if they are both infected and express the appropriate class I antigen. Recently OKT4-positive cytotoxic T-cells have been described[5] and, predictably, these only lyse targets expressing specific antigen in association with class II molecules.

Class II antigens are expressed by the classical antigen presenting cells (APC), macrophages, and play a major role in antigen recognition by helper T-cells, which can only be stimulated or primed by co-recognition of the antigen and class II molecule on the APC. Thereafter the T-cell will only respond to antigen in association with the same class II molecule. Whether the subgroups of class II antigens, like DP, DQ and DR, have similar or distinct roles in antigen presentation is currently unclear[6]. It should also be mentioned that *in vitro*, class II molecules themselves (on monocytes and B-cells) seem capable of stimulating certain autologous OKT4-positive T-cells to proliferate; this is termed an autologous mixed lymphocyte reaction (AMLR). However, the freedom of these systems from contamination with foreign antigens, introduced during cell manipulations, and their *in vivo* relevance have been questioned.

The possession of certain class II antigens is associated with the degree of immune responsiveness the individual mounts to particular antigens. In mice the genes controlling such idiosyncrasies were mapped to the I region and called immune response (Ir) genes. While it seems true that genes encoding class II antigens are indeed Ir genes, there are likely to be other Ir genes outside the MHC. How might class II antigens be linked to the determination of immune responsiveness? Two possible mechanisms are *determinant selection* and *clonal deletion*[7]. If a particular strain of animal responds to antigen X but not Y, determinant selection proposes that it is the combination of Y and the MHC antigen on an APC which fails to stimulate Y-specific T-cells; the combination of X and the same MHC molecule, however, can stimulate X-specific T-cells. In effect the failure to respond is at the level of the class II antigen on the APC. Clonal deletion implies that in a non-responder strain, the animal has antigen X-specific T-cells but not antigen Y-specific T-cells. The missing clones of T-cells are absent as the result of some Ir gene effect on the T-cell repertoire, and the failure to respond is at the level of the T-cell. It is probable that both mechanisms operate *in vivo*.

## ANTIGEN PRESENTATION

Studies, primarily using murine macrophages, have shown that these cells function optimally as APC when they bear class II molecules, process the antigen to render it immunogenic and release interleukin-1 (IL-1)[8,9]. Class II antigen expression by macrophages is not constant and therefore modulation by various stimuli can affect subsequent antigen presentation. It is also apparent that other Ia-positive cells besides macrophages can function as APC. These features of antigen presentation will be considered in turn.

### Antigen processing

Many studies have shown that for efficient presentation a wide range of antigens, from whole bacteria to soluble proteins, require endocytosis, processing in acid vesicles and re-expression on the macrophage surface (possible in direct conjunction with Ia molecules)[8]. Blockage at any stage of antigen processing with pharmacological agents will prevent subsequent T-cell stimulation. Conversely, if an antigen is degraded by enzymes in the absence of APC, immunogenic fragments can be obtained which require no further intracellular processing for presentation. However, some antigens may not require any processing at all. In particular, Unanue and co-workers have suggested that membrane-bound antigens which persist for a long time may be recognized in their native state[9], a concept of singular relevance to endocrine autoimmunity as discussed below.

### Interleukin 1

This monokine is released by macrophages in response to a variety of signals and in turn has many effects[10]. In the present context, it is pertinent that presentation of antigen by a macrophage causes T-cell activation and proliferation, which depends upon the elaboration of interleukin-2 (IL-2) and IL-2 receptors by the T-cell. The release of IL-1 by macrophages, probably in response to an initial signal from T-cells, stimulates IL-2 production, thereby enhancing the stimulating effect of antigen presentation (Figure 8.4). How critical a role IL-1 plays is not clear. It may only be essential in antigen presentation to memory T-cells or to unprimed T-cells, which have never encountered antigen before[9]. In other situations, IL-1 may only be facilitatory or indeed may not be required.

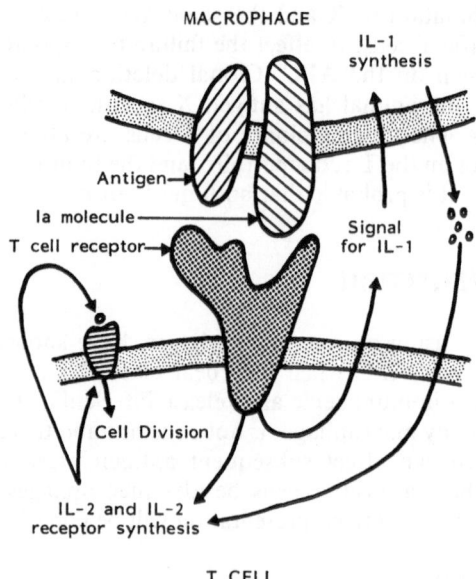

**Figure 8.4** Sequence of events during antigen presentation by a macrophage. Antigen, in suitably processed form, is presented in association with appropriate Ia molecule to the T-cell. This triggers IL-1 and IL-2 production, leading to T-cell division

## Modulation of macrophage Ia expression

Basal levels of macrophage Ia expression vary between tissues and are dependent on a continuous influx of young Ia-positive macrophages[8]. Ia antigens are subsequently lost but can be induced again on the cells during an immune response. The stimulus for this is provided by lymphokines released by activated T-cells. The most potent of these lymphokines in the mouse and in man is $\gamma$-interferon ($\gamma$-IFN) but the existence of other lymphokines with this property has not been excluded. Thus a major function of $\gamma$-IFN release is to enhance the immune response locally by increasing the number of macrophages available with antigen-presenting capacity. Class I MHC antigen expression is enhanced by $\gamma$-IFN as well as $\alpha$-IFN and $\beta$-IFN;

however, these other interferons alone have no effect on class II antigen expression and may actually inhibit it, if added to macrophages *in vitro* at the same time as $\gamma$-IFN[11].

Furthermore, several compounds decrease murine macrophage Ia expression, including prostaglandin $E_2$, $\alpha$-fetoprotein, dibutyryl cyclic AMP and glucocorticoids[8]. The first two of these may be responsible for the low levels of Ia-positive macrophages found in all neonatal tissues (except thymus), which in turn may contribute to the ease of inducing antigen tolerance at this stage of development. It should also be noted that hydrocortisone enhances, rather than diminishes, human monocyte HLA-DR antigen expression; HLA-DQ remains unchanged[12]. This species difference highlights the need for great caution in extrapolating any results derived from mice to man.

## Other antigen presenting cells

The foregoing discussion has been confined to the macrophage and its blood-borne precursor, the monocyte. However, other cells also normally express Ia antigens and their capacity to present antigen has been extensively examined. Class II antigens on B-cells can be increased by cross-linking the cell surface immunoglobulin with anti-$\mu$ chain antibodies and by unidentified T-cell-derived lymphokines[13,14]. No effect of IL-2 or $\gamma$-IFN on B-cell Ia antigen-expression was found in these studies. Murine splenic B-cells, B-cell tumours and human EBV-transformed B-cells can all present antigen, and have been shown to process and present it in a way similar to macrophages[8,15].

An essential difference, however, is that B-cells recognize antigen in a specific manner by means of their surface immunoglobulins; macrophages do not discriminate between antigens. Thus at the beginning of a response to an antigen, X, very few X-specific B-cells will be present and only these B-cells can present X to T-cells. At this stage macrophages would have a major role in initiating the response. However, as the reaction proceeds, X-specific helper T-cells will stimulate the clonal expansion of X-specific B-cells and these will then act as APC to enhance the response to X. In effect the B-cell is an APC which captures, or focuses, antigen[4]. The large number of auto-antigen-specific B-cells infiltrating the target organs involved in auto-immunity could clearly be important in the perpetuation of disease by such a mechanism. The efficiency of antigen presentation by B-cells correlates quantitatively with the amount of Ia antigen they express[16], and presentation may be enhanced by exogenous IL-1 in some circumstances[8]. Indeed, an absolute requirement for IL-1 has been demonstrated, if B-cells are to act as APC for resting T-cells[17].

Langerhans cells found in the skin and dendritic cells found throughout the body are strongly Ia-positive[8,9]. They are very effective in stimulating a MLR and producing antigen-specific T-cell proliferation. However, they may be limited in their ability to process antigen and recent experiments have shown that dendritic cells were unable to activate helper T-cells using soluble antigens; that is, they could not act as APC for those T-cells which stimulate B-cells to make antibody[18]. Thus these cells may have a different role to macrophages in antigen presentation. Epithelial cells of the thymic cortex and some myeloid cells are also Ia positive under normal conditions[19,20]. Their role as APC has not been elucidated.

## ABERRANT EXPRESSION OF Ia ANTIGENS

It is now clear that a wide variety of cells besides the APC just discussed are capable of expressing class II antigens under particular conditions *in vivo* and *in vitro*. Rat epidermal and gut epithelial cells express Ia antigens during the course of a graft-versus-host reaction[21] and renal transplant rejection induces HLA-DR antigens on kidney tubule cells[22]. Moreover, $\gamma$-IFN can induce Ia antigens on melanoma cells, fibroblasts, endothelial cells and astrocytes[23-25] and mammary gland epithelium expresses class II antigens during lactation, under the positive control of oestrogen and prolactin and the negative control of androgen[26]. In some cases, cells expressing Ia antigens aberrantly have been shown to stimulate T-cells, suggesting their capability of functioning as APC[24,27]. Furthermore, deliberate transfection of HLA-DQ genes into mouse fibroblasts leads to DQ antigen expression; these cells are then capable of presenting antigen in a suitably DQ-restricted fashion to T-cell clones[28].

### Ia antigen expression by thyroid follicular cells

The thyroid has been the main endocrine organ investigated for aberrant Ia antigen expression. Normal human thyroid cells are class II antigen-negative *in vivo* or in primary cell culture but Ia antigens can be induced *in vitro* using lectins like phytohaemagglutinin (PHA) and concanavalin A (Con A)[29]. Furthermore, thyroid follicles from patients with Graves' disease and Hashimoto's thyroiditis are spontaneously HLA-DR positive *in vivo*[30]. Species differences are again important since freshly dissociated thyroid cells from normal mice are Ia positive[31], yet rat thyroid cells neither express Ia antigens constitutively, nor become Ia positive *in vitro* with lectins[29].

The results with human thyroid cells led to the hypothesis that if HLA-DR antigens were induced on a thyroid cell it could then act as an APC and present surface autoantigens to helper T-cells. In this manner autoimmune thyroid disease could be initiated or perpetuated, provided other features, such as an agent which induced Ia antigen expression, a source of IL-1 and a relative suppressor cell deficiency, were also present[32].

### Regulation of thyroid Ia antigen expression

HLA-DR antigens can be induced on normal thyroid cells using lymphokines generated by Con A stimulation of T-cells; $\gamma$-IFN is an even better stimulus (Figure 8.5)[33,34]. In our experience, high basal levels of HLA-DR expression only occur in a minority of primary thyroid cell cultures from Graves' and Hashimoto's patients, but the antigen can be induced on these cells by $\gamma$-IFN with the same time and dose response as normal thyroid cells. HLA-DQ antigens can also be induced by PHA or $\gamma$-IFN[33].

Thus thyroid cells express Ia antigens exactly as do other non-lymphoid

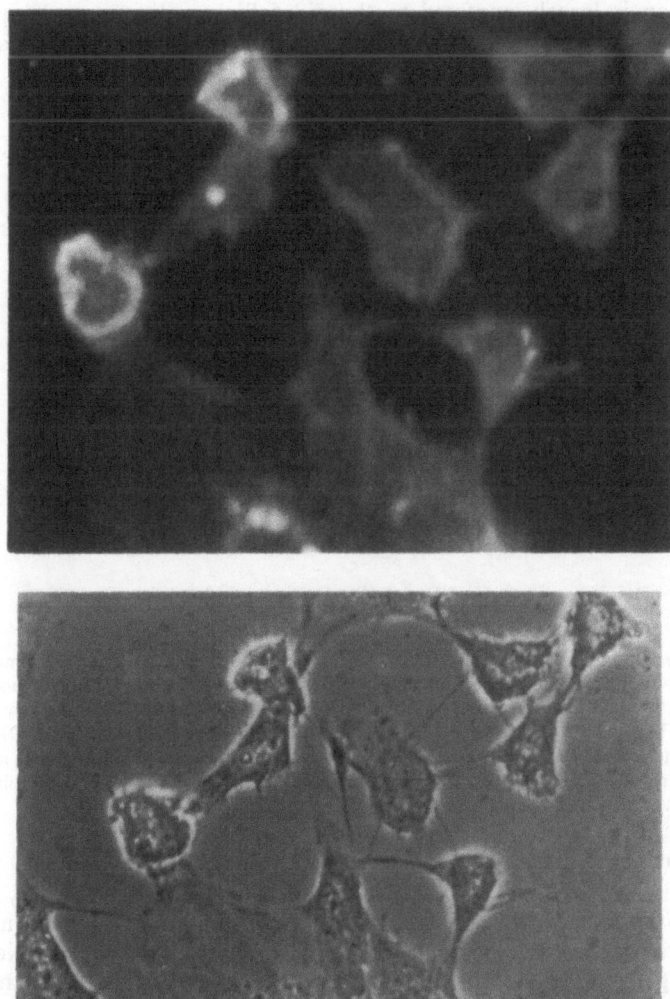

**Figure 8.5** Photomicrograph of thyroid follicular cells in monolayer culture for 6 days with 10 U γ-IFN/ml (upper) and immunofluorescence of the same cells following staining with anti-HLA-DR monoclonal antibody (lower) (magnification × 960)

cells in response to γ-IFN, but the response to lectins is novel. A likely explanation is that PHA and Con A work indirectly, stimulating γ-IFN production by contaminating lymphocytes in thyroid cell cultures. Support for this is provided by use of cyclosporin A which acts on T-cells and prevents γ-IFN and IL-2 synthesis. Addition of cyclosporin A with PHA to thyroid cell cultures prevented HLA-DR expression, yet cyclosporin A had no effect on HLA-DR induction by exogenous γ-IFN[33]. Moreover, *in vivo* HLA-DR expression is largely confined to thyroid follicles adjacent to lymphocytic infiltrates[35], supporting the idea that lymphokines, like $\gamma$-IFN, have a central role in aberrant HLA-DR expression (Figure 8.6).

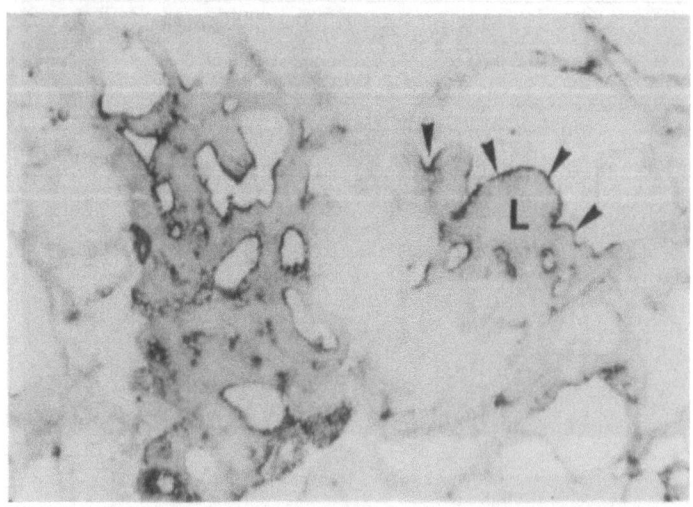

**Figure 8.6** Frozen section of a Graves' thyroid gland stained with anti-HLA-DR monoclonal antibody and the glucose oxidase immunocytochemical technique. Activated lymphocytes and adjacent thyroid follicular cells are shown to be HLA-DR positive (identified by the dark staining). This is seen most clearly in the follicle in the upper right quarter; HLA-DR-positive epithelium is highlighted by the arrow heads and is adjacent to a lymphoid aggregate marked L. The remaining follicular cells are HLA-DR-negative. Magnification × 26. (Photograph courtesy of Dr J. B. Margolick)

An intriguing question is: what prevents Ia antigen expression by normal human thyroid (and indeed other) cells? Perhaps $\gamma$-IFN, produced by normal blood lymphocytes *in vitro* without stimulation[36], is at too low a serum concentration *in vivo*, or may not have access to thyroid cells. Normally occurring thyroidal T-cells[37] presumably are not activated and therefore would not release $\gamma$-IFN locally. Finally, there may be inhibitors which actually suppress class II antigen expression. However, prostaglandin $E_2$ and dibutyryl cAMP, known to inhibit murine macrophage Ia expression, have no effect on thyroidal HLA-DR expression induced by $\gamma$-IFN[33]. This could be another species difference or a phenomenon peculiar to the thyroid.

## Antigen presentation by thyroidal cells

*In vitro* experiments have supported the possibility that HLA-DR-positive thyroid cells could act as APC in the autoimmune response. Normal thyroid cells treated with PHA to induce HLA-DR antigens were able to stimulate proliferation of autologous peripheral blood T-cells in an AMLR; T-cells from Graves' patients were stimulated by autologous thyroid cells, spontaneously HLA-DR-positive[38]. A proportion of OKT4-positive T-cell clones obtained from the thyroids of Graves' patients proliferated in response to autologous thyroid cells but did not display an AMLR with other Ia-positive cells[39]. The proliferation was blocked by anti-Ia antibodies. This indicates that both a class II molecule and a thyroid cell surface antigen were required to stimulate the T-cell clones, implying true APC function by the thyroid cells.

Furthermore we have found that certain OKT4-positive thyroidal T-cell lines from patients with Graves' disease proliferated in response to autologous thyroid cells only when HLA-DR was induced by γ-IFN; untreated, DR-negative thyroid cells or γ-IFN alone had no stimulatory effect (Figure 8.7)[40]. Monocytes were unable to present thyroglobulin or thyroid microsomal antigen to these lines. This suggests that either the lines recognized these surface autoantigens preferentially when expressed by HLA-DR-positive thyroid cells or the lines responded to a different autoantigen on the thyroid cells.

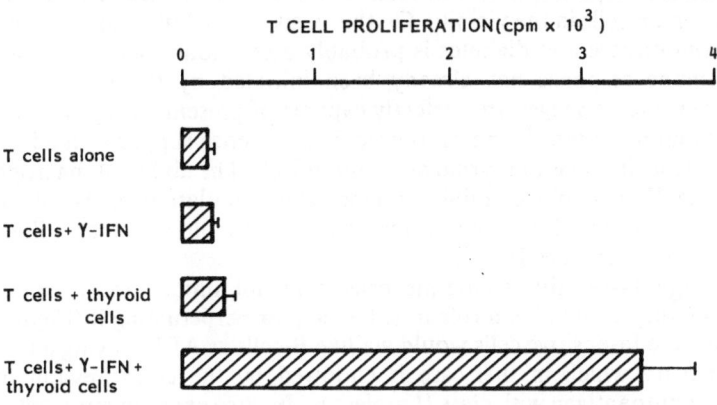

**Figure 8.7** T-cell line proliferation in response to HLA-DR positive thyroid follicular cells. A T-cell line was derived from a Graves' thyroid by culture with IL-2. This line only proliferated in the presence of γ-IFN-treated, DR-positive autologous thyroid follicular cells. The bar is the SEM

## Ia antigen expression in other diseases

There has been a single case report of aberrant HLA-DR antigen expression by pancreatic cells in a newly diagnosed diabetic child, but the exact nature of these cells is unclear[41]. In pre-diabetic BB rats which develop autoimmune insulitis, only the pancreatic capillary endothelium is Ia-positive; β-cells express Ia antigens late in the disease[42]. Alopecia areata and Sjögren's syndrome are associated with organ-specific autoimmune diseases and HLA-DR-positive hair follicles and salivary gland epithelium have been found in the respective condition[43,44]. In primary biliary cirrhosis, the intrahepatic bile ducts may become Ia-positive[45]. In Sjögren's syndrome and primary biliary cirrhosis, but not alopecia areata, the presence of aberrant Ia-positive cells appears to correlate with the extent of lymphocytic infiltration around the site of HLA-DR antigen expression. Finally a role for Ia-positive astrocytes as APC in multiple sclerosis has been suggested by animal studies, in which these cells have been shown to present myelin basic protein to encephalitogenic T-cell lines[27]. Of interest is the fact that astrocytes were also able to elaborate an IL-1-like factor.

## ROLE OF Ia ANTIGEN EXPRESSION IN AUTOIMMUNITY

From the foregoing it is apparent that thyroid and probably other endocrine epithelia share with many other tissues the ability to express class II antigens. A common thread in most of these studies has been the link between ongoing immunological responses and the induction of Ia antigens: $\gamma$-IFN appears to be the key mediator. It seems likely that when T-cells are activated, for example during transplantation rejection, a graft-versus-host reaction or an autoimmune response, they will release $\gamma$-IFN and induce class II antigen expression on cells in the vicinity. On this basis, HLA-DR antigen expression in thyroid disease and diabetes is probably a secondary phenomenon – the autoimmune response has already been initiated by the time it occurs. Moreover, macrophages are perfectly capable of presenting thyroid antigens to the immune system[46], and morphological evidence supports an additional role for dendritic cells in thyroid autoimmunity[47]. The ability of macrophages to secrete IL-1 would certainly enhance the stimulation of T-cells at the initiation of the autoimmune response, whereas thyroid follicular cells do not appear able to produce IL-1[33].

Although Ia-positive endocrine cells may not initiate the autoimmune response, they could play a role in enhancing or perpetuating it (Figure 8.8). In a way, the Ia-positive cells would act like B-cells as APC, having a measure of specificity which in this case is endowed by the co-expression of the pertinent autoantigen with class II molecule. *In vitro* experiments cited above support this concept but the exact nature of the autoantigens recognized by T-cells is unknown. It also remains to be explained why such antigens apparently do not require processing. Could the autoimmune response itself modulate the way antigen is expressed on the cell surface, or does persistence of antigen on the cell surface allow it to escape the need for processing[9]?

Other important aspects of aberrant class II antigen expression need to be addressed. The first is to investigate why Ia antigens cannot be induced on rat thyroid cells[29], a fact we have confirmed using both primary cell cultures and the FRTL5 thyroid cell line treated with lectins or with T-cell-derived lymphokines (Weetman and Kohn, unpublished). Autoimmune thyroiditis is readily induced in rats and it will be important to see whether thyroid cells then become Ia antigen-positive; the existence of a model for thyroid autoimmunity in which aberrant class II antigen expression is not found would argue strongly against a key role for this phenomenon in generating disease.

A second area of uncertainty concerns the physiological regulation of Ia antigen expression. Is there a regulatory mechanism to decrease as well as increase expression? Such a molecule could have therapeutic potential. How

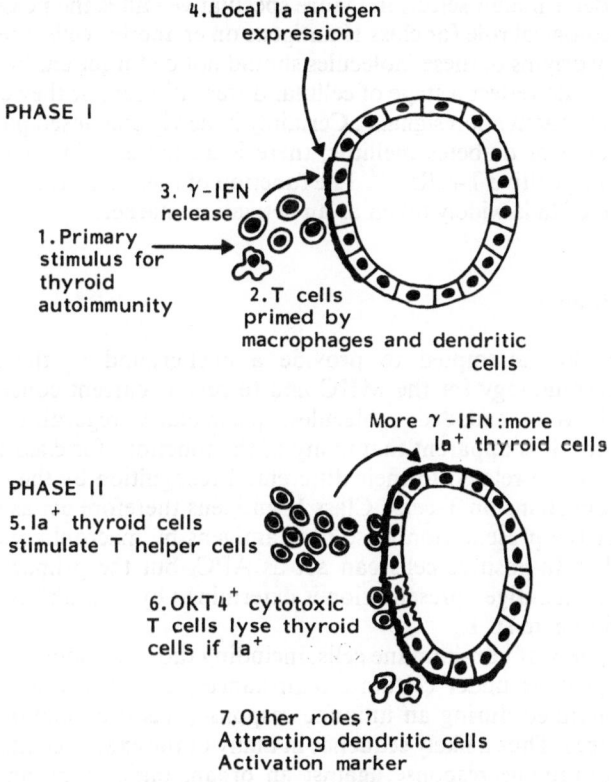

**Figure 8.8** Summary of the induction and function of Ia-positive thyroid follicular cells in Hashimoto's thyroiditis or Graves' disease

does $\gamma$-IFN stimulate Ia antigen synthesis? One possibility is via an action on an MHC-unlinked regulator gene, controlling all class II genes[6]. If this is correct, $\gamma$-IFN should produce coordinate expression of HLA-DP, -DQ and -DR antigens. Is this always the case and do these molecules have similar or distinct functions?

Finally, could Ia antigen expression have a role besides converting an epithelial cell into an 'auto-APC'? Certainly class II antigen expression would make these cells targets for destruction by OKT4-positive cytotoxic cells. Expression of Ia antigen by keratinocytes seems to act as an attractant to Langerhans cells in the skin[48], raising the possibility that Ia-positive endocrine cells may alter the migration of neighbouring lymphoid cells. Is aberrant expression of class II antigens related to Ir gene function and the HLA-DR associations recognized in autoimmunity? The fact that normal thyroid cells can become Ia-positive with $\gamma$-IFN treatment does not refute this possibility; for instance it may be that autoimmunity is associated with a particular configuration of aberrantly expressed Ia antigen with autoantigen. Thus abnormal class II antigen expression by certain cells adds a new twist to the concept of determinant selection. More speculative still is the possibility of a non-immunological role for class II antigens on endocrine cells: the proposed evolutionary origins of these molecules should not be forgotten. For instance, Ia antigens could reflect a stage of cellular differentiation, or they could serve as receptors for activation signals[6]. Certainly in newly diagnosed patients with Graves' disease or diabetes mellitus, there is an increase in the number of circulating Ia-positive T-cells[49,50]. The function of these cells is unknown, but the presence of Ia is widely taken as an activation marker.

## CONCLUSIONS

This review has attempted to provide a background to the somewhat confusing terminology for the MHC and to review current concepts of the function of MHC-encoded molecules, particularly regarding endocrine autoimmunity. It is apparent that many of the functions for class I and class II antigens can be related to their differential recognition by the OKT8 and OKT4 glycoproteins on T-cells. Class II antigens therefore act as restriction elements for the presentation of soluble antigens by macrophages to helper T-cells. Other Ia-positive cells can act as APC, but the primary status of macrophages in antigen presentation is determined by their ability to process antigen and secrete IL-1.

A wide variety of non-immune cells, including those in endocrine epithelia, become Ia-positive under certain circumstances; a central role for $\gamma$-IFN, which is generated during an immune response, has been demonstrated in many instances. Thus a likely sequence in many of the examples cited above is that an autoimmune response against an organ, initiated by an unknown process, generates autoreactive T-cells which accumulate in the organ and release lymphokines. Target cells then become Ia-positive and may exacerbate the autoimmune response by acting as additional APC, presenting autoantigen on their surfaces (Figure 8.8). This is supported by recent work performed *in vitro* with T-cell lines and clones. However, since conventional APC, such as macrophages and dendritic cells, are present in diseased target organs, together with B-cells which can act as specific APC, the exact contribution made by Ia-positive glandular epithelia to autoantigen presentation remains to be elucidated. The possibility also exists that aberrant Ia antigen expression may have a non-immunological function. In this rapidly moving section of endocrine immunology, we should not have too long to wait for these issues to be settled.

## ACKNOWLEDGEMENTS

The author is a Wellcome Senior Research Fellow in Clinical Science. I am grateful to Mrs Jane Pearson for expert secretarial assistance.

# References

1. Paul, W. E. (ed.) (1984). *Immunogenetics* (New York: Raven Press)
2. Bodmer, J. and Bodmer, W. E. (1984). Histocompatibility 1984. *Immunol. Today*, 5, 251–4
3. Thorsby, E. (1984). The role of HLA in T cell activation. *Human Immunol.*, 9, 1–7
4. Howard, J. C. (1985). Immunological help at last. *Nature (London)*, 314, 494–5
5. Meuer, S. C., Acuto, O., Hercend, T., Schlossman, S. F. and Reinherz, E. L. (1984). The human T cell receptor. *Ann. Rev. Immunol.*, 2, 23–50
6. Kinde, T. J., Mach, B., Sogn, J. A., Robinson, M. A., Kulaga, H., Moller, E., Carlsson, B., Wallin, J. and Bach, F. H. (1984). Identical or distinct functional roles for products of the HLA-DR, DC and SB loci. *Scand. J. Immunol.*, 20, 471–91
7. Heber-Katz, E., Hansburg, D. and Schwartz, R. H. (1983). The Ia molecule of the antigen presenting cell plays a critical role in immune response gene regulation of T cell activation. *J. Mol. Cell Immunol.*, 1, 3–14
8. Unanue, E. R. (1984). Antigen presenting function of the macrophage. *Ann. Rev. Immunol.*, 2, 395–428
9. Unanue, E. R., Beller, D. I., Yu, C. L. and Allen, P. M. (1984). Antigen presentation: comments on its regulation and mechanism. *J. Immunol.*, 132, 1–5
10. Gery, I. (1982). Production and assay of interleukin 1 (IL-1). In Fathman, C. G. and Fitch, F. W. (eds.) *Isolation, Characterization and Utilization of T Lymphocyte Clones*, pp. 42–56. (New York: Academic Press)
11. Ling, P. D., Warren, M. K. and Vogel, S. N. (1985). Antagonistic effect of interferon-$\beta$ on the interferon $\gamma$-induced expression of Ia antigen in murine macrophages. *J. Immunol.*, 135, 1857–63
12. Gerrard, T. L., Cupps, T. R., Jurgensen, C. H. and Fauci, A. S. (1984). Increased expression of HLA-DR antigens in hydrocortisone-treated monocytes. *Cell Immunol.*, 84, 311–6
13. Kehrl, J. H., Muraguchi, A. and Fauci, A. S. (1985). The modulation of membrane Ia on human B lymphocytes. *Cell Immunol.*, 92, 391–403
14. Roehm, N. W., Leibson, H. J., Zlotnik, A., Kappler, J., Marrack, P. and Cambier, J. C. (1984). Interleukin-induced increase in Ia expression by normal mouse B cells. *J. Exp. Med.*, 160, 679–94
15. Lanzavecchia, A. (1985). Antigen-specific interaction between T and B cells. *Nature (London)*, 314, 537–9
16. Bekkhoucha, F., Naquet, P., Pierres, A., Marchetto, S. and Pierres, M. (1984). Efficiency of antigen presentation to T cell clones by (B cell × B cell lymphoma) hybridomas correlates quantitatively with cell surface Ia antigen expression. *Eur. J. Immunol.*, 14, 807–14
17. Chu, E. T., Lareau, M., Rosenwasser, L. J., Dinarello, C. A. and Geha, R. S. (1985). Antigen presentation by EBV-B cells to resting and activated T cells: role of interleukin 1. *J. Immunol.*, 134, 1676–81
18. Ramila, G., Sklenar, I., Kennedy, M., Sunshine, G. H. and Erb, P. (1985). Evaluation of accessory cell heterogeneity. II. Failure of dendritic cells to activate antigen-specific T helper cells to soluble antigens. *Eur. J. Immunol.*, 15, 189–92
19. Janossy, G., Thomas, J. A., Bollum, J. J., Granger, S., Pizzdo, G., Brandstock, K. F., Wong, K., McMichael, A., Ganeshaguru, K. and Hoffbrand, A. V. (1980). The human thymic microenvironment: an immunohistologic study. *J. Immunol.*, 125, 202–12
20. Winchester, R. J., Ross, C. D., Jarowski, C. I., Wang, C. Y., Halper, J. and Broxmeyer, H. E. (1977). Expression of Ia-like antigen molecules on human granulocytes during early phases of differentiation. *Proc. Natl. Acad. Sci. USA*, 74, 4012–6
21. Mason, D. W., Dullman, M. and Barclay, A. N. (1981). Graft-versus-host disease induces expression of Ia antigen in rat epidermal cells and gut epithelium. *Nature (London)*, 293, 150–1
22. Hall, B. M., Bishop, G. A., Duggin, G. G., Horvath, J. S., Phillips, J. and Tiller, D. J. (1984). Increased expression of HLA-DR antigens on renal tubular cells in renal transplants: relevance to the rejection response. *Lancet*, 2, 247–57
23. Basham, T. Y. and Merigan, T. C. (1983). Recombinant interferon-$\gamma$ increases HLA-DR synthesis and expression. *J. Immunol.*, 130, 1492–4
24. Parker, J. S., Collins, T., Gimbrone, M. A., Cotran, R. S., Gitlin, J. D., Fiers, W.,

Clayberger, C., Krensky, A. M., Burakoff, S. J. and Reiss, C. S. (1983). Lymphocytes recognize human vascular endothelial and dermal fibroblast Ia antigens induced by recombinant immune interferon. *Nature (London)*, **305**, 726–9

25. Hirsch, M. R., Wietzerbin, J., Pierres, M. and Gordis, C. (1983). Expression of Ia antigens by cultured astrocytes treated with gamma-interferon. *Neurosci. Lett.*, **41**, 199–204

26. Klareskog, L., Forsum, U. and Peterson, P. A. (1980). Hormonal regulation of the expression of Ia antigens on mammary gland epithelium. *Eur. J. Immunol.*, **10**, 958–63

27. Fontana, A., Fierz, W. and Wekerle, H. (1984). Astrocytes present myelin basic protein to encephalitogenic T cell lines. *Nature (London)*, **307**, 273–6

28. Austin, P., Trowsdale, J., Rudd, C., Bodmer, W., Feldmann, M. and Lamb, J. (1985). Functional expression of the HLA-DP genes transfected into mouse fibroblasts. *Nature (London)*. **313**, 61–4

29. Pujol-Borrell, R., Hanafusa, T., Chiovato, L. and Bottazzo, G. F. (1983). Lectin-induced expression of DR antigen on human cultured follicular thyroid cells. *Nature (London)*, **304**, 71–3

30. Hanafusa, T., Pujol-Borrell, R., Chiovato, L., Russell, R. C. G., Doniach, D. and Bottazzo, G. F. (1983). Aberrant expression of HLA-DR antigen on thyrocytes in Graves' disease; relevance for autoimmunity. *Lancet*, **2**, 1111–5

31. Salamero, J., Michel-Bechet, M. and Charreire, J. (1983). Expression of H-2 antigens and thyroglobulin (Tg) on freshly dissociated and *in vitro* cultured monolayers of mouse thyroid epithelial cells (TEC). *Tissue Antigens*, **22**, 231–8

32. Bottazzo, G. F., Pujol-Borrell, R., Hanafusa, T. and Feldmann, M. (1983). Role of aberrant HLA-DR expression and antigen presentation in induction of endocrine autoimmunity. *Lancet*, **2**, 1115–9

33. Weetman, A. P., Volkman, D. J., Burman, K. D., Gerrard, T. L. and Fauci, A. S. (1985). The *in vitro* regulation of human thyrocyte HLA-DR antigen expression. *J. Clin. Endocrinol. Metab.*, **61**,

34. Todd, I., Pujol-Borrell, R., Hammond, L., Bottazzo, G. F. and Feldmann, M. (1985). Interferon-γ induces HLA-DR expression by thyroid epithelium. *Clin. Exp. Immunol.*, **61**, 265–73

35. Jansson, R., Karlsson, A. and Forsum, U. (1984). Intrathyroidal HLA-DR expression and T lymphocyte phenotypes in Graves' thyrotoxicosis, Hashimoto's thyroiditis and nodular colloid goitre. *Clin. Exp. Immunol.*, **58**, 264–72

36. Martinez-Maza, O., Andersson, U., Andersson, J., Britton, S. and De Ley, M. (1984). Spontaneous production of interferon-γ in adult and newborn humans. *J. Immunol.*, **132**, 251–5

37. Margolick, J. B., Hsu, S. M., Volkman, D. J., Burman, K. D. and Fauci, A. S. (1984). Immunohistochemical characterization of intrathyroid lymphocytes in Graves' disease. *Am. J. Med.*, **76**, 815–21

38. Davies, T. F. (1985). The role of human thyroid cell Ia (DR) antigen in thyroid autoimmunity. In Walfish, P. G., Wall, J. R. and Volpé, R. (eds.) *Autoimmunity and the Thyroid.* pp. 57–65. (Orlando: Academic Press)

39. Londei, M., Bottazzo, G. F. and Feldmann, M. (1985). Human T-cell clones from autoimmune thyroid glands: specific recognition of autologous thyroid cells. *Science*, **228**, 85–9

40. Weetman, A. P., Volkman, D. J., Burman, K. D., Margolick, J. B., Petrick, P., Weintraub, B. D. and Fauci, A. S. (1986). The production and characterisation of thyroid-derived T cell lines in Graves' disease and Hashimoto's thyroiditis. *Clin. Immunol. Immunopathol.* (In press)

41. Bottazzo, G. F. (1984). Cell damage in diabetic insulitis: are we approaching a solution? *Diabetologia*, **26**, 241–9

42. Janeway, C. (1985). The immune destruction of pancreatic beta cells. *Immunol. Today*, **6**, 229–32

43. Messenger, A. G., Bleehen, S. S., Slater, D. N. and Rooney, N. (1984). Expression of HLA-DR in hair follicles in alopecia areata. *Lancet*, **2**, 287–8

44. Lindahl, G., Hedfors, E., Klareskog, L. and Forsum, U. (1985). Epithelial HLA-DR expression and T lymphocyte subsets in salivary glands in Sjögren's syndrome. *Clin. Exp. Immunol.*, **61**, 475–82

45. Ballardini, G., Mirakian, R., Bianchi, F. B., Pisi, E., Doniach, D. and Bottazzo, G. F. (1984). Aberrant expression of HLA-DR antigens on bile duct epithelium in primary biliary cirrhosis: relevance to pathogenesis. *Lancet*, **2**, 1009–13

46. Weetman, A. P., McGregor, A. M. and Hall, R. (1983). Thyroglobulin uptake and presentation by macrophages in experimental autoimmune thyroiditis. *Immunology*, **50**, 315–8

47. Drexhage, H. A., Voorbij, H. A. M., van der Gaag, R. D. and Wiersinga, W. M. (1985). Antigen presenting dendritic cells in autoimmune thyroid disease. *Proceeding of the 9th International Thyroid Congress*. Sao Paulo, 1985 (Plenum Press, in press)

48. Roberts, L. K., Krueger, G. G. and Daynes, R. A. (1985). Correlation between the inducible keratinocyte expression of Ia and the movement of Langerhans cells into the epidermis. *J. Immunol.*, **134**, 3781–4

49. Jackson, R., Morris, M., Haynes, B. and Eisenbarth, G. (1982). Type I diabetes mellitus: Ia antigen-bearing T cells. *N. Engl. J. Med.*, **306**, 785–8

50. Jackson, R., Haynes, B., Burch, W. M., Shimizu, K., Bowring, M. A. and Eisenbarth, G. S. (1984). Ia$^+$ T cells in new onset Graves' disease. *J. Clin. Endocrinol. Metab.*, **59**, 187–90

# 9
# Observations on Graves' Ophthalmopathy; Pathology and Pathogenesis

## R. M. POPE, M. E. LUDGATE AND A. M. McGREGOR

Recognition of a link between the thyroid and the eye as is seen in Graves' ophthalmopathy (GO) has been attributed to Parry, Graves and von Basedow but observations relating exophthalmos to goitre can be found as early as the 12th century. Despite the growth of a vast literature, considerable uncertainty exists regarding many aspects of this potentially distressing and disfiguring clinical condition, particularly with regard to its pathogenesis and hence to the management of patients with the problem. Many excellent reviews providing an historical perspective and emphasizing the clinical aspects of GO have appeared in recent years[1-3]. This chapter will therefore focus particularly on information relating to the pathogenesis of GO.

A number of difficulties face workers in this field and before reviewing the available information it would seem appropriate to attempt to identify these to highlight their importance in the context of our understanding (or perhaps lack of understanding) of the pathogenesis of GO. A fundamental problem is the identification of patients with the disease. Although there is no doubt that it is relatively easy to recognize on clinical grounds the 3–5% of patients with severe or congestive ophthalmopathy who present with typical clinical features, reliable recognition of milder forms of the condition using purely clinical criteria such as those suggested by the American Thyroid Association (Table 9.1) is open to question. Using such criteria, it has been suggested that ophthalmopathy is detectable in between 25 and 50% of patients with Graves' disease. However, use of sensitive diagnostic aids such as ultrasound[4] and CT scanning[5] has shown that over 90% of all Graves' patients studied show evidence of extraocular muscle involvement, which, as will be discussed below is one of the hallmarks of the pathology of this condition. In addition, Gamblin and his colleagues[6] reported that in 40 out of 59 (68%) patients with Graves' disease and no apparent eye disease, an abnormal increase in intraocular pressure was detectable on upward gaze, perhaps suggesting that these patients had subclinical ophthalmopathy. These data will be discussed

**Table 9.1** Classification of the eye changes of Graves' disease

| Grade | Suggestions for grading |
|---|---|
| Class 0 | No physical signs or symptoms |
| Class 1 | Only signs (signs limited to upper lid retraction, stare, and lid lag) |
| Class 2 | Soft-tissue involvement with symptoms and signs |
| 0 | Absent |
| a | Minimal |
| b | Moderate |
| c | Marked |
| Class 3 | Proptosis 3 mm or more in excess of upper normal limits, with or without symptoms |
| 0 | Absent |
| a | 3–4 mm increase over upper normal |
| b | 5–7 mm increase |
| c | 8 mm or more increase |
| Class 4 | Extraocular muscle involvement (usually with diplopia, other symptoms, and other signs) |
| 0 | Absent |
| a | Limitation of motion of extreme gaze |
| b | Evident restriction of motion |
| c | Fixation of globe or globes |
| Class 5 | Corneal involvement (primarily due to lagophthalmos) |
| 0 | Absent |
| a | Stippling of cornea |
| b | Ulceration |
| c | Clouding, necrosis, perforation |
| Class 6 | Sight loss (due to optic nerve involvement) |
| 0 | Absent |
| a | Disc pallor or choking, or visual field defect; vision 20/20 to 20/60 |
| b | Same, but vision 20/70 to 20/200 |
| c | Blindness, i.e. failure to perceive light, vision 20/200 |

After Werner (1977). *J. Clin. Endocrinol. Metab.*, **44**, 203

in more depth later in the context of the relationship between Graves' disease *per se* and ophthalmopathy. However, they serve for the present to illustrate that selection of patients on clinical grounds alone may provide an unrepresentative population of patients for study, with all the attendant implications for the interpretation of data resulting from such studies.

The second major difficulty in the study of GO patients has been that of obtaining adequate, representative tissue samples. In the vast majority of cases, samples for study have come from the orbital contents of patients either undergoing decompressive surgery for severe or congestive ophthalmopathy, from patients undergoing squint surgery with stable 'burnt out' eye disease or at autopsy. The latter source was particularly used in many of the early studies involving collection of data from both controls and patients dying from untreated thyrotoxicosis. Whilst all three sources of tissue have proved useful and a great deal of worthwhile data has been obtained from them, one point that should be stressed is that their use has resulted in examination of patients with advanced disease, in whom one might expect to find only the relatively non-specific end-stage features of the condition. The important and large group of patients who at present defy adequate study in this way are those with early but progressive disease, the very group that must be looked at in more depth in order to appreciate underlying pathogenetic mechanisms with any clarity.

These problems together with the fact that to date, no satisfactory animal model of the condition exists, must somewhat temper our interpretation of the available data. Bearing these points in mind it is appropriate to consider the pathological features which have been recognized in GO before considering current thoughts on the pathogenesis itself.

## PATHOLOGY

### Extraocular muscle histology

Histological changes are present in a number of orbital tissues, though the most significant pathological changes are seen in the extraocular eye muscles themselves. These muscles are macroscopically characteristically enlarged by anything up to 8 times their normal size, with a rubbery firm texture (Figure 9.1). Studies of the muscle at a light microscopic level have shown this enlargement to be secondary to a combination of features, including interstitial oedema, together with a cellular infiltrate. In those cases of early disease which have been studied this is sparse and composed to a large extent of mature lymphocytes with a few plasma cells and macrophages (Figure 9.2). Focal collections of cells are present and there may also be a diffuse cellular infiltrate. In addition, small numbers of mast cells can be found, often in a perivascular distribution[7]. Detailed information regarding the nature of cellular subsets of lymphocytes etc. is, to date, not available. As the disease progresses and the lymphocytic infiltrate increases, enlargement and proliferation of interstitial fibroblasts occur and it seems likely that these latter cells are the source of increased amounts of glycosaminoglycans (GAG) which are present in the oedema fluid[8]. As hydrated forms of GAG occupy between 100 and 1000 times the volume of non-hydrated molecules, it becomes tempting to propose that it is the increase in extracellular fluid volume resulting from accumulation of these compounds in their hydrated form which is responsible for the increase in the volume of the muscles themselves. With progression of disease activity, involving further fibroblast proliferation and collagen production within the perimysium, muscle fibre bundles become progressively compressed and as a result atrophy. Extension of fibrous tissue from the muscles into the periorbital fat has been recognized and the overall histological appearances are of dense orbital scarring by the time the so-called 'end stage' of the disease is reached.

The degree of involvement of extraocular muscle appears to be rather variable as, although histological changes such as those described above are

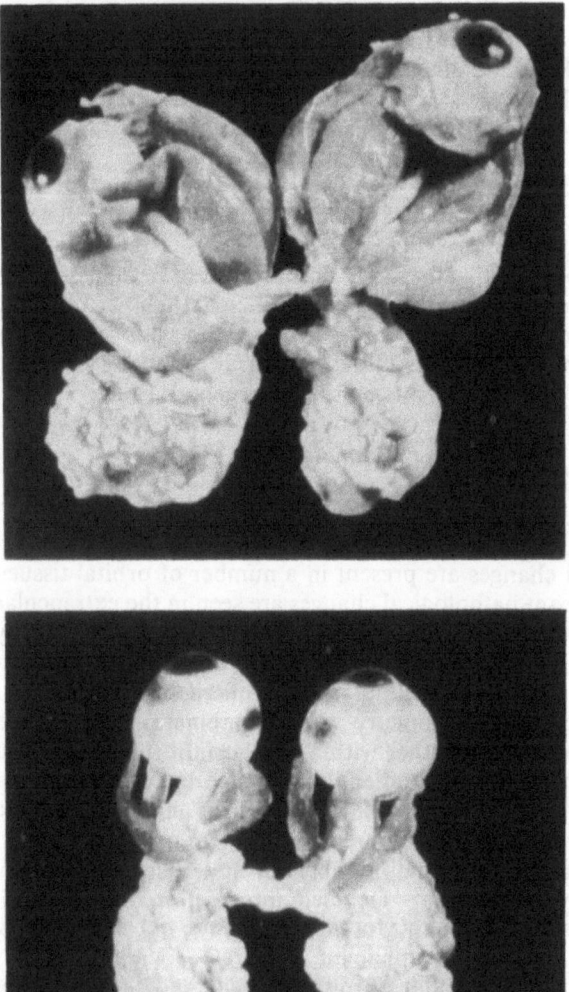

**Figure 9.1** Extraocular muscle enlargement (top) at postmortem in a patient with Graves' ophthalmopathy as compared with a normal control (bottom). Reproduced with permission from Jacobson, D. H. *et al.*, (1984). *Endocrine Rev.*, **5**, 200

usually present in all muscles, the inferior and medial recti show both the earliest and most severe changes, and in addition there may be considerable differences between the degree of involvement of the right and left eyes in any given individual.

Although a number of early reports suggested that extraocular muscle fibres showed definite degenerative changes with such features as loss of muscle striations and the presence of giant fibres with irregular and equal staining, these findings were in retrospect probably artifactual to a large

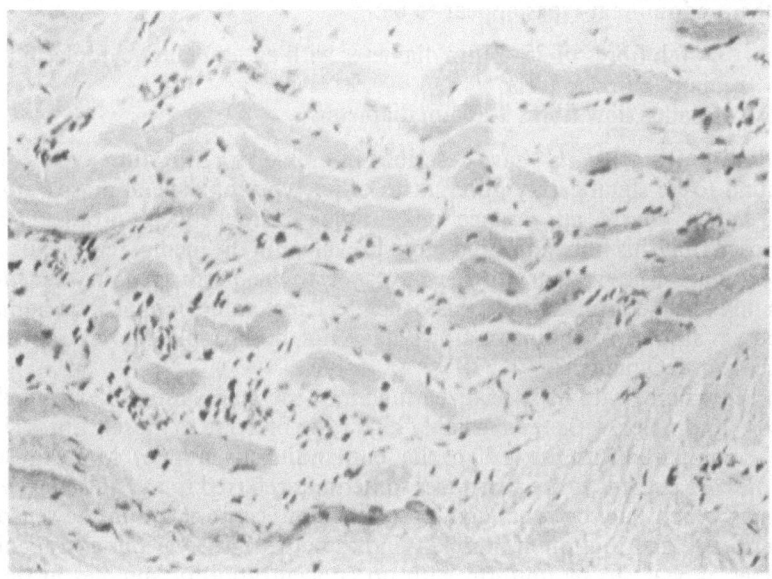

**Figure 9.2** Immune cell infiltration of extraocular muscle tissue from a patient with Graves' ophthalmopathy on light microscopy

extent. More recent light and electron microscopic studies of extraocular muscle[9,10] show that in the vast majority of cases, there is no abnormality of the muscle cell itself, with good preservation of muscle striations and only occasional cells showing disordered architecture or destruction of the sarcolemmal membrane. There is considerable muscle fibre atrophy but this seems likely therefore to be a secondary phenomenon resulting from the presence of fibrosis within the extraocular muscle as a whole, rather than to a primary destructive process affecting the muscle cells themselves.

The significance of these morphological observations remains unclear but the overall picture is one of enlargement of the extraocular muscles which show characteristic interstitial histological changes and further, probably secondary changes in other orbital tissues.

Histological changes are present in the lacrimal gland (which shows similar but less marked changes to those seen in the eye muscles) and in orbital fat, which may show a variable degree of thickening of connective tissue septa between lobules and a mild focal mononuclear cell infiltrate. These changes are, however, felt by the majority of workers to represent secondary rather than primary effects.

### Extraocular muscle characteristics

There are many features of extraocular muscle which may be responsible for their unique involvement in GO. Extraocular muscle is derived embryologically from neuroectoderm rather than from the mesoderm which forms other skeletal muscle[11]. A number of fibre types have been described in eye muscle but the predominant types appear to be:

(1)　twitch fibres of 25–50 μm diameter with an abundant cytoplasm and many mitochondria;

(2)　smaller slow fibres 9–15 μm diameter.

In addition Ringel *et al.*[12] have described in monkeys a third fibre type which is found to be significantly different to other types of skeletal muscle fibre. This has a coarse appearance and unique histochemical profile. They proposed that this fibre appeared more prevalent in the medial rectus muscle. Unfortunately equivalent studies have yet to be performed in man and certainly the detailed modern histochemical techniques applied to human tissues in studies of the myopathies have not been applied to extraocular tissue from GO patients.

In accordance with its specialized functions the innervation of extraocular muscle is complex with a remarkably high ratio of nerve to muscle fibres (1: 5 or 6 as compared with the 1: 50 of the semitendinosus muscle). Many muscle spindles are present as are structures sometimes referred to as pallisade nerve endings which may be functioning as mechanoreceptors within the sensory system. The distribution of muscle spindles between the various extraocular muscles appears to be uniform with no concentration of spindles in those muscles most severely affected in GO[13].

Physiological differences between extraocular and other skeletal muscles have also been demonstrated once again in accordance with specialized functions of eye muscle. A rapid twitch response is seen as is a high tetanic fusion frequency with rapid recruitment of fibres.

Other workers have shown that extraocular muscles have an extraordinarily profuse and variable blood supply and have also convincingly demonstrated the presence of a lymphatic system within the orbit, though this does not involve the eye itself, which as an extension of the central nervous system is therefore without lymphatics.

## Clinical consequences of extraocular muscle involvement

There are therefore several embryological, morphological and functional reasons why extraocular muscle may be preferentially involved in GO. Many of the clinical features of this condition are readily explained by the pathological changes which have been described. Thus any pathological process which results in an increase in the volume of the orbital contents, which are confined posteriorly by the bony orbit itself results in anterior movement of the globe. Postmortem studies performed by Rundle in 1944 showed that an increase of as little as 4 ml in the volume of the tissues within the orbit produced up to 6 mm of proptosis. When one appreciates that the average total volume of the six extraocular muscles in each orbit is 4 ml and that potential exists for considerable enlargement of each extraocular muscle, a mechanism for the production of proptosis becomes clear. In addition, the occurrence of such changes at the apex of the orbit can compress the optic nerve and result in the well-recognized forms of optic neuropathy seen in severe cases of GO. Diplopia is of course a well-recognized clinical feature of

GO and this is related to tethering of extraocular muscles by fibrosis which is occurring within and around them. Recent work correlating the risk of developing optic neuropathy with eye movements and the volume of retro-orbital muscles in fact suggests that a combination of these two measurements provides the best clinical index of risk for optic nerve damage. Earlier theories that the muscles were frankly myopathic have been rendered less tenable following electromyographic studies and saccadic velocity tests which show no evidence of a myopathy on formalized testing[3]. Inflammation and oedema may result in conjunctival injection with swelling, and a combination of these two features may produce corneal exposure and irritation, manifested by discomfort (often described as a gritty sensation in the eyes) and in the early stages, excessive lacrimation.

## NATURAL HISTORY

Considerable controversy has surrounded the important question of (1) whether GO and autoimmune thyroid disease represent differing presentations of the same problem, or (2) the two conditions are in fact separate entities which tend to frequently occur together. If the latter situation is the case, we must consider what the nature of the association is. Does thyroid dysfunction ever exist without some evidence of ophthalmopathy (or vice versa)? The importance of achieving an understanding of these two points is clear, as by defining the true relationship between these two problems it may prove possible to clarify the presently poor appreciation of the natural history of ophthalmopathy and direct future research appropriately. Computerized tomography of the orbit[5] has been shown in several studies to be valuable not only in evaluating the orbital muscles in GO (Figures 9.3, 9.4), but also in helping to resolve what may be a difficult differential diagnosis between GO and other causes of exophthalmos. In Enzman's series of 13 patients with Graves' disease who had no clinical signs of orbital involvement, five (40%) had orbital CT evidence of muscle enlargement. In addition 50% of a group of patients with what appeared clinically to be unilateral ophthalmopathy had CT evidence of bilateral disease.

Functional impairment (with tethering secondary to fibrosis) of the extraocular muscles, particularly involving the inferior and medial recti, is believed to be responsible not only for the characteristic ophthalmoplegia of GO which was discussed earlier but also for the abnormal rise in intraocular pressure on upward gaze which is seen in a percentage of patients with eye disease. In one series similar pressure changes were seen in 68% of 59 patients without clinical evidence of ophthalmopathy[6] but other workers report changes in 20–25% of all Graves' patients studied[14]. Clear evidence from a number of sources therefore shows the presence of eye disease in a percentage of Graves' patients who show no outward signs of ocular problems.

In addition, a normal distribution of the degree of proptosis in Graves' patients has been reported from Japan[15] (Figure 9.5) which is not in keeping with the concept that two populations of Graves' patients exist, one with and

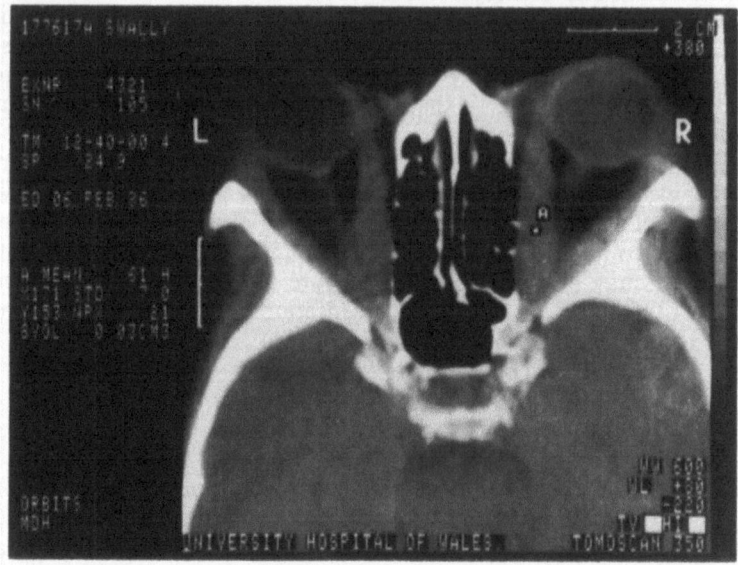

**Figure 9.3** Computerized tomographic scan of the orbits in a patient with Graves' ophthalmopathy showing in particular the enlarged medial recti muscles with crowding of the apex of both orbits in the area of the optic nerve

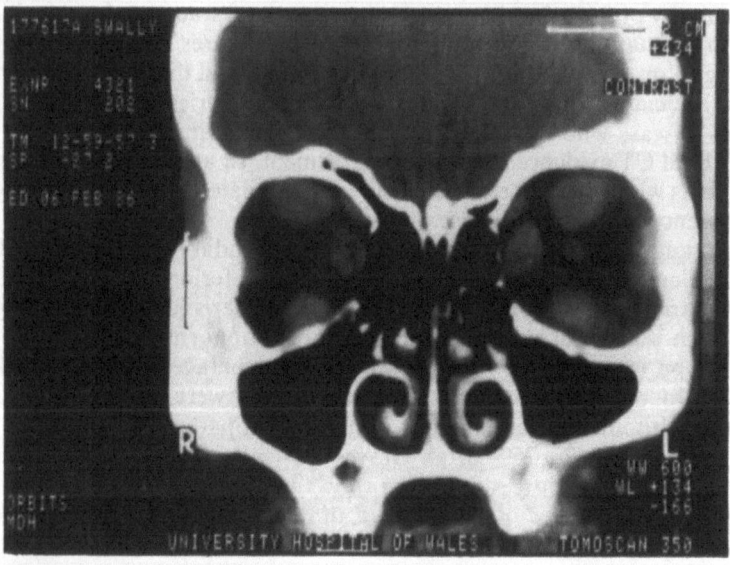

**Figure 9.4** Computerized tomographic scan in the coronal plane of the orbits of a patient with Graves' ophthalmopathy demonstrating enlargement of the extraocular muscles

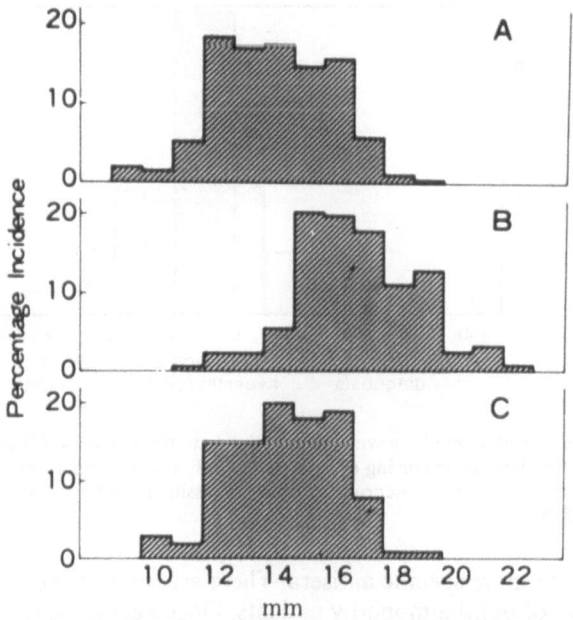

**Figure 9.5** The frequency of distribution of eye protrusion in healthy subjects (A), and patients with Graves' disease (B) and Hashimoto's thyroiditis (C). Reproduced with permission from Amino, N. *et al.* (1980). *J. Clin. Endocrinol. Metab.*, **51**, 1233

one without eye disease. There also appears to be a symmetrical distribution of the time of onset of eye symptoms around the time of diagnosis of hyperthyroidism[16] (Figure 9.6). However, there remains a group of Graves' patients who appear not to have evidence of eye involvement at the time of study, despite the use of a variety of diagnostic aids. It is not known whether this group would, if followed for a sufficient period of time, develop ophthalmopathy. Further studies in this area are needed before one can confirm the belief of many clinicians, that ophthalmopathy is an invariable event in Graves' patients.

There is also debate regarding the possibility that ophthalmopathy exists without thyroid dysfunction. Many groups have published series of patients showing no apparent evidence of thyroid dysfunction in the presence of ophthalmopathy, but there is a growing body of evidence to suggest that such patients may develop thyroid dysfunction if sufficiently sensitive tests of thyroid function are used and the patients are followed for long enough[17,18].

If Graves' disease and GO are part of the same disease spectrum then one might expect to see a similar pattern of inheritance between the two conditions. This on present evidence seems not to be the case with a female/male ratio of 6:1 being seen in Graves' disease and a ratio which may be closer to 2:1 in ophthalmopathy. However, detailed studies of the HLA associations of Graves' disease *per se* are limited[19] and require further work,

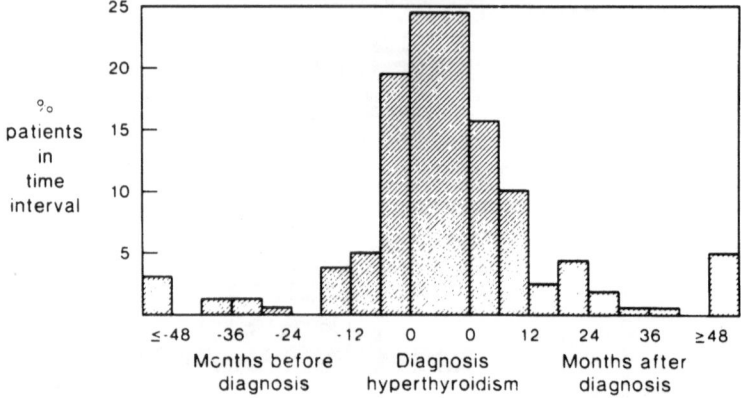

**Figure 9.6** The time of onset of eye symptoms in relation to the diagnosis of hyperthyroidism with the number of patients experiencing eye symptoms within each 6-month period expressed as a percentage of the whole group. Reproduced with permission from Gorman, C. A. (1983). *Mayo Clin. Proc.*, **58**, 517

possibly using more specific antisera. There are, to date, no published large-scale studies of ophthalmopathy patients. Once again, the spectre of patient definition and diagnosis rears its head as such studies could only be made truly comprehensive with the use of an as yet undefined diagnostic test which will reliably identify all patients with both clinical and subclinical disease.

Although the above comments refer to patients with Graves' disease, it is well recognized that the same ocular problems may occur in patients with Hashimoto's thyroiditis who may be hypothyroid, again perhaps implying that ophthalmopathy is a distinct condition which is almost invariably found in association with one of a variety of forms of autoimmune thyroid dysfunction.

Insufficient data currently exist to dogmatically favour the concept of either one or two diseases.

## PATHOGENESIS

Graves' ophthalmopathy is a condition in which the histological features, clinical course (particularly in terms of its response to immunosuppressive treatment) and close association with autoimmune thyroid disease (AITD) very strongly suggest an autoimmune aetiology. It is, however, true to say that not all the criteria for defining a disease as being autoimmune have been met (Table 9.2). Considerable effort over a number of years has centred on the investigation of a variety of possible pathogenetic mechanisms. Two lines of thought have emerged.

Firstly, is the eye disease causally related to events occurring in the thyroid gland and secondly, might there be specific pathogenetic mechanisms involving the orbital tissues in an unique fashion and independently of events

**Table 9.2** Autoimmune disease; criteria for establishment of a disease as autoimmune

---

(1)  Association with other autoimmune diseases

(2)  Autoantibodies or immune cell-mediated events

(3)  Target organ lymphocytic infiltration

(4)  Autoantigen isolated and characterized

(5)  Animal model produced with autoantigen

(6)  Disease transferred with serum or cells

(7)  Disease responsive to immunosuppression

---

occurring within the thyroid itself? The following discussion will follow these two theories separately, accepting that this is an artificial situation and will then attempt to draw together such conclusions as can be made from each section.

## Thyroid–eye association

Possible ways in which thyroidal disease might influence the orbit include:

(1)  The effect of alterations in thyroid hormone status;

(2)  An anatomical connection between thyroid and orbit;

(3)  Circulating thyroid-directed autoantibodies and their corresponding antigens may be deposited in orbital tissues in either native or complexed form and initiate damage;

(4)  True cross-reaction between thyroid-directed antibodies and putative orbital antigens may occur;

(5)  The effect of cell-mediated responses which, although directed against thyroidal antigens, have an effect on the orbit.

### Effects of alteration in thyroid status

Thyroid status has been implicated in the pathogenesis of autoimmune disease via an effect on suppressor T-cell function (Volpé in ref. 3). Early suggestions that a specific immunological defect resulted from such changes have, however, not been borne out by several recent studies[20]. There is debate regarding the consequences of hypo- or hyperthyroidism on eye status. The majority of GO patients have either treated or untreated hyperthyroidism but there is no significant correlation between severity of hyperthyroidism and severity of eye disease. In addition, many reports exist documenting the worsening of eye disease in patients who have become hypothyroid. An inhibitory effect of $T_3$ levels on glycosaminoglycans production from skin fibroblasts in culture has also been reported[21]. This may be of relevance in such cases, but is clearly not the complete explanation. It is, therefore, the practice of many physicians to aim to rapidly achieve and maintain the euthyroid state in all individuals with GO in the belief that abnormal thyroid status will tend to accelerate the progression of ophthalmopathy, though evidence for a causal relationship between the two is at present anecdotal only.

## An anatomical connection

Well-known work exists suggesting a role for radiographically demonstrated lymphatic connections between the deep cervical nodes and both thyroid and orbit[22]. Whilst this connection (which has not been demonstrated anatomically) could provide a means whereby antigen, antibody and lymphocyte transfer could take place between thyroid and orbit with resulting orbital damage, lymphatic flow in this direction has been said to depend on negating the effects of gravity by assuming the recumbent position and the relevance of this link remains unclear.

## Antigen, antibody or immune complex deposition and cross-reactivity between thyroid and putative orbital antigens

The presence of many autoantigens and their respective autoantibodies in AITD raises the possibilities that (1) circulating antibodies, antigens or immune complexes may be deposited in the orbit and initiate immunologically mediated damage, or (2) there may be immunological cross-reaction between thyroid-directed autoantibodies and either a normal or in some way modified component of the orbital tissues. Many authors have presented data to show an affinity of eye muscle for thyroglobulin (Tg) or Tg-antiTg complexes[23,24], and Kriss' group[25] demonstrated that vesicles which had been synthesized and contained Tg were lysed by patients' lymphocytes. However, these effects were also produced by lymphocytes from controls and are likely to be non-specific. Subsequent work by Feldt-Rasmussen and others[26] failed to show any correlation between ophthalmopathy and the presence or levels of either Tg or anti-Tg. Wall's group[27] have used Tg-specific monoclonal antibodies (McAbs) to show that Tg could not be identified in normal eye muscle and that immune complexes did not bind specifically to their eye muscle membrane preparation. More recently these workers, using similar Tg-specific McAbs[28] have studied the relationship between Tg and an orbital connective tissue (OCT) membrane preparation. These antibodies bound to both Tg and the OCT preparation, suggesting that a Tg-like antigenic site was present in the preparation, though this was not felt to be Tg itself, as the activity was not present in the cytosol fraction of OCT and could not be solubilized. Sera from 50% of patients also reacted with the preparation and this activity correlated closely with the level of Tg antibodies. Whilst this is an interesting observation it is unlikely to be of pathogenic significance in GO since no correlation between serum binding to OCT membrane and the presence, duration or severity of ophthalmopathy was observed. The present balance of evidence would therefore support the thesis that Tg or anti-Tg do not play a pathogenetic role in GO.

## Thyroid directed autoantibodies and TSH

A number of other antibodies have also been studied in this context. There is no relationship between LATS, TSI, TBII or thyroid microsomal antibody and ophthalmopathy[26,29]. TSH itself has also been studied in detail. There is no evidence that TSH itself causes ophthalmopathy but fragments of TSH in association with a serum immunoglobulin from patients with GO have been reported to stimulate GAG production in the mouse Harderian gland[30]. The validity of this model is questioned by many since the Harderian gland is not represented in man and the work has not been confirmed by other groups. There has been one report of a monoclonal antibody to the TSH receptor which stimulates both thyroid activity and collagen synthesis from fibroblasts which, if confirmed, provides an interesting potential mechanism for the stimulation of orbital fibroblasts in GO. It seems reasonable to state that those antibodies which are currently regularly identified in AITD and are directed against thyroidal antigens do not play a pathogenic role in GO. The concept of cross-reactivity between thyroid/orbital shared antigens and as yet undefined autoantibody remains valid and merits further study.

## Cell-mediated responses

That cell-mediated immune responses (CMI) play an important role in AITD is unequivocal, though many details of the mechanisms involved are not understood, and there is controversy over some central issues, particularly in relation to proposed defects in specific suppressor T-cell subsets[31]. These have been demonstrated by the results of modified Migration Inhibition Factor (MIF) tests which are regarded by their proponents as central to an explanation of the pathogenesis of AITD and yet have proved difficult to reproduce in the hands of others[32]. In view of the potential errors and difficulties involved in performing such tests without a pure antigen preparation (and none are currently available), it has not been possible to study the suggestion that T-cell responses may be directed against orbital tissues by 'thyroid-specific' T-cells, though evidence for orbital tissue-specific CMI will be discussed later.

Finally, if thyroid directed immune responses have an effect on orbital tissues one might expect to see in the orbital tissues a dramatic response to the removal of the thyroid gland, either surgically or by radioablation with [131]I. Difficulties arise in the assessment of response to such measures, however, as the natural history of GO is variable. The majority of patients tend to have relatively mild disease which does not progress rapidly, but a small proportion (perhaps 2–5%) have rapidly progressive ocular changes and prove a difficult management problem. In both groups, however, there is a pronounced tendency for the eyes to become quiescent after a period of years. In addition the difficulties of accurate assessment of the severity of ophthalmopathy have already been discussed, and it is not ethical to conduct controlled studies of such treatment modes in patients with anything but the very mildest disease. With these caveats, data from Werner[33] and Pequegnat[34] failed to show a reduction of progression of eye disease with either surgery or adequate radioablation. Many clinicians also have anecdotal evidence in individual patients of a rapid worsening of ophthalmopathy following both modes of treatment. This view is, however, not held by all[35].

## Ophthalmopathy as a non-thyroid-related disease process

What is the evidence that ophthalmopathy occurs in response to an immune response directed at orbital tissue-specific antigens? From an historical viewpoint the first experimental data came in 1968 from Pisarev and later from Singh and McKenzie[36], whose work suggested that a serum Ig from some patients with GO could promote histological changes and GAG synthesis in mouse Harderian gland. This activity was distinct from LATS activity in over 50% of the Ig-positive patients studied. These findings stimulated a search for orbital tissue-directed humoral and cell-mediated responses which continues to date. The advent of modern immunological methodology, particularly with respect to the development of improved immunoassay techniques and the use of monoclonal antibodies, has facilitated work in this area but it remains fraught with potential pitfalls.

### Cell-mediated immune responses

Many groups have studied CMI using the MIF test, which measures the production of lymphokines by sensitized T-cells in the presence of their specific antigen. Mahieu and Winand first reported MIF production using a preparation of orbital muscle and fat in 1972 and their work was extended by Munro et al.[31] who found MIF production in response to a crude orbital muscle antigen preparation and suggested that this did not correlate with MIF production in response to a thyroid antigen preparation. They inferred from this that a specific retro-orbital antigen was being recognized by their patients' lymphocytes and that it was likely that a different lymphocyte population was involved in recognition of thyroidal antigen. This finding supported the concept that the ophthalmopathy and thyroid disease were separate entities. One perhaps surprising feature, given the very crude nature of the antigen preparation, was the remarkable separation of results between controls and patients with exophthalmos in this study ($p < 0.0005$).

Other indices of lymphocyte activity have also been studied. Inhibition of leukocyte adherence has been assessed with conflicting results[37,38] and blastogenesis has been reported after in vitro incubation of lymphocytes from GO patients with a lacrimal gland preparation.

To date the information relating to T-cell subsets in peripheral blood in GO is limited. We have reported two cases with active ophthalmopathy who had increased numbers of activated (Ia+) T-cells and abnormal helper/suppressor ratios (2.5 and 3.2 in the respective patients; normal 1.9 ± 0.2). These changes reverted to normal during therapy with cyclosporin. In contrast, in a series of 55 patients[40], an elevation of suppressor/cytotoxic OKT8+ cells was found in cases with severe ophthalmopathy; once again the changes reverting to normal when immunosuppression (in this case with corticosteroids) was instituted. There is still other data which suggests a decrease in numbers of peripheral activated T-cells in Graves' patients with or without ophthalmo-pathy[41] and clearly more work is needed to clarify the true position in this important area. It may well be, of course, that the most relevant information will only be obtained from studies of lymphocytes obtained from within the eye muscles of GO where the presumably small numbers of antigen-specific T-cells may be concentrated. The difficulties of obtaining such tissue seem almost insurmountable, particularly as tissue would be required from patients with recent onset, active ophthalmopathy. A promising attempt to at least partially solve this problem has been the use of human extraocular muscle cells in an *in vitro* culture system to study the effects of GO patients' lymphocytes[42]. To date only very preliminary data has been published showing Tg-independent muscle cell lysis by lymphocytes from one patient with GO. It is important that parameters of immune activity other than cell lysis be studied in this system, perhaps particularly looking for production (in a specific manner by GO patients' lymphocytes) of lymphokines which stimulate fibroblast activity. Further reports from this group are awaited with considerable interest. One problem with the use of cloned eye muscle cells (at least in our hands) is their frustratingly slow growth rate; this may partially explain the lack of new data in this field. The system could also be extended to study CMI to a variety of other orbital tissues in an attempt to define the nature of the orbital antigens and in this context the work of Sissons[43] should be recalled. Lymphocytes from patients and controls stimulated GAG production from orbital fibroblasts in culture. This work needs to be repeated using HLA-matched tissue and lymphocytes to minimize non-relevant interactions.

The evidence which currently exists for the presence of CMI to orbital antigens continues to be debated. The reproducibility and relevance of these findings will remain unclear until the precise antigen(s) involved are defined. The question of whether such phenomena represent primary or secondary events in pathogenetic terms has not been answered. In the light of recent advances in our understanding of the relevance of HLA class II antigen expression in autoimmune states there is scope for a great deal of work using a variety of orbital tissues as targets, in an attempt to answer these questions.

## Humoral aspects

The relevance of thyroid-directed antibodies in relation to GO was discussed earlier in this article. It has been thought for some time that orbital autoantigens existed and that corresponding autoantibodies should be identifiable in patients.

Kodama *et al.*[44] were the first to use McAbs prepared against a variety of orbital tissues to try and identify autoantigens and hence (using an ELISA-based system) the corresponding autoantibodies in patients' serum. Although their initial results appeared most encouraging they subsequently showed a high degree of non-specific binding between their ELISA antiserum enzyme conjugate and blood-derived IgG contaminating their eye muscle preparation. A variety of biochemical manipulations of the antigen were required to try and eliminate these responses and the resulting ELISA data showed a marked reduction in specific activity. They have since published showing inability to identify specific human eye muscle-binding activity in GO patients' sera despite the use of a variety of techniques, and concluded that the sera of patients with GO does not contain eye muscle-specific antibodies. However, more recent data from this group[28] suggests that sera from 50% of patients with GO reacted with a binding site in an orbital CT membrane preparation and that the activity correlated closely with Tg activity, despite the finding that the OCT membrane-binding site did not appear to be Tg itself. This work was discussed earlier.

There have been other reports of the detection of retro-orbital antigen-specific antibodies in GO patients. Atkinson et al.[29] described an Ig (which they termed ophthalmopathic immunoglobulin) using an ELISA assay system and a $100000 \times g$ porcine eye muscle membrane preparation. This was detected in 64% of patients with active, untreated GO, in 25% of patients with active disease on steroid treatment and in only 16% of those with inactive disease. Only one of 22 patients without clinical evidence of eye disease reacted in the assay. In defining the specificity of binding using membrane preparations from other tissues the authors showed that there was specific binding only to the eye muscle membrane preparation. In addition there was no correlation with TBII, microsomal or Tg antibodies, and the putative immunoglobulin did not react with Tg itself. It was suggested that the assay might be useful as a marker of disease activity and hence in further studies into the pathogenesis of the condition. Another attempt to identify HEMMemb-specific antibodies used an immunoprecipitation technique with $^{125}$I Staph. protein A[47]. The results of this study were expressed as an index which took account of non-specific binding of the radio-labelled protein A directly to the sample and highly significant differences were seen between patients and controls ($p < 0.001$). No such differences were seen when skeletal muscle membrane was used and the addition of anti-Tg antibodies in a wide range of dilutions produced no change in the results, suggesting that the binding was Tg-independent. The authors have subsequently correlated the level of antibody with disease activity and have also attempted to purify their antigen preparation prior to assessing the effects of treatment on antibody levels. The results of these studies are awaited with interest but it should be stressed that once again, other workers have reported difficulties in reproducing these findings[48].

Many of the difficulties encountered in the demonstration of eye tissue-specific antibodies result from the crude nature of the antigen preparation and the resulting strong possibility that different preparations contain varying antigenic determinants. Until a uniform purified antigen preparation can be prepared it remains difficult to interpret the above data and to draw any conclusions in terms of the pathological relevance of humoral activity against retro-orbital tissues as measured in the serum.

## Infectious agents as potential sources of cross-reacting antigens

Evidence that antigenic determinants may be shared between two apparently unrelated tissues is available from other sources, particularly with regard to cross-reacting determinants between micro-organisms and human tissues. Weiss and Ingbar[45] have shown a saturable binding site for bovine TSH on a number of micro-organisms and other workers have demonstrated the appearance of thyroid epithelium-binding antibodies in patients who have suffered infection with *Yersinia enterocolitica* organisms. The occurrence of *Yersinia* reactive antibodies in animals immunized against human thyroid epithelium membranes provides further support for this thesis, and increasing numbers of reports describe the appearance of bacterial antigens in a number of autoimmune diseases[46]. Whether or not these observations have pathogenic significance remains to be investigated, but the potential implications are clear. Similar studies should be carried out to assess their relevance to ophthalmopathy.

## CONCLUSIONS

Despite accumulation of a considerable literature on GO we still remain remarkably ignorant about the underlying pathogenetic processes and the link with AITD. Limited access to relevant pathological tissue has undoubtedly been the major problem. This may be resolved by recent developments in tissue culture techniques. Until such time as the relevant antigenic determinants against which the autoimmune assault is directed are defined, the present confusion and controversy surrounding GO will continue. Efforts therefore need to be directed urgently, with techniques that are already available, towards attempting to define the tissues against which the autoimmune process is directed and, in particular, the relevant autoantigenic constituents within these tissues.

### References

1. Jacobson, D. H. and Gorman, C. A. (1984). Endocrine ophthalmopathy: current ideas concerning aetiology, pathogenesis and treatment. *Endocrine Rev.*, 5, 200–20
2. Lewis, M., Topliss, D. J., Okita, N., How, J., Row, V. V. and Volpé, R. (1983). The etiology of endocrine exophthalmos. In Franklin, E. C. (ed.) *Clinical Immunology Update. Reviews for Physicians.* pp. 261–80. (New York: Elsevier Biomedical)
3. Gorman, C. A., Waller, R., Dyer, J. A. (eds.) (1984). *The Eye and Orbit in Thyroid Disease.* (New York: Raven Press)
4. Werner, S. C., Coleman, D. J. and Franzen, L. A. (1974). Ultrasonographic evidence of a consistent orbital involvement in Graves' disease. *N. Engl. J. Med.*, 290, 1447–50
5. Enzmann, D. R., Donaldson, S. S. and Kriss, J. P. (1979). Appearance of Graves' disease on orbital computed tomography. *J. Computer Assisted Tomography*, 3, 815–9
6. Gamblin, G. T., Harper, D. G., Galentine, P., Buck, D. R., Chernow, B. and Eil, C. (1983). Prevalence of increased intraocular pressure in Graves' disease – evidence of frequent subclinical ophthalmopathy. *N. Engl. J. Med.*, 308, 420–4
7. Rundle, F. F., Finlay-Jones, L. R. and Noad, K. B. (1953). Malignant exophthalmos: a quantitative analysis of the orbital tissues. *Aust. Ann. Med.*, 2, 128–35
8. Wegelius, O., Asboe-Hansen, G. and Lamberg, B. A. (1957). Retrobular connective tissue changes in malignant exophthalmos. *Acta Endocrinol. (Copenh).* 25, 452–6
9. Kroll, A. J. and Kuwabara, T. (1966). Dysthyroid ocular myopathy; anatomy, histology and electron microscopy. *Arch. Ophthalmol.*, 76, 244–57
10. Hufnagel, T. J., Hickey, W. F., Cobbs, W. H., Jakobiec, F. A., Iwamoto, T. and Eagle, R. C. (1984). Immunohistochemical and ultrastructural studies on the exenterated orbital

tissues of a patient with Graves' disease. *Ophthalmology*, **91**, 1411–9

11. Sevel, D. (1981). A reappraisal of the origin of the human extraocular muscles. *Ophthalmology*, **88**, 1330–8

12. Ringel, S. R., Engel, W. K., Bender, A. N., Peters, N. D. and Yee, R. D. (1978). Histochemistry and acetylcholine receptor distribution in normal and denervated monkey extraocular muscles. *Neurology*, **28**, 55–63

13. Cooper, S. and Daniel, P. M. (1949). Muscle spindles in human extrinsic eye muscles. *Brain*, **72**, 1–24

14. Allen, C., Stetz, D., Roman, S. H., Podos, S., Som, P. and Davies, T. F. (1985). Prevalence and clinical associations of intraocular pressure changes in Graves' disease. *J. Clin. Endocrinol. Metab.*, **61**, 183–7

15. Amino, N., Yuasa, T., Yabu, Y., Miyai, K. and Kumahara, Y. (1980). Exophthalmos in autoimmune thyroid disease. *J. Clin. Endocrinol. Metab.*, **51**, 1232–4

16. Gorman, C. A. (1983). Temporal relationship between onset of Graves' ophthalmopathy and diagnosis of thyrotoxicosis. *Mayo Clin. Proc.*, **58**, 515–9

17. Tamai, H., Nakagawa, T., Ohsako, N., Fukino, O., Takahashi, H., Matsu-Zuka, F., Kuma, K. and Nagataki, S. (1980). Changes in thyroid function in patients with euthyroid Graves' disease. *J. Clin. Endocrinol. Metab.*, **50**, 108–2

18. Teng, C. S. and Yeo, P. P. B. (1977). Ophthalmic Graves' disease: natural history and detailed thyroid function studies. *Br. Med. J.*, **1**, 273–5

19. Farid, N. R., Sampson, L., Noel, E. P. *et al.*, (1979). A study of human leukocyte D locus related antigens in Graves' disease. *J. Clin. Invest.*, **63**, 108–13

20. Weetman, A. P., McGregor, A. M., Ludgate, M. and Hall, R. (1984). Effect of triiodothyronine on normal human lymphocyte function. *J. Endocrinol.*, **101**, 81–6

21. Smith, T. J., Horowitz, A. L. and Refetoff, S. (1981). The effect of thyroid hormone on glycosaminoglycans accumulation in skin fibroblasts. *Endocrinology*, **108**, 2997–9

22. Kriss, J. P. (1970). Radioisotopic thyroidolymphography in patients with Graves' disease. *J. Clin. Endocrinol. Metab.*, **40**, 872–85

23. Mullin, B. R., Levinson, R. E., Friedman, A., Hanson, D. E., Winand, R. J. and Kohn, L. D. (1977). Delayed hypersensitivity in Graves' disease and exophthalmos; identification of thyroglobulin in normal human orbital muscle. *Endocrinology*, **100**, 351–66

24. Konishi, J., Herman, M. M. and Kriss, J. P. (1974). Binding of thyroglobulin and thyroglobulin-antithyroglobulin complex to extraocular muscle membrane. *Endocrinology*, **95**, 434–66

25. Kriss, J. P., Konishi, J. and Herman, M. (1975). Studies on the pathogenesis of Graves' ophthalmopathy (with some related observations regarding therapy). *Recent Prog. Horm. Res.*, **3**, 533–66

26. Feldt-Rasmussen, U., Kemp, A., Bech, K., Madsen, S. N. and Date, J. (1981). Serum thyroglobulin; its autoantibody and thyroid stimulating antibodies in the endocrine exophthalmos. *Acta Endocrinol.*, **96**, 192–8

27. Kodama, K., Sikorska, H., Bayly, R., Bandy-Dafoe, P. and Wall, J. R. (1984). Use of monoclonal antibodies to investigate a possible role of thyroglobulin in the pathogenesis of Graves' ophthalmopathy. *J. Clin. Endocrinol. Metab.*, **59**, 67–73

28. Kuroki, T., Ruf, J., Whelan, L., Miller, A. and Wall, J. R. (1985). Antithyroglobulin monoclonal and autoantibodies cross-react with an orbital connective tissue membrane antigen: a possible mechanism for the association of ophthalmopathy with autoimmune thyroid disorders. *Clin. Exp. Immunol.*, **62**, 361–70

29. Atkinson, S., Holcombe, M., Taylor, J. and Kendall-Taylor, P. (1984). Ophthalmopathic immunoglobulin in patients with Graves' ophthalmopathy. *Lancet*, **2**, 374–6

30. Winand, R. J. and Kohn, L. D. (1975). Stimulation of adenylate cyclase activity in retro-orbital tissue membranes by thyrotropin and an exophthalmogenic factor derived from thyrotropin. *J. Biol. Chem.*, **250**, 6522–6

31. Munro, R. E., Lamki, L., Row, V. V. and Volpé, R. (1973). Cell mediated immunity in the exophthalmos of Graves' disease as demonstrated by the Migration Inhibition Factor (MIF) test. *J. Clin. Endocrinol. Metab.*, **37**, 286–92

32. Ludgate, M. E., Ratanachaiyavong, S., Weetman, A. P., Hall, R. and McGregor, A. M. (1985). Failure to demonstrate cell mediated immune responses to thyroid antigens in Graves' disease using *in vitro* tests of lymphokine-mediated migration inhibition. *J. Clin.*

*Endocrinol. Metab.*, **60**, 98–102

33. Werner, S. C., Feind, C. R. and Aida, M. (1967). Graves' disease and total thyroidectomy: progression of severe eye changes and decrease in serum long acting thyroid stimulator after operation. *N. Engl. J. Med.*, **276**, 132–8

34. Pequegnat, E. P., Mayberry, W. E., McConahey, W. M. and Wyse, E. P. (1967). Large doses of radioiodine in Graves' disease: effect on ophthalmopathy and long-acting thyroid stimulation. *Mayo Clin. Proc.*, **42**, 802–11

35. Gwinup, G., Elias, A. N. and Ascher, M. S. (1982). Effect on exophthalmos of various methods of treatment of Graves' disease. *J. Am. Med. Assoc.*, **247**, 2135–8

36. Singh, S. P. and McKenzie, J. M. (1971). $^{35}$S-sulphate uptake by mouse Harderian gland: effect of serum from patients with Graves' disease. *Metabolism*, **20**, 422–7

37. Silverberg, J., Trokoudes, K., Sugenoya, A., Row, V. V. and Volpé, R. (1978). Leukocyte adherence inhibition in thyroid disease. *Clin. Invest. Med.*, **1**, 93

38. Wall, J. R., Walters, B. A. J. and Grant, C. (1979). Leukocyte adherence inhibition in response to human orbital and lacrimal extracts in patients with Graves' ophthalmopathy. *J. Endocrinol. Invest.*, **2**, 375

39. Weetman, A. P., McGregor, A. M., Ludgate, M., Beck, L., Mills, P. V., Lazarus, J. H. and Hall, R. (1983). Cyclosporin improves Graves' ophthalmopathy. *Lancet*, **2**, 486–9

40. Felberg, N. T., Sergott, R. C., Savino, P. J., Blizzard, J. J., Schatz, N. J. and Amsel, J. (1985). Lymphocyte subpopulations in Graves' ophthalmopathy. *Arch. Ophthalmol.*, **103**, 656–9

41. Wall, J. R., Gray, B. and Greenwood, D. M. (1977). Total and 'activated' peripheral blood T lymphocytes in patients with thyroid disorders. *Acta Endocrinol. (Copenh).*, **85**, 753–9

42. Blau, H. M., Kaplan, I., Tao, T.-W. and Kriss, J. P. (1983). Thyroglobulin independent cell mediated cytoxicity of human eye muscle cells in tissue culture by lymphocytes of a patient with Graves' ophthalmopathy. *Life Sci.*, **32**, 45–53

43. Sissons, J. C., Kothary, P. and Kirchick, H. (1971). The effect of lymphocytes, sera and long-acting thyroid stimulator from patients with Graves' disease on retrobulbar fibroblasts. *J. Clin. Endocrinol. Metab.*, **37**, 17–24

44. Kodama, K., Sikorska, H., Bandy-Defoe, P., Bayly, R. and Wall, J. R. (1982). Demonstration of a circulating autoantibody against a soluble eye muscle antigen in Graves' ophthalmopathy. *Lancet*, **2**, 1353–6

45. Weiss, M., Kasper, D. and Ingbar, S. H. (1983). Antigenic cross-reactivity of thyroid membranes and certain Gram negative bacteria. Presented at the *65th Annual Meeting of the Endocrine Society*, San Antonio, Texas, June 8–10

46. Winbald, S. (1973). The clinical panorama of human *Yersiniosis enterocolitica. Contrib. Microbiol. Immunol.*, **2**, 129

47. Farnya, M., Nauman, J. and Gardas, A. (1985). Measurement of autoantibodies against human eye muscle plasma membranes in Graves' ophthalmopathy. *Br. Med. J.*, **290**, 191–2

48. Sikorska, H. and Wall, J. R. (1985). Failure to detect eye muscle membrane specific autoantibodies in Graves' ophthalmopathy (letter). *Br. Med. J.*, **291**, 604

# 10
# Autoimmune Thyroid Disease in Pregnancy and the Postpartum Period

**R. JANSSON AND A. KARLSSON**

Pregnancy represents a specific immunologic situation because the fetus is recognized by the maternal immune system as an allograft which needs protection from being rejected by the mother. Numerous factors have been proposed as possible mediators of an immunosuppressive effect on an antifetal allograft response[1,2]. These include local mechanisms in the placenta, presence of serum inhibitory factors and/or maternal cellular hyporeactivity (Table 10.1). However, the primary events behind the development of tolerance against the fetal allograft are still largely unknown.

**Table 10.1** Factors that have been implicated in the suppression of the immune response during pregnancy

Hormones (oestrogens, progesterone, HCG, placental lactogen)
Pregnancy-associated plasma proteins (e.g. PZ-protein)
Immune complexes
$\alpha$-Fetoprotein
Prostaglandins
Lymphokines
Fetal suppressor lymphocytes
Maternal blocking antibodies
Reduction of T-helper and B-cell numbers in maternal circulation

Understanding the mechanisms of immunological tolerance during pregnancy is of importance for the study of reproduction. However, knowledge in this field may be even more important to the understanding of the course and cure of autoimmune diseases, which are characterized by an abnormal regulation of immunological tolerance. Studies of autoimmune thyroid diseases have provided us with an understanding of autoimmune processes not only in the thyroid but in other organs as well. Similarly, it may be assumed that the expanding research on autoimmune thyroid disease in pregnancy will contribute to our knowledge of autoimmunity in general.

In this chapter three aspects (Table 10.2) of the influence of pregnancy on autoimmune thyroid disease will be presented and discussed: (1) maternal disease activity during pregnancy; (2) fetal disease due to transplacental transfer of autoantibodies; and (3) transient maternal disease in the postpartum period. First, however, a short review of autoimmune thyroid disease will be given. The normal physiological alterations in thyroid hormone levels and iodine metabolism that occur during pregnancy will not be considered. For this topic the interested reader is referred to some recent reviews[3,4].

**Table 10.2** Aspects of autoimmune thyroid disease in relation to pregnancy

---

Reduced activity of maternal disease in pregnancy

Fetal disease due to transplacental passage of autoantibodies

Transient aggravation of maternal disease in the postpartum period

---

## AUTOIMMUNE THYROID DISORDERS

Autoimmune disorders in general are characterized by the presence of autoaggressive lymphocytes and the production of autoantibodies. The relative pathogenetic importance of the cellular and humoral immune responses may differ in various disorders. In autoimmune thyroid disease the production of autoantibodies seems fundamental[5,6]. The most important autoantibodies are directed against the TSH receptor, thyroglobulin and the thyroid microsomal antigen (Figure 10.1).

TSH receptor antibodies produce *Graves' thyrotoxicosis* by mimicking the effect of pituitary TSH on specific receptors localized in the surface membrane of thyroid follicular cells. This leads to an overproduction of thyroid hormones and a breakdown of the pituitary feedback regulation of thyroid function. High levels of thyroid hormones are found in the circulation and a high thyroidal turnover rate of iodine can be demonstrated by radioiodine uptake measurements.

*Autoimmune thyroiditis* is characterized by lymphocytic infiltration of the thyroid gland. This may cause goitre (Hashimoto's thyroiditis) and/or destruction of the thyroid epithelium (atrophic thyroiditis). In both cases thyroid function may be impaired leading to hypothyroidism. Autoantibodies in autoimmune thyroiditis are generally directed against the thyroid microsomal antigen and/or thyroglobulin (Figure 10.1). Some observations suggest that autoantibodies against the thyroid microsomal antigen may have a functional role in the development of autoimmune thyroiditis[7]. The microsomal antigen is localized in the membrane of endocytic vesicles that carry uniodinated thyroglobulin from the endoplasmic reticulum to the apical surface of the thyroid follicular cell. Recent data suggest that the microsomal antigen is identical to or at least closely attached to the thyroid peroxidase enzyme[8]. This enzyme is exposed on the apical surface and necessary for iodination of thyroglobulin. Thus it is possible that the microsomal antigen–

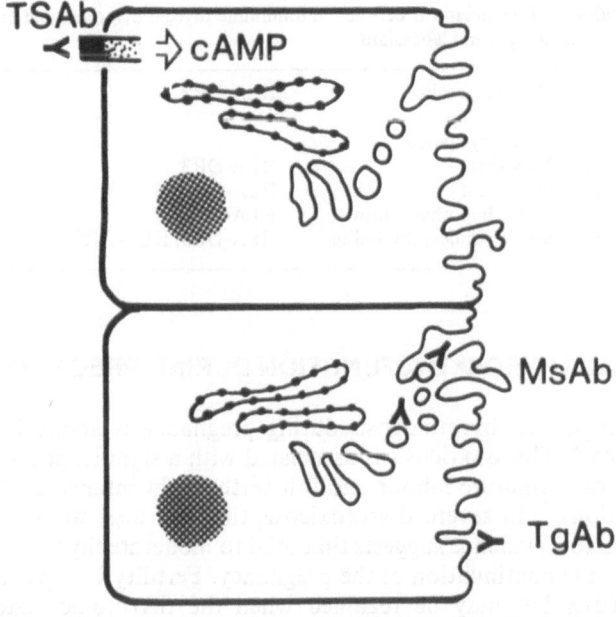

**Figure 10.1** Thyroid autoantibodies of importance in autoimmune thyroid disease. Antibodies bind to the receptor and thereby activate a membrane-bound adenylate cyclase to generate cAMP – thyroid-stimulating antibodies (TSAb). This signal causes a biochemical cascade stimulating thyroid hormone production and secretion, and eventually leads to Graves' thyrotoxicosis. The thyroid microsomal antigen is localized in the membrane of endocytotic vesicles which carry thyroglobulin from the endoplasmic reticulum to the apical cell surface, where thyroglobulin is being iodinated. Antibodies against the thyroid microsomal antigen (MsAb) and thyroglobulin (TgAb) are found in autoimmune thyroiditis

antibody reactions can impair iodination and thereby thyroid hormone production.

Most autoimmune disorders are associated with certain haplotypes of HLA-DR (class II) antigens. The HLA-DR3 antigen is over-represented among patients with Graves' disease, whereas in autoimmune thyroiditis the picture is more complex (Table 10.3)[9]. The atrophic variant of autoimmune thyroiditis seems to be associated with HLA-DR3, whereas HLA-DR5 has been found to be over-represented among individuals with the goitrous (Hashimoto) variant. However, cross-reactivity between HLA-DR4 and HLA-DR5 antisera (N. R. Farid, personal communication) may cast doubt on the validity of such observations in some of the older studies. In a recent population study it was found that the HLA-DR4 antigen was prevalent among euthyroid women with thyroid microsomal antibodies and this association was even stronger in those of the women who developed postpartum hypothyroidism[10]. The molecular basis for the genetic linkage between HLA-DR haplotypes and disease is not completely understood. The recent observation of HLA-DR antigen expression on thyrocytes in autoimmune thyroid disease, but not in normal thyroids, seems to provide a clue for our understanding of the autoimmune process[11].

**Table 10.3** Associations between autoimmune thyroid disorders and HLA-DR haplotypes in Caucasians

| | |
|---|---|
| Graves' thyrotoxicosis | HLA-DR3 |
| Autoimmune thyroiditis | |
| atrophic variant | HLA-DR3 |
| goitrous variant | HLA-DR5 (?) |
| postpartum hypothyroidism | HLA-DR4 |
| postpartum painless thyroiditis | HLA-DR3, HLA-DR5 (?) |

## MATERNAL THYROID DYSFUNCTION DURING PREGNANCY

The prevalence of thyrotoxicosis during pregnancy is about 1–2 per 1000 pregnancies[3,4]. Thyrotoxicosis is associated with a significant increase in the frequency of premature labour and low birthweight infants[3] and congenital malformations[12]. In severe thyrotoxicosis the fetal loss rate is increased as well[4]. Available evidence suggests that mild to moderate thyrotoxicosis is not harmful to the continuation of the pregnancy. Fertility is impaired in severe thyrotoxicosis but may be regained when the thyrotoxic state has been brought under control by treatment. The patient should therefore be told of an increased risk of pregnancy after initiation of treatment.

Hypothyroidism during pregnancy is probably more common than thyrotoxicosis and mild cases may remain undetected due to lack of typical symptoms. Severe hypothyroidism is a cause of infertility whereas mild to moderate hypothyroidism appears to have a minimal effect on the reproductive capacity. The reports on the outcome of pregnancy in hypothyroid women with respect to fetal loss rate and the fetal development are contradictory[13,14]. The diagnostic methods used in many of the older studies are not accepted today and, secondly, iodine deficiency may have been more important than maternal hypothyroidism for the outcome of the pregnancy. It is well established that iodine deficiency is one very important cause of cretinism and intellectual disability in areas with endemic goitres[15].

The *fetal thyroid* begins to produce hormones at about the 12th week of gestation but the pituitary–thyroid axis is not established until the fourth or fifth month of gestation[16]. It appears that the normal fetal development depends upon adequate amounts of fetal as well as maternal thyroid hormones. Fetal thyroid hormone production is of the greatest importance. Athyreotic infants of euthyroid mothers show some lack of thyroid hormones, and may have impaired fetal development[17]. The transplacental passage of thyroid hormones is minimal and the extent to which maternal thyroid hormones are necessary for fetal development is not yet clear. However, a role also of maternal hypothyroxinaemia in causing congenital neurological damage in iodine deficiency states is increasingly suspected. Recent experimental studies in rats have shown that maternal iodine deficiency is associated with embryonic thyroid hormone deficiency throughout gestation[18]. Further, maternal hypothyroxinaemia in rats on normal diet results in abnormally low triiodothyronine and thyroxine tissue concentrations throughout gestation, and the reduction is most pronounced prior to the onset of fetal thyroid hormone production[19].

With respect to the human situation it appears that maternal hypothyroidism compatible with fertility is unlikely to be severe enough to harm the fetus. Fetal thyroid hormone production is the most important factor and iodine deficiency should thus be avoided. Irrespective of these considerations it is certainly desirable to give thyroxine to a hypothyroid woman during pregnancy. Elevations in serum TSH alone with normal levels of $T_4$ and $T_3$ probably have no effect on the fetus since TSH does not cross the placenta (Table 10.4).

**Table 10.4** Placental transfer of substances that are of importance for the course and treatment of autoimmune thyroid disease in pregnancy

Transplacental passage without difficulty
  Iodide
  Antithyroid drugs
  Maternal IgG, e.g. TSH receptor antibodies
  TRH

Minimal passage
  $T_3$
  $T_4$

No passage
  TSH

## INFLUENCE OF PREGNANCY ON AUTOIMMUNE ACTIVITY

It has been well known to the clinician for many years that some patients with autoimmune disorders, as for example rheumatoid arthritis, may improve considerably during pregnancy[20]. The frequent amelioration of symptoms in pregnant women with Graves' disease was reported already in the 1920s[21] and a similar remission of goitrous hypothyroidism was reported in 1975[22].

Systematic studies on maternal disease activity in women with autoimmune thyroid disease during pregnancy have been performed by Amino *et al.* (Figure 10.2)[23]. These investigations have shown that mild cases of hypothyroidism spontaneously remit, which incorrectly had been attributed to transplacental transfer of fetal thyroxine to the mother in previous reports. Similarly, there is a spontaneous improvement of thyrotoxicosis in late pregnancy[21,24]. This usually leads to a reduction of the dose of antithyroid drug required and sometimes the treatment may even be stopped.

Some women with inactive thyrotoxicosis may experience a transient mild activation of the disease in early pregnancy[24]. Further, hyperemesis gravidarum, which may occur early in pregnancy, has been associated with transient thyrotoxicosis (Figure 10.3). This may involve a stimulating effect of placental HCG on the thyroid[25,26].

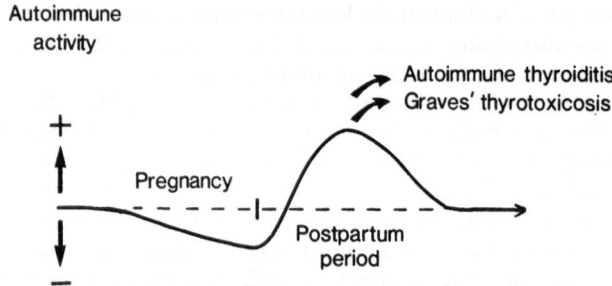

**Figure 10.2** The relation between pregnancy and autoimmune disease activity as typically found in thyroid disorders. (Adapted from Amino *et al.*[23])

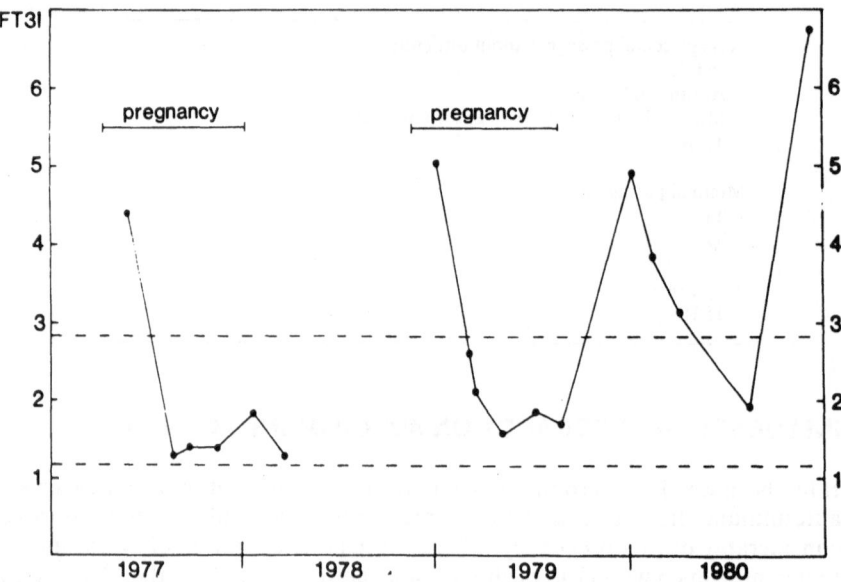

**Figure 10.3** A case with recurrent thyrotoxicosis and hyperemesis gravidarum during two pregnancies. The woman was first seen early in her first pregnancy when she suffered from hyperemesis gravidarum. Thyrotoxic thyroid hormone values were found and the condition remitted without treatment. She remained euthyroid during pregnancy and was lost to follow-up in the early postpartum period. In her second pregnancy hyperemesis recurred. Again she was found to be thyrotoxic and again a spontaneous remission occurred during pregnancy. A transient flare-up was observed in the postpartum period. Finally, 1½ year after the second pregnancy, permanent thyrotoxicosis developed. FT3I = serum-free triiodothyronine index (reference range 1.2–2.8)

Thyroid microsomal and thyroglobulin antibody titres fall in women with autoimmune thyroid disease during pregnancy[27,28]. A similar decline in thyroid-stimulating activity has been reported in women with Graves' thyrotoxicosis[29]. Also, a reduction of total IgG (but not IgA, IgE or IgM) levels, albeit much smaller than that of the autoantibody titres, is observed both in women with autoimmune thyroid disease and in healthy pregnant women[2].

## FETAL AND NEONATAL THYROID DISEASE DUE TO TRANSPLACENTAL PASSAGE OF AUTOANTIBODIES

Thyroid autoantibodies are typically of IgG class and thus may cross the placental barrier to reach the fetal circulation (Table 10.4). The passage of thyroid microsomal and/or thyroglobulin antibodies does not seem to have any harmful effect on the thyroid development in the fetus, as women with autoimmune thyroiditis give birth to healthy children[30].

TSH receptor antibodies may, on the other hand, have severe effects in the fetus and neonatal infant. TSH receptor-stimulating antibodies cause *fetal thyrotoxicosis* by stimulating the fetal thyroid. This may lead to retarded growth, goitre, cardiac failure and intrauterine death[3,4]. In the neonatal period the thyrotoxic state continues, *neonatal thyrotoxicosis*, and treatment with antithyroid drugs may be required for 1–3 months. Eventually the disease subsides in parallel with the disappearance of antibodies from the circulation of the neonate (Figure 10.4).

If the mother is treated with an antithyroid drug during pregnancy the fetus will be treated as well, as these drugs cross the placenta easily (Table 10.4). The placental passage is higher for methimazole than for propylthiouracil. It is important to avoid unnecessarily high doses of the antithyroid drug, as otherwise the fetus becomes hypothyroid and may develop a goitre. For this reason some clinicians prefer propylthiouracil to methimazole. For the same reason many give antithyroid drugs without adding thyroxine (which crosses the placental barrier poorly) to the treatment schedule since this enables the lowest possible dose of the antithyroid drug to be administered. However, empirical data do not confirm that these theoretical considerations are clinically important[31]. The aim of the treatment should be to keep the mother on the borderline between euthyroidism and thyrotoxicosis[3,4].

The neonatal thyrotoxicosis may not develop until several days after delivery because of a residual effect of antithyroid drugs received during the fetal period. Children born to mothers treated for thyrotoxicosis should therefore be kept under close observation for the first 7–10 days after delivery. Features suggesting neonatal thyrotoxicosis are an initial weight loss that is greater than normal, irritability, tachycardia, goiter and exophthalmos. Treatment should be given immediately, since without treatment the mortality rate is over 10%. Premature craniosynostosis is another serious complication[32].

Most cases of fetal and neonatal thyrotoxicosis develop in women with active Graves' thyrotoxicosis. It has been estimated that one out of 70 pregnant women with thyrotoxicosis will deliver a child with neonatal thyrotoxicosis. It should, however, be observed that TSH receptor-stimulating antibodies may be present in high concentrations also in an euthyroid woman who previously has been treated with thyroidectomy or radioiodine because of Graves' thyrotoxicosis (Figure 10.4) or in a woman with coexisting autoimmune thyroiditis, which may prevent the development

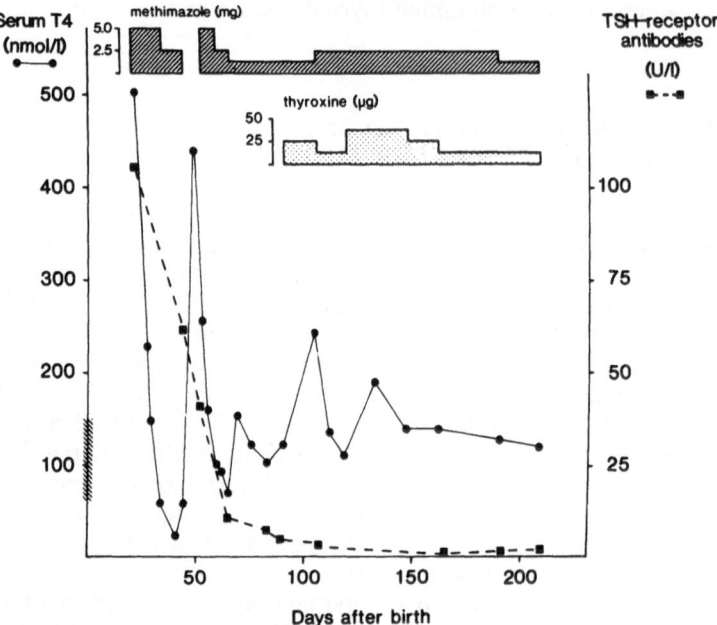

**Figure 10.4** TSH receptor antibody levels and thyroid hormone values (T₄) in a case of neonatal thyrotoxicosis. (Courtesy of Dr I. Tessin, Mölndal Hospital, Sweden). The disease was detected 3 weeks after delivery. The mother had a history of subtotal thyroidectomy for Graves' thyrotoxicosis 10 years earlier. She was not on any drug treatment.

The infant was treated with methimazole and later thyroxine was added. The methimazole treatment was interrupted 41 days after delivery and within a few days the disease recurred. The analyses of TSH receptor antibodies, which were done in retrospect with a radioreceptor assay (TRAK, Henning Berlin Gmbh, Berlin, West Germany; reference range <3 U/l), still showed a high level at that time. Probably the duration of treatment could have been shortened since later the antibody levels were normalized

of thyroid overactivity. In such rare cases monitoring of fetal heart rate can be of help to decide if the mother should be treated with an antithyroid drug (and thyroxine to prevent maternal hypothyroidism) in order to protect the fetus from thyrotoxicosis. A fetal heart rate over 160 beats per minute is suggestive of active fetal thyrotoxicosis[33].

A prerequisite for the development of fetal or neonatal thyrotoxicosis is very high levels of TSH receptor-stimulating antibodies[34,35]. We now have access to convenient assay methods based on competitive inhibition by receptor antibodies of labelled TSH binding to solubilized TSH receptors. It has been suggested that TSH receptor antibodies should be checked in the third trimester of pregnancy in all women with autoimmune thyroid disease[36]. Certainly such a determination is desirable in women with Graves' disease, and in women with autoimmune thyroiditis accompanied by very high levels of thyroid microsomal antibodies (Table 10.5). In such cases there may be a coexisting Graves' disease not manifesting itself due to autoimmune destruction (or inhibition?) of the thyroid gland.

**Table 10.5** Women with autoimmune thyroid disease in whom there is a risk of fetal or neonatal thyrotoxicosis in the offspring, due to transplacental passage of TSH receptor-stimulating antibodies

---

Active Graves' thyrotoxicosis (especially if exophthalmos and/or pretibial myxoedema is present)

Inactive Graves' thyrotoxicosis after previous treatment with surgery or radioiodine*

Autoimmune thyroiditis with coexisting Graves' thyrotoxicosis*

---

*These women may be on treatment with thyroxine

Not all TSH receptors have stimulatory properties. Some may bind to but not stimulate, the receptor and antagonize the effect of TSH. Such antibodies have been found in rare cases of autoimmune thyroiditis and have been implicated in the development of transient *neonatal hypothyroidism*[37,38]. As with neonatal thyrotoxicosis, the hypothyroidism remits spontaneously as the maternal antibodies disappear from the circulation of the infant. These children are detected in the national screening programmes for congenital hypothyroidism and they will receive thyroxine therapy, as it is important to start treatment as soon as possible in congenital hypothyroidism. Usually all infants are treated for 1–3 years until a trial off treatment is made to determine if hypothyroidism is permanent or transient.

Complex alterations in fetal and neonatal thyroid function may occur in the rare cases where combinations of stimulating and blocking TSH receptor antibodies are present in the same individual. Depending on the affinities and the relative titres of these antibodies the infant can develop alternating periods of hypothyroidism and thyrotoxicosis until euthyroidism is finally reached as the antibodies disappear from the circulation of the neonate[39].

Recently it was suggested that congenital hypothyroidism could be caused by transplacental passage of maternal antibodies having thyroid growth inhibitory action[40]. The investigators claimed that such growth-blocking antibodies were found in the serum of 15 out of 34 women who had given birth to children with congenital hypothyroidism. Surprisingly, the mothers showed no signs of thyroid dysfunction and had no history of thyroid autoimmunity. These remarkable findings must await confirmatory reports from other laboratories.

## POSTPARTUM THYROID DISEASE

Already in 1948 a detailed report was published by Dr H. E. W. Roberton on women developing clinical hypothyroidism following pregnancy[41]. In Christchurch, New Zealand, Roberton had observed the common occurrence of this condition, which could be ameliorated by giving thyroid extracts. Often, however, a spontaneous remission was seen. Although it was associated with endemic goitre due to iodine deficiency, Roberton noticed that in two women it had developed in England before they settled in New Zealand and he anticipated that 'if looked for, it would be found in the goitre-free countries in women who have undergone thyroidectomy and in families with a history of goitre'.

In the years following a few patients with postpartum primary myxoedema were described but otherwise the 'Roberton syndrome' remained unknown. It was rediscovered in 1976 when Amino et al. published their first report on six Japanese women with transient postpartum hypothyroidism[42]. At about the same time a new form of thyroid inflammatory disease, 'painless' or 'silent thyroiditis', was described from North America. This syndrome was characterized by thyrotoxicosis with a low radioiodine uptake in the thyroid (in contrast to Graves' thyrotoxicosis with a high uptake) and it was found to have a predilection for the postpartum period[43].

In recent years a number of case reports and a few systematic prevalence studies have disclosed the common occurrence of thyroid dysfunction in the postpartum period. In Japanese and Swedish prevalence studies on unselected groups of women who were followed in the year following delivery, thyroid dysfunction (thyrotoxicosis and/or hypothyroidism) was found in 5.5% and 6.5%, respectively, of the women tested[44,45]. In both these studies thyroid microsomal antibodies were detected in most of the women who developed hypothyroidism. Secondly, TSH receptor-stimulating antibodies (TSAb) were found in some women with thyrotoxicosis alone[45]. Amino et al. later suggested that in women who experience a relapse of Graves' thyrotoxicosis in the postpartum period, the TSAb assays may not be sensitive enough to allow early detection of these antibodies[23]. Thus, in almost all women who develop postpartum thyroid dysfunction an underlying autoimmune thyroiditis and/or Graves' thyrotoxicosis is to be suspected.

The symptoms of the postpartum thyroid dysfunction may be mistaken for postpartum fatigue and a consequence of lactation and therefore may go unrecognized. The transient nature of the disease adds to the diagnostic difficulty. The development of postpartum hypothyroidism is accompanied by goitre development in most cases. Often a history of previous goitre and/or thyroid dysfunction or a family history of autoimmune thyroid disease is present. Usually the disease recurs after a subsequent pregnancy (Figure 10.5) and sometimes even after a miscarriage or abortion.

In some populations (for example in some parts of North America and in Japan) postpartum hypothyroidism is preceded by clinical thyrotoxicosis with a low radioiodine uptake. The severity of this 'destruction-induced' thyrotoxic phase may differ and depend on the amount of thyroid iodoproteins that are released. Thyroid iodine contents differ in various populations because of iodine intake. In populations with a high iodine intake (as in North America and in Japan) the thyrotoxic phase may be more pronounced causing the clinical syndrome of 'painless' or 'silent thyroiditis'[46]. When carefully looked for a similar but mostly subclinical thyrotoxic phase is found also in a population with a lower iodine intake (as in Sweden) prior to the development of postpartum hypothyroidism[47]. Taken together these observations suggest that autoimmune postpartum thyroiditis is character-

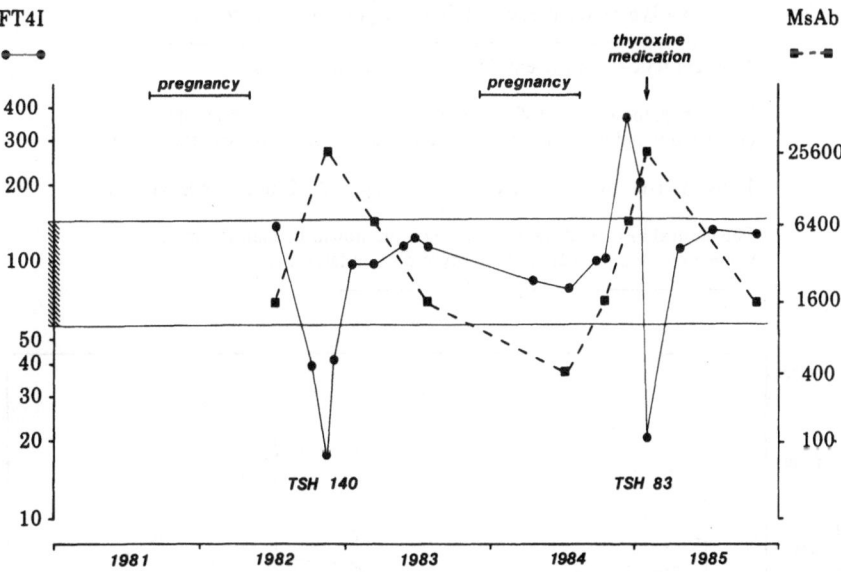

**Figure 10.5** Recurrent autoimmune postpartum thyroiditis. The woman was first investigated 2 months after delivering her first baby, a boy. A thyrotoxic phase with thyroid hormones within the reference range was followed by goitrous hypothyroidism (TSH 140 mU/l; reference range <5 mU/l). No treatment was instituted and the woman became euthyroid within a year postpartum. She remained euthyroid during her second pregnancy. Four months after giving birth to a girl she again was found to be thyrotoxic. Six weeks later she was hypothyroid (TSH 83 mU/l) and thyroxine was instituted. Withdrawal of the medication has not yet been attempted. FT4I = serum-free thyroxine index (reference range 57–145). MsAb = serum thyroid microsomal antibodies (by Thymune-M haemaglutination assay, Wellcome, Beckenham, UK)

ized by an initial destructive phase 1–5 months postpartum followed by the subsequent development of hypothyroidism (Table 10.6 and Figure 10.5).

In the typical case the degree of hypothyroidism correlates well with the titre levels of thyroid microsomal antibodies, not only in the postpartum period but also in early pregnancy (Figure 10.6). Thus, the early pregnancy titre may be used to predict the development of postpartum hypothyroidism[23,45]. The predictive value of thyroid microsomal antibodies may be strengthened further by analysis of microsomal antibody IgG subclasses[48]. Thus, postpartum hypothyroidism was associated with the IgG1 subclass, whereas the level of the IgG4 subclass was similar in women who developed postpartum hypothyroidism and those who did not. Microsomal antibodies of subclasses IgG2 and IgG3 were of low concentrations in all women. It is of interest that antibodies of subclass IgG1 have the ability to fix complement, in contrast to antibodies of subclass IgG4. Thyroglobulin antibody titres have been low or undetectable in women with postpartum thyroiditis and are accordingly of no predictive value[23,45,46].

A complex pattern may be found in women with a predisposition for both autoimmune thyroiditis and Graves' thyrotoxicosis. In these patients the

**Table 10.6** Typical features of autoimmune postpartum thyroiditis

---

Transient flare-up of pre-existing autoimmune thyroiditis

Initial thyrotoxic phase (often symptomless) that occurs 1–5 months postpartum and is characterized by a low radioiodine uptake in the thyroid

Transient hypothyroidism and goitre developing 3–12 months postpartum

The natural history of the disease is still unknown. Probably some of the women develop permanent hypothyroidism in later life.

---

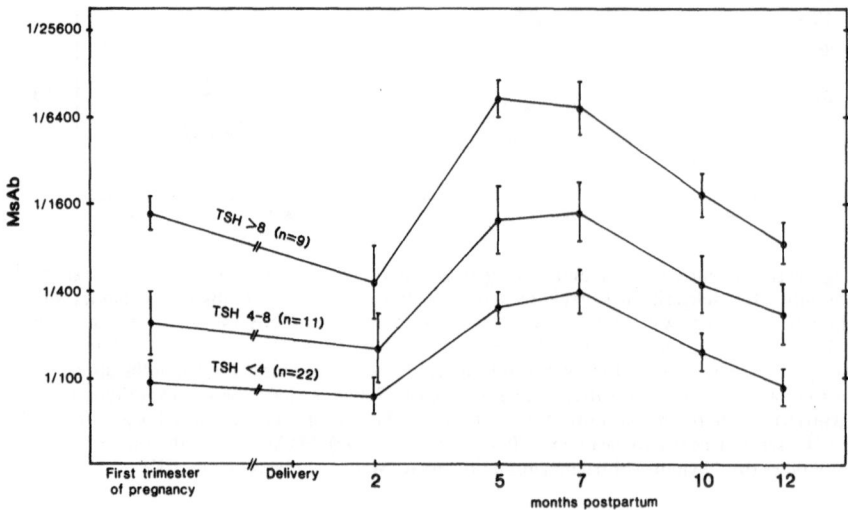

**Figure 10.6** Changes in serum thyroid microsomal antibody (MsAb) titres (log scale) in pregnancy and the postpartum period. Results (mean ± SEM) are presented for three groups of women divided according to the maximal postpartum TSH observed. (Adapted from Jansson *et al.*[45] with permission from the Journal of Clinical Endocrinology and Metabolism)

destructive and hypothyroid effects associated with the microsomal antibodies sometimes seem to be counteracted by the stimulatory effect of TSH receptor-stimulating antibodies. This could explain why euthyroidism may be maintained after delivery in a woman with high titres of thyroid microsomal antibodies, and why occasionally an initial episode of low radioiodine uptake thyrotoxicosis may be followed by high radioiodine uptake thyrotoxicosis[49]. Finally, women previously treated for Graves' thyrotoxicosis with antithyroid drugs or surgery may, following delivery, develop hypothyroidism if they have thyroid microsomal antibodies[45].

The accumulated evidence supports the assumption that postpartum thyroid disease results from an altered immunotolerance following pregnancy-induced immunosuppression in women with latent or subclinical autoimmune thyroid disease (Figure 10.2). Thus, thyroid microsomal antibody titres change in a typical way in pregnancy and the postpartum period (Figure 10.6). A decrease during pregnancy is followed by an increase after delivery[28,45]. A peak level is reached around 6 months postpartum before the titres decline again. One year postpartum the titres have reached a steady state level which is similar to the titre before pregnancy. At the same time hypothyroidism and goitre have decreased or disappeared in most cases. Interestingly, parallel changes are observed in total IgG and IgG subclass levels both in these women and in healthy postpartum women with no signs of autoimmune thyroid disease[47]. Thus, the changes of thyroid microsomal antibody titres may reflect a general immunoregulatory rebound phenomenon after delivery. Probably the activation of Graves' thyrotoxicosis in the postpartum period is due to similar changes of TSH receptor antibody titres, since the temporal occurrence of thyrotoxicosis coincides with that of hypothyroidism in women with thyroid microsomal antibodies[45].

The data presented above suggest that autoantibodies (predominantly thyroid microsomal antibodies and in some cases TSH receptor-stimulating antibodies) have important roles in the development of the postpartum thyroid syndromes. In postpartum autoimmune thyroiditis (but not postpartum Graves' thyrotoxicosis) the number of circulating K-lymphocytes increases at the time of the postpartum aggravation[23]. The number of B-lymphocytes has been reported to increase at time of thyrotoxicosis in both postpartum autoimmune thyroiditis and Graves' thyrotoxicosis but no consistent changes in the number of total T-lymphocytes or helper or suppressor/cytotoxic phenotypic T-cells have been observed in peripheral blood[23]. Within the thyroid a local accumulation of B-lymphocytes and T-lymphocytes with the helper phenotype but a low number of T-lymphocytes with the suppressor-cytotoxic phenotype has been found[50]. Taken together, these findings indicate that autoantibodies produced within the thyroid also might act in conjunction with K-cells and complement to cause cytotoxic destruction of thyrocytes.

## CONCLUSIONS

Pregnancy is an important regulator of disease activity both in autoimmune thyroid disease and in other autoimmune disorders. Typically, amelioration of disease activity during pregnancy is followed by a rebound in the postpartum period, which may cause a transient disorder in otherwise apparently healthy women with a subclinical state of disease and/or a genetic disposition for disease. Therefore autoimmune disease is much more prevalent in the postpartum period than during pregnancy. On the other hand, autoimmune disorders are more troublesome to manage during gestation due to fetal considerations and transplacental passage of thyroid antibodies that may cause thyroid dysfunction in the fetus and the neonatal infant.

Future research in this field will provide insight into the regulatory mechanisms involved in immune tolerance in pregnancy and the rebound of the postpartum period. Prospective studies will delineate the natural history of the postpartum thyroid disorders, and clarify which women are likely to develop permanent disease later in life. From a practical point of view it should be stressed that we have already learned, by screening for autoantibodies, to predict the development of maternal thyroid disease during and after pregnancy and to detect infants at risk for fetal and neonatal thyroid disease.

## References

1. Gleicher, N. and Siegel, I. (1983). Pregnancy and the immune state. In Davies, T. F. (ed.) *Autoimmune Endocrine Disease* pp. 225–45 (New York: John Wiley & Sons)
2. Gall, S. A. (1983). Maternal adjustments in the immune system in normal pregnancy. *Clin. Obstet, Gynecol.*, **26**, 521–36
3. Burrow, G. N. (1985). The management of thyrotoxicosis in pregnancy. *N. Engl. J. Med.*, **313**, 562–5
4. Davies, T. F. and Cobin, R. (1985). Thyroid disease in pregnancy and the postpartum period. *Mt. Sinai. J. Med.*, **52**, 59–77
5. Weetman, A. P. and McGregor, A. M. (1984). Autoimmune thyroid disease: developments in our understanding. *Endocr. Rev.*, **5**, 309–55
6. Burman, K. D. and Baker Jr., J. R. (1985). Immune mechanisms in Graves' disease. *Endocr. Rev.*, **6**, 183–232
7. Tunbridge, W. M. G., Brewis, M., French, J. M., Appleton, D., Bird, T., Clark, F., Evered, D. C., Grimley Evans, J., Hall, R., Smith, P., Stephenson, J. and Young, E. (1981). Natural history of autoimmune thyroiditis. *Br. Med. J.*, **282**, 258–62
8. Portmann, L., Hamada, N., Heinrich, G. and DeGroot, L. J. (1985). Anti-thyroid peroxidase antibody in patients with autoimmune thyroid disease: possible identity with antimicrosomal antibody. *J. Clin. Endocrinol. Metab.*, **61**, 1001–3
9. Walfish, P. G. and Farid, N. R. (1985). The immunogenetic basis of autoimmune thyroid disease. In Walfish, P. G., Wall, J. R. and Volpé, R. (eds). *Autoimmunity and the Thyroid.* pp. 9–36. (Orlando: Academic Press)
10. Jansson, R., Säfwenberg, J. and Dahlberg, P. A. (1985). Influence of the HLA-DR4 antigen and iodine status on the development of autoimmune postpartum thyroiditis. *J. Clin. Endocrinol. Metab.*, **60**, 168–73
11. Bottazzo, G. F., Pujol-Borrell, R., Hanafusa, T. and Feldmann, M. (1983). Role of aberrant HLA-DR expression and antigen presentation in induction of endocrine autoimmunity. *Lancet*, **2**, 1115–9
12. Momotani, N., Ito, K., Hamada, N., Ban, Y., Nishikawa, Y. and Mimura, T. (1984). Maternal hyperthyroidism and congenital malformations in the offspring. *Clin. Endocrinol.*, **20**, 695–700
13. Montoro, M., Collea, J. V., Frasier, S. D. and Mestman, J. H. (1981). Successful outcome of pregnancy in women with hypothyroidism. *Ann. Intern. Med.*, **94**, 31–4
14. Man, E. B., Jones, W. S., Holden, R. H. and Mellits, D. E. (1971). Thyroid function in human pregnancy. VIII. Retardation of progeny aged 7 years; relationship to maternal age and maternal thyroid function. *Am. J. Obstet. Gynecol.*, **111**, 905–16
15. Hetzel, B. (1983). Iodine deficiency disorders (IDD) and their eradication. *Lancet.*, **2**, 1126–9
16. Fisher, D. A. (1983). Maternal-fetal thyroid function in pregnancy. *Clin. Perinatol.*, **10**, 615–26
17. Glorieux, J., Dussault, J. H., Letarte, J., Guyda, H. and Morisette, J. (1983). Preliminary results on the mental development of hypothyroid infants detected by the Quebec screening program. *J. Pediatr.*, **102**, 19–22
18. Escobar del Rey, F., Pastor, R., Mallol, J. and Morreale de Escobar, G. (1985). Effects of maternal iodine deficiency on T4 and T3 contents of rat concepta, before and after onset of fetal thyroid function. Presented at the *9th International Thyroid Congress*, September 1–6, Sao Paolo, Brazil
19. Morreale de Escobar, G., Pastor, R., Obregon, M. J. and Escobar del Rey, F. (1985). Effects of maternal thyroidectomy on rat embryonic T4 and T3 contents and development

before and after onset of fetal thyroid function. Presented at the *9th International Thyroid Congress*, September 1–6, Sao Paolo, Brazil

20. Oka, M. (1953). Effect of pregnancy on the onset and course of rheumatoid arthritis. *Ann. Rheum. Dis.*, **12**, 227

21. Gardiner-Hill, H. (1929). Pregnancy complicating simple goitre and Graves' disease. *Lancet*, **1**, 120–4

22. Nelson, J. C. and Palmer, F. J. (1974). A remission of goitrous hypothyroidism during pregnancy. *J. Clin. Endocrinol. Metab.*, **40**, 383–6

23. Amino, N. and Miyai, K. (1983). Postpartum autoimmune endocrine syndromes. In Davies, T. F. (ed.) *Autoimmune Endocrine Disease*, pp. 247–72 (New York: J. Wiley and Sons)

24. Amino, N., Tanizawa, O., Mori, H., Iwatani, Y., Yamada, T., Kurachi, K., Kumahara, Y. and Miyai, K. (1982). Aggravation of thyrotoxicosis in early pregnancy and after delivery in Graves' disease. *J. Clin. Endocrinol. Metab.*, **55**, 108–12

25. Bovillon, R., Naesens, M., Van Assche, F. A., De Keyser, L., De Moor, P., Renaer, M., De Vos, P. and De Roo, M. (1982). Thyroid function in patients with hyperemesis gravidarum. *Am. J. Obstet. Gynecol.*, **143**, 922–6

26. Jeffcoate, W. J. and Bain, C. (1985). Recurrent pregnancy-induced thyrotoxicosis presenting as hyperemesis gravidarum. Case report. *Br. J. Obstet. Gynaecol.*, **92**, 413–5

27. Parker, R. H. and Beierwaltes, W. H. (1961). Thyroid antibodies during pregnancy and in the newborn. *J. Clin. Endocrinol. Metab.*, **21**, 792–8

28. Amino, N., Kuro, R., Tanizawa, O., Tanaka, F., Hayashi, C., Kotani, K., Kawashima, M., Miyai, K. and Kumahara, Y. (1978). Changes of serum antithyroid antibodies during and after pregnancy in autoimmune thyroid diseases. *Clin. Exp. Immunol.*, **31**, 30–7

29. Hardisty, C. A. and Munro, D. S. (1983). Serum long acting thyroid stimulator protector in pregnancy complicated by Graves' disease. *Br. Med. J.*, **286**, 934–5

30. Dussault, J. H., Letarte, J., Guyda, H. and Laberge, C. (1980). Lack of influence of thyroid antibodies on thyroid function in the newborn infant and on a mass screening program for congenital hypothyroidism. *J. Pediatr.*, **96**, 385–9

31. Ramsay, I., Kaur, S. and Krassas, G. (1983). Thyrotoxicosis in pregnancy: results of treatment by antithyroid drugs combined with T4. *Clin. Endocrinol.*, **18**, 73–85

32. Daneman, D. and Howard, N. J. (1980). Neonatal thyrotoxicosis, intellectual impairment and craniosynostasis in later years. *J. Pediatr.*, **97**, 257–9

33. Cove, D. H. and Johnston, P. (1985). Fetal hyperthyroidism: experience of treatment of four siblings. *Lancet*, **1**, 430–2

34. Munro, D. S., Dirmikis, S. M., Humphries, H., Smith, T. and Broadhead, G. D. (1978). The role of thyroid stimulating immunoglobulins of Graves' disease in neonatal thyrotoxicosis. *Br. J. Obstet. Gynaecol.*, **85**, 837–43

35. Zakarija, M. and McKenzie, J. M. (1983). Pregnancy-associated changes in the thyroid-stimulating antibody of Graves' disease and the relationship to neonatal hyperthyroidism. *J. Clin. Endocrinol. Metab.*, **57**, 1036–40

36. McGregor, A. M., Hall, R. and Richards, C. (1984). Autoimmune thyroid disease and pregnancy. *Br. Med. J.*, **288**, 1780–1

37. Matsuura, N., Yamada, Y., Nohara, Y., Konishi, J., Kasagi, K., Endo, K., Kojima, H. and Wataya, K. (1980). Familial neonatal transient hypothyroidism due to maternal TSH-binding inhibitor immunoglobulins. *N. Engl. J. Med.*, **303**, 737–41

38. Karlsson, F. A., Dahlberg, P. A. and Ritzén, E. M. (1984). Thyroid blocking antibodies in thyroiditis. *Acta Med. Scand.*, **215**, 461–6

39. Zakarija, M., McKenzie, J. M. and Munro, D. S. (1983). Immunoglobulin G inhibitor of thyroid-stimulating antibody is a cause of delay in the onset of neonatal Graves' disease. *J. Clin. Invest.*, **72**, 1352–6

40. Van der Gaag, R.D., Drexhage, H. A. and Dussault, J. H. (1985). Role of maternal immunoglobulins blocking TSH-induced thyroid growth in sporadic forms of congenital hypothyroidism. *Lancet*, **1**, 246–50

41. Roberton, H. E. W. (1948). Lassitude, coldness, and hair changes following pregnancy, and their response to treatment with thyroid extract. *Br. Med. J.*, **2**, 93–4

42. Amino, N., Miyai, K., Onishi, T., Hashimoto, T., Arai, K., Ishibashi, K. and Kumahara, Y. (1976). Transient hypothyroidism after delivery in autoimmune thyroiditis. *J. Clin.*

*Endocrinol. Metab.*, **42**, 296–301

43. Ginsberg, J. and Walfish, P. G. (1977). Post-partum transient thyrotoxicosis with painless thyroiditis. *Lancet*, **1**, 1125–8

44. Amino, N., Mori, H., Iwatani, Y., Tanizawa, O., Kawashima, M., Tsuge, I., Ibaragi, K., Kumahara, Y. and Miyai, K. (1982). High prevalence of transient postpartum thyrotoxicosis and hypothyroidism. *N. Engl. J. Med.*, **306**, 849–52

45. Jansson, R., Bernander, S., Karlsson, A., Levin, K. and Nilsson, G. (1984). Autoimmune thyroid dysfunction in the postpartum period. *J. Clin. Endocrinol. Metab.*, **58**, 681–7

46. Walfish, P. G. and Chan, J. Y. C. (1985). Post-partum hyperthyroidism. *Clin. Endocrinol. Metab.*, **14**, 417–47

47. Jansson, R. (1984). Autoimmune thyroiditis – a clinical, epidemiological and immunological study with special reference to transient aggravation in the postpartum period. (Thesis). *Acta Univ. Ups.*, **492**, 1–73

48. Jansson, R., Thompson, P. M., Clark, F. and McLachlan, S. M. (1985). Association between thyroid microsomal antibodies of subclass IgG1 and hypothyroidism in autoimmune postpartum thyroiditis. *Clin. Exp. Immunol.*, **62**

49. Taylor, H. C. and Sheeler, L. R. (1982). Recurrence and heterogeneity in painless thyrotoxic lymphocytic thyroiditis. Report of five cases. *J. Am. Med. Assoc.*, **248**, 1085–8

50. Jansson, R., Tötterman, T. H., Sällström, J. and Dahlberg, P. A. (1984). Intrathyroidal and circulating lymphocyte subsets in different stages of autoimmune postpartum thyroiditis. *J. Clin. Endocrinol. Metab.*, **58**, 942–6

# Index